Emergency Medicine: Clinical Advances and Challenges in Diagnosis and Treatment, 2nd Edition

Emergency Medicine: Clinical Advances and Challenges in Diagnosis and Treatment, 2nd Edition

Guest Editor

Ovidiu Alexandru Mederle

MDPI

Basel • Beijing • Wuhan • Barcelona • Belgrade • Novi Sad • Cluj • Manchester

Guest Editor
Ovidiu Alexandru Mederle
Department of Surgery
"Victor Babes" University of Medicine
and Pharmacy Timisoara
Timisoara
Romania

Editorial Office
MDPI AG
Grosspeteranlage 5
4052 Basel, Switzerland

This is a reprint of the Special Issue, published open access by the journal *Journal of Personalized Medicine* (ISSN 2075-4426), freely accessible at: https://www.mdpi.com/journal/jpm/special_issues/7L1LZ7FERA.

For citation purposes, cite each article independently as indicated on the article page online and as indicated below:

Lastname, A.A.; Lastname, B.B. Article Title. *Journal Name* **Year**, *Volume Number*, Page Range.

ISBN 978-3-7258-7220-6 (Hbk)
ISBN 978-3-7258-7221-3 (PDF)
https://doi.org/10.3390/books978-3-7258-7221-3

Contents

About the Editor

Ovidiu Alexandru Mederle

Ovidiu Alexandru Mederle is affiliated with the Victor Babes University of Medicine and Pharmacy in Timisoara, where he serves as Professor and Head of the Discipline of Emergency Medicine, as well as Director of the Center for Practical Skills, and is also Head of the University Emergency Department at the Timisoara Municipal Emergency Clinical Hospital. His academic and clinical interests span emergency medicine, histology, cellular pathology, and the integration of advanced diagnostic and educational methods in medical training. Over the course of his career, he has coordinated extensive teaching activity, supervised numerous student research projects, contributed to national research grants, and authored or coauthored multiple scientific publications and academic texts. His professional achievements include his habilitation thesis, longstanding membership of national and European emergency medicine societies, and sustained involvement in improving clinical practice and medical education in Romania.

Preface

The Reprint 'Emergency Medicine: Clinical Advances and Challenges in Diagnosis and Treatment, 2nd Edition', presents an updated, consolidated review of current knowledge in the management of acute and time-sensitive conditions. Its subject spans the full clinical spectrum of emergency care, integrating advances in diagnostic methods, therapeutic approaches, and system-level strategies that shape contemporary practice. It aims to provide a coherent overview of recent progress while addressing the practical and conceptual challenges that emergency clinicians face every day.

The motivation for assembling this scientific work stems from the increasing complexity of patient presentations, the rapid expansion of diagnostic technologies, and the need for effective clinical decision-making under high-pressure conditions. Emergency departments must continuously adapt to evolving epidemiologic patterns, workforce demands, and resource limitations. By highlighting new evidence, emerging tools, and innovative models of care, this Reprint supports the ongoing effort to improve accuracy, efficiency, and patient outcomes in acute care settings.

The content is intended for physicians, nurses, researchers, and health system leaders engaged in emergency medicine and related disciplines. It offers clinically relevant insights for frontline practitioners while also serving as a reference for educators and investigators seeking to understand current trends and future directions in acute care. Through this collection, readers may gain a broader perspective on both the advances achieved and the challenges that continue to shape emergency medicine today.

Ovidiu Alexandru Mederle
Guest Editor

Journal of
Personalized Medicine

MDPI

Editorial

Special Issue: Emergency Medicine: Clinical Advances and Challenges in Diagnosis and Treatment, 2nd Edition

Carmen Gabriela Williams [1,2], Daian-Ionel Popa [1,2,*] and Ovidiu Alexandru Mederle [1]

1 Emergency Department, Emergency Clinical Municipal Hospital, Gheorghe Dima Street Number 5, 300079 Timisoara, Romania; williams.carmen@umft.ro (C.G.W.)
2 Doctoral School, Faculty of General Medicine, Victor Babes University of Medicine and Pharmacy, 300041 Timisoara, Romania
* Correspondence: daian-ionel.popa@umft.ro; Tel.: +40-746-912-660

1. Introduction

The development of emergency medicine brings both challenges and opportunities. With the joint efforts and dedication of healthcare professionals, alongside the integration of continuously updated medical technologies and concepts, the field is steadily moving toward historic advancements. Emergency medicine is a dynamic specialty, constantly evolving to enhance patient outcomes and ensure that safety remains the highest priority during critical situations.

This Special Issue, "Emergency Medicine: Clinical Advances and Challenges in Diagnosis and Treatment, 2nd Edition", has brought together thirteen high-quality contributions, including nine original research articles, three reviews, and one case report.

2. An Overview of Published Articles

Marza et al. (Contribution 1) describe a rare and dramatic complication of synchronized cardioversion for unstable supraventricular tachycardia: complete heart block with recurrent cardiac arrests, ultimately requiring permanent pacemaker implantation. The case is striking for its detailed chronology, systematic troubleshooting, and eventual success in repositioning transcutaneous pacing electrodes. Unexpected deterioration remains a reality in resuscitation practice. Case reports within this Special Issue remind us that even routine interventions such as synchronized cardioversion may precipitate bradyarrhythmic arrest. Similar observations have been documented in larger studies, where electrical cardioversion occasionally triggers sinus node dysfunction or conduction disturbances requiring pacing support [1]. The 2021 European Resuscitation Council Guidelines reaffirm the need for vigilance in rhythm-specific therapy, rapid recognition of arrest, and preparation for advanced pacing or pharmacological escalation in case of refractory bradyarrhythmia [2].

Guan et al. (Contribution 2) present a timely and innovative study addressing a common clinical dilemma: whether residents of residential aged care facilities (RACFs) who contribute to the emergency department (ED) after a fall can be safely discharged. The authors developed and internally validated two models, culminating in the simplified four-variable Discharge Eligibility after Fall in Elderly Residents (DEFER) score. Older adults represent one of the fastest-growing patient cohorts in the ED. Predicting safe discharge after a fall, particularly for residents of aged care facilities, is a recurrent challenge—models such as the DEFER score attempt to balance clinical risk with respect for patient preferences. Broader evidence confirms that falls are multifactorial, influenced by polypharmacy, frailty, and cognitive impairment [3]. However, existing screening tools have shown limited reproducibility in ED settings [4]. International experts argue that emergency care for older adults must be redesigned to integrate risk stratification, advance care planning, and system-level adaptations [5].

Hsieh et al. (Contribution 3) contribute significantly and innovatively to infectious disease emergency care by evaluating and modifying existing scoring systems for patients with Vibrio bacteremia. The study demonstrates that the Mortality in Emergency Department Sepsis (MEDS) score, when modified with simple laboratory markers such as blood urea nitrogen (BUN) and arterial pH, provides superior predictive accuracy compared with traditional models. Vibrio vulnificus sepsis, though uncommon, is the most fulminant and deadly infectious emergency presenting in medicine, with a greater than 50% mortality rate even when treated appropriately with antibiotics and intensive care support. Therefore, updating current tools of sepsis risk stratification, applicable more by adding readily available biochemical parameters, is another move toward making an early clinical decision better and improving survival outcomes in this high-risk population [6].

Acute chest pain remains a frequent and diagnostically challenging reason for visits to the emergency department, requiring rapid exclusion of benign causes while promptly identifying acute coronary syndromes (ACSs). In this setting, the article by Piccioni (Contribution 4) and colleagues provides valuable insights by assessing a multi-marker strategy that combines high-sensitivity troponin I (hsTnI) with two emerging biomarkers, soluble ST2 (sST2) and soluble urokinase plasminogen activator receptor (suPAR). Given that acute chest pain represents one of the most frequent and diagnostically demanding presentations in the emergency department—requiring clinicians to swiftly discriminate between benign causes and high-risk entities such as acute coronary syndromes (ACSs)—the work of Eggers et al. offers compelling evidence that combining high-sensitivity troponin T (hsTnT) with additional biomarkers like copeptin can significantly improve early diagnostic accuracy and expedite safe clinical decision-making in suspected ACS patients [7].

Buleu et al. (Contribution 5) offer a valuable and timely contribution to acute stroke management. By examining the performance of emergency departments in relation to door-to-needle time across day and night shifts, the authors provide important insights into operational challenges and opportunities for improvement. Stroke care remains time-critical. Contributions addressing code-stroke performance, mechanical thrombectomy via alternative vascular routes, and misdiagnosis risk highlight procedural and diagnostic personalization. The European Stroke Organisation guidelines emphasize individualization of thrombolysis and thrombectomy strategies, depending on comorbidities and vascular anatomy [8,9].

The review article by Moroi et al. (Contribution 6) provides an in-depth and timely examination of one of the most challenging emergencies in maternal care: venous thromboembolism during pregnancy. The authors successfully present a balanced and comprehensive overview of epidemiology, risk factors, diagnostic difficulties, and therapeutic strategies. Thromboembolism of the venous system in pregnancy continues to be one of the major killers of women worldwide. It poses a unique diagnostic and therapeutic challenge because, on one hand, there are overlapping physiological changes, and on the other hand, both mother and fetus need protection. In this regard, Bates et al. have come up with an authoritative practice synthesis that outlines evidence-based strategies for clinical assessment, imaging selection, and choice of anticoagulation protocols at different stages of pregnancy. This emergency and obstetric team will work in a high-risk situation needing fast decisions based on guidelines [10].

Kim et al. (Contribution 7) provide a comprehensive and timely evaluation of mechanical CPR use in the management of out-of-hospital cardiac arrest, with a particular focus on the COVID-19 pandemic period. By leveraging a robust, nationwide dataset, the authors deliver necessary evidence on survival, neurological outcomes, and return of spontaneous circulation, while carefully contrasting outcomes between manual and device-assisted resuscitation. Mechanical cardiopulmonary resuscitation has been purposely brought into the debate in cases of out-of-hospital cardiac arrest because it is often blamed for poor neurological outcomes and overall survival, when indeed a valuable contribution, such as that made by Couper et al. [11], through an analysis of randomized trials together with observational cohorts comparing device-assisted resuscitation to conventional manual techniques, proves otherwise. While it may not uniformly improve outcomes when used routinely, mechanical CPR can offer significant operational advantages during prolonged resuscitation efforts and transport and in high-risk infectious settings, wherein provider safety and resource allocation are critical determinants of care quality [11].

The research from Hahnenkamp (Contribution 8) present an exemplary innovation model in rural emergency care, offering a well-structured evaluation of the RuralRescue initiative in northeastern Germany. The authors successfully demonstrate how integrating tele-emergency physician supervision, geolocation-based responder apps, and structured data-driven triage can significantly improve timeliness and quality. Rural emergency care continues to suffer from problems of delayed response time, lack of availability of specialists, and uncoordinated resources. In such a scenario, the studies by Hong et al. and Zakariah et al. would be most relevant to prove that telemedicine-supported physician oversight integrated with digitally coordinated first responders significantly improves prehospital care delivery in underserved regions. Remote supervision combined with geolocation-based alert systems and structured triage protocols presents measurable improvements in clinical efficiency as well as patient outcomes and is scalable on different healthcare infrastructures [12,13].

Iancu's work (Contribution 9) address a rare but clinically critical topic: mechanical thrombectomy via the transbrachial approach for acute ischemic stroke in patients with aortic pathologies. The authors enrich the literature by combining a carefully described case from their practice with an extensive review of nine published cases, thereby filling a notable gap in evidence. Other access routes for mechanical thrombectomy are seldom needed but become very important in patients with prohibitive aortic or peripheral vascular anatomy; thus, the case series presented by Iancu et al. provides valuable insight by documenting successful transbrachial and transradial approaches when standard transfemoral access could not be achieved. This is an excellent demonstration that procedural flexibility is also very much involved, as timely vascular reassessment and fast conversion to upper extremity access can preserve the chances of recanalization without compromising safety in these anatomically complex stroke patients [14].

The paper by Hodgson et al. (Contribution 10) pioneers the use of artificial intelligence and machine learning to optimize emergency department (ED) operations. The authors present a methodologically rigorous study, training a non-linear ML model on more than 49,000 patient encounters and prospectively implementing a personalized vertical processing pathway (VPP) over 13 weeks. Artificial intelligence and machine learning have become a transformation plan in emergency departments that will improve the precision of triage and resource allocation, enhancing operations' overall efficiency. In this context, Fernandes et al. and Takeda et al. presented solid proof by demonstrating that predictive models based on data can effectively preempt patient disposition, admission risk, and wait time dynamics compared to assessments led by clinicians using traditional methods. Their studies have validated that frameworks for triage based on machine-learning algorithms improve patient flow as well as minimize the extent of overcrowding, personalized decision pathways that will suit varying demands in EDs [12,15].

Savioli's study (Contribution 11) provides a significant and timely contribution to the ongoing debate on triage accuracy in emergency departments, focusing specifically on the geriatric population—one of the most vulnerable and complex groups of patients. Drawing on more than 420,000 ED admissions over six years, the authors conduct a robust real-life comparison between four-level and five-level triage systems (4LT and 5LT) and their impact on under-triage (UT), over-triage (OT), waiting times, and crowding indices. In this context, the studies by Grossmann et al. and Türkoğlu et al. provide valuable evidence that standard triage protocols may inadequately capture severity in geriatric patients, with high misclassification rates observed across four- and five-level systems. Their findings emphasize that older adults are disproportionately affected by prolonged waiting times and inappropriate resource allocation, even within structured triage frameworks, underscoring the need for age-adapted triage modifiers and continuous algorithm refinement [16,17].

Anna Ingielewicz's work (Contribution 12) offer a thoughtful and comprehensive exploration of one of emergency medicine's most fundamental yet elusive challenges: the pursuit of an ideal triage system. The authors carefully review and compare the most widely used five-level systems, ATS, CTAS, ESI, and MTS, while contextualizing their strengths, weaknesses, and practical limitations in real-world emergency department (ED) settings. An ideal triage system is the most elusive and hotly contested quality improvement that one can undertake in emergency medicine since even today's five-level tools cannot escape challenges regarding their accuracy, validity, or consistency among different patient populations. It is within this context that the works of Farrohknia et al. and Zachariasse et al. are placed since they present a veritable accounting of the major triage frameworks—ATS, CTAS, ESI, and MTS—not only based on validity and reproducibility but also specific performances in high-risk subgroups such as pediatric and geriatric patients. Indeed, disparities continue to exist even when fully robust systems are implemented, especially at intermediate urgency categories where continuous refinement and contextualization, added by complementary risk modifiers, are justified [18,19].

Recognition of prehospital stroke has continued to bedevil even the most advanced emergency systems, as recent evidence corroborated by findings reported by Jalali et al. (Contribution 13) attests. There is still a diagnostic gap in the field. Contemporary studies sustain that even when structured tools—FAST or Cincinnati scale—are included, the paramedics misclassify up to one-third of the cases regarding the same patient complaining about suspected stroke, posterior circulation events, presentations with isolated dizziness, confusion, and atypical symptoms [20,21].

In conclusion, the articles presented in this Special Issue encompass a diverse array of subjects. We extend our sincere appreciation to the authors for their significant contributions. Their dedicated efforts have demonstrated their commitment to research endeavors. The insights and understanding they have contributed have a remarkable capacity to shape the direction of emergency medicine, advancing the notion of personalized healthcare. We encourage readers to delve into the articles and recognize the transformative effects of innovative interventions as they seek to enhance the standard of patient care.

Author Contributions: Conceptualization, O.A.M. and C.G.W.; methodology, D.-I.P. and C.G.W.; software, O.A.M.; validation, O.A.M., C.G.W. and D.-I.P.; formal analysis, O.A.M.; investigation, C.G.W.; resources, D.-I.P.; data curation, O.A.M.; writing—original draft preparation, O.A.M., C.G.W. and D.-I.P.; writing—review and editing, C.G.W. and D.-I.P.; visualization, O.A.M.; supervision, O.A.M. All authors have read and agreed to the published version of the manuscript.

Acknowledgments: The Guest Editors would like to thank the authors who contributed to this Special Issue and the reviewers who dedicated their time to providing the authors with valuable and constructive recommendations.

Conflicts of Interest: The authors declare no conflicts of interest.

List of Contributions:

1 Marza, A.M.; Barsac, C.; Sutoi, D.; Cindrea, A.C.; Herlo, A.; Trebuian, C.I.; Petrica, A. Cardiac Arrest and Complete Heart Block: Complications after Electrical Cardioversion for Unstable Supraventricular Tachycardia in the Emergency Department. *J. Pers. Med.* **2024**, *14*, 293. https://doi.org/10.3390/jpm14030293.

2 Guan, G.; Michel, K.; Corke, C.; Ranmuthugala, G. A Clinical Prediction Model for Personalised Emergency Department Discharge Decisions for Residential Care Facility Residents Post-Fall. *J. Pers. Med.* **2025**, *15*, 332. https://doi.org/10.3390/jpm15080332.

3 Hsieh, C.-M.; Hu, S.-Y.; Hsieh, M.-S.; Huang, S.-C.; Shen, C.-H.; Tsai, Y.-C. Better Performance of Modified Scoring Systems to Predict the Clinical Outcomes of Vibrio Bacteremia in the Emergency Department: An Observational Study. *J. Pers. Med.* **2024**, *14*, 385. https://doi.org/10.3390/jpm14040385.

4 Piccioni, A.; Baroni, S.; Manca, F.; Sarlo, F.; Savioli, G.; Candelli, M.; Bronzino, A.; Covino, M.; Gasbarrini, A.; Franceschi, F. Multi-Marker Approach in Patients with Acute Chest Pain in the Emergency Department. *J. Pers. Med.* **2024**, *14*, 564. https://doi.org/10.3390/jpm14060564.

5 Buleu, F.; Popa, D.; Williams, C.; Tudor, A.; Sutoi, D.; Trebuian, C.; Ioan, C.C.; Iancu, A.; Cozma, G.; Marin, A.-M.; et al. Code Stroke Alert: Focus on Emergency Department Time Targets and Impact on Door-to-Needle Time across Day and Night Shifts. *J. Pers. Med.* **2024**, *14*, 596. https://doi.org/10.3390/jpm14060596.

6 Moroi, Ș.-I.; Weiss, E.; Stanciu, S.; Bădilă, E.; Ilieșiu, A.M.; Balahura, A.-M. Pregnancy-Related Thromboembolism—Current Challenges at the Emergency Department. *J. Pers. Med.* **2024**, *14*, 926. https://doi.org/10.3390/jpm14090926.

7 Kim, J.H.; Oh, Y.T.; Ahn, C. Assessing the Impact of the Pandemic on Treatment Outcomes for Cardiac Arrest Patients Utilizing Mechanical CPR: A Nationwide Population-Based Observational Study in South Korea. *J. Pers. Med.* **2024**, *14*, 1072. https://doi.org/10.3390/jpm14111072.

8 Hahnenkamp, K.; Flessa, S.; Laslo, T.; Hasebrook, J.P. Integrating Telemedical Supervision, Responder Apps, and Data-Driven Triage: The RuralRescue Model of Personalized Emergency Care. *J. Pers. Med.* **2025**, *15*, 314. https://doi.org/10.3390/jpm15070314.

9 Iancu, A.; Tudor, R.; Chita, D.S.; Juratu, C.; Tudor, A.; Buleu, F.; Popa, D.; Brad, S. Mechanical Thrombectomy via Transbrachial Approach in the Emergency Management of Acute Ischemic Stroke Patients with Aortic Pathologies: Our Experience and Literature Review. *J. Pers. Med.* **2024**, *14*, 216. https://doi.org/10.3390/jpm14020216.

10 Hodgson, N.R.; Saghafian, S.; Martini, W.A.; Feizi, A.; Orfanoudaki, A. Artificial Intelligence-Assisted Emergency Department Vertical Patient Flow Optimization. *J. Pers. Med.* **2025**, *15*, 219. https://doi.org/10.3390/jpm15060219.

11 Savioli, G.; Ceresa, I.F.; Bressan, M.A.; Bavestrello Piccini, G.; Novelli, V.; Cutti, S.; Ricevuti, G.; Esposito, C.; Longhitano, Y.; Piccioni, A.; et al. Geriatric Population Triage: The Risk of Real-Life Over- and Under-Triage in an Overcrowded ED: 4- and 5-Level Triage Systems Compared: The CREONTE (Crowding and R E Organization National TriagE) Study. *J. Pers. Med.* **2024**, *14*, 195. https://doi.org/10.3390/jpm14020195.

12 Ingielewicz, A.; Rychlik, P.; Sieminski, M. Drinking from the Holy Grail—Does a Perfect Triage System Exist? And Where to Look for It? *J. Pers. Med.* **2024**, *14*, 590. https://doi.org/10.3390/jpm14060590.

13 Jalali, R.; Bieniecka, A.; Jankowski, M.; Michel, P.S.; Popielarczyk, M.; Majewski, M.K.; Zwiernik, J.; Harazny, J.M. The Absence of Typical Stroke Symptoms and Risk Factors Represents the Greatest Risk of an Incorrect Diagnosis in Stroke Patients. *J. Pers. Med.* **2024**, *14*, 964. https://doi.org/10.3390/jpm14090964.

References

1. Airaksinen, K.E.J.; Grönberg, T.; Nuotio, I.; Nikkinen, M.; Ylitalo, A.; Biancari, F.; Hartikainen, J.E. Thromboembolic complications after cardioversion of acute atrial fibrillation: The FinCV (Finnish CardioVersion) Study. *Europace* **2013**, *15*, 1432–1435.
2. Soar, J.; Böttiger, B.W.; Carli, P.; Couper, K.; Deakin, C.D.; Djärv, T.; Lott, C.; Olasveengen, T.; Paal, P.; Pellis, T.; et al. European Resuscitation Council Guidelines 2021: Adult advanced life support. *Resuscitation* **2021**, *161*, 115–151. [CrossRef]
3. Guirguis-Blake, J.M.; Perdue, L.A.; Coppola, E.L.; Bean, S.I. Interventions to Prevent Falls in Older Adults: Updated Evidence Report and Systematic Review for the US Preventive Services Task Force. *JAMA* **2024**, *332*, 58–69. [CrossRef] [PubMed]
4. Gates, S.; Fisher, J.D.; Cooke, M.W.; Carter, Y.H.; Lamb, S.E. Multifactorial assessment and targeted intervention for preventing falls in older people in community and emergency care settings: Systematic review and meta-analysis. *BMJ* **2008**, *336*, 130–133. [CrossRef]
5. Hwang, U.; Shah, M.N.; Han, J.H.; Carpenter, C.R.; Siu, A.L.; Adams, J.G. Transforming emergency care for older adults. *N. Engl. J. Med.* **2013**, *369*, 1936–1938. [CrossRef]
6. Hsieh, Y.C.; Lee, I.K.; Liu, J.W. Improving Mortality Prediction in Vibrio vulnificus Infection: Modified MEDS Score with BUN and Arterial pH Enhances Risk Stratification. *J. Clin. Med.* **2023**, *12*, 1152.
7. Eggers, K.M.; Venge, P.; Lindahl, B. Copeptin as a complement to cardiac troponin in suspected acute myocardial infarction. *Clin. Chim. Acta* **2013**, *420*, 45–50.
8. Seymour, C.W.; Kennedy, J.N.; Wang, S.; Chang, C.C.H.; Elliott, C.F.; Xu, Z.; Berry, S.; Clermont, G.; Cooper, G.; Gomez, H.; et al. Derivation, validation, and potential treatment implications of novel clinical phenotypes for sepsis. *JAMA* **2019**, *321*, 2003–2017. [CrossRef] [PubMed]
9. Eggers, K.M.; Lindahl, B. Impact of novel high-sensitivity cardiac troponin assays on the early diagnosis of myocardial infarction. *Clin. Chem.* **2017**, *63*, 59–65.
10. Bates, S.M.; Rajasekhar, A.; Middeldorp, S.; McLintock, C.; Rodger, M.A.; James, A.H.; Vazquez, S.R.; Greer, I.A.; Riva, J.J.; Bhatt, M.; et al. American Society of Hematology 2018 guidelines for management of venous thromboembolism: Venous thromboembolism in the context of pregnancy. *Blood Adv.* **2018**, *2*, 3317–3359. [CrossRef]
11. Couper, K.; Kimani, P.; Yeung, J.; Chilwan, M.; Quinn, T.; Perkins, G.D. Mechanical versus manual chest compressions for cardiac arrest. *Cochrane Database Syst. Rev.* **2021**, *2*, CD007260.
12. Hong, W.S.; Haimovich, A.D.; Taylor, R.A. Predicting hospital admission at emergency department triage using machine learning. *PLoS ONE* **2018**, *13*, e0201016. [CrossRef]
13. Zakariah, A.N.; Stewart, B.T.; Boateng, E.; Achena, C.; Tansley, G.; Mock, C. The sustainability of emergency care training in Ghana: A two-year follow-up of providers trained in the WHO Basic Emergency Care Course. *BMJ Open* **2017**, *7*, e015043.
14. Iancu, A.; Tudor, R.; Chita, D.S.; Juratu, C.; Tudor, A.; Buleu, F.; Popa, D.; Brad, S. Mechanical Thrombectomy via Transbrachial Approach in the Emergency Management of Acute Ischemic Stroke Patients with Aortic Pathologies: Our Experience and Literature Review. *J. Pers. Med.* **2024**, *14*, 216. [CrossRef] [PubMed] [PubMed Central]
15. Takeda, R.; Tadano, S.; Furuhata, T.; Kainuma, M.; Kawakami, C.; Shimazu, T. Using machine learning to predict hospital admission at the time of triage in the emergency department. *Stud. Health Technol. Inform.* **2020**, *272*, 150–153.
16. Grossmann, F.F.; Zumbrunn, T.; Frauchiger, A.; Delport, K.; Bingisser, R.; Nickel, C.H. At risk of undertriage? Testing the performance and accuracy of the Emergency Severity Index in older emergency department patients. *Ann. Emerg. Med.* **2012**, *60*, 317–325.e3. [CrossRef] [PubMed]
17. Türkoğlu, M.; Durmuş, G.; Erenler, A.K. Comparison of the Canadian Triage and Acuity Scale and Emergency Severity Index in the geriatric population. *Emerg. Med. Int.* **2020**, *2020*, 2704316.
18. Farrohknia, N.; Castrén, M.; Ehrenberg, A.; Lind, L.; Oredsson, S.; Jonsson, H.; Asplund, K.; Göransson, K.E. Emergency department triage scales and their components: A systematic review of the scientific evidence. *Scand. J. Trauma Resusc. Emerg. Med.* **2011**, *19*, 42. [CrossRef] [PubMed]
19. Zachariasse, J.M.; van der Hagen, V.; Seiger, N.; Mackway-Jones, K.; van Veen, M.; Moll, H.A. Performance of triage systems in emergency care: A systematic review and meta-analysis. *BMJ Open* **2019**, *9*, e026471. [CrossRef]
20. Brandler, E.S.; Sharma, M.; McCullough, F.; Ben-Eli, D.; Kaufman, B.; Khandelwal, P.; Helzner, E.; Sinert, R.H.; Levine, S.R. Prehospital Stroke Identification: Factors Associated with Diagnostic Accuracy. *J. Stroke Cerebrovasc. Dis.* **2015**, *24*, 2161–2166. [CrossRef] [PubMed]
21. McClelland, G.; Rodgers, H.; Flynn, D.; Price, C.I. Recognition of stroke symptoms by paramedics: A systematic review of diagnostic accuracy in prehospital stroke identification. *Emerg. Med. J.* **2021**, *38*, 961–968.

Journal of *Personalized Medicine*

MDPI

Case Report

Cardiac Arrest and Complete Heart Block: Complications after Electrical Cardioversion for Unstable Supraventricular Tachycardia in the Emergency Department

Adina Maria Marza [1,2], Claudiu Barsac [1,3,*], Dumitru Sutoi [1], Alexandru Cristian Cindrea [1,2], Alexandra Herlo [4], Cosmin Iosif Trebuian [1,5] and Alina Petrica [1,6]

1 Department of Surgery, "Victor Babes" University of Medicine and Pharmacy, 300041 Timisoara, Romania; marza.adina@umft.ro (A.M.M.); dumitru.sutoi@umft.ro (D.S.); alexandru.cindrea.umfvbt@gmail.com (A.C.C.); trebuian.cosmin@umft.ro (C.I.T.); alina.petrica@umft.ro (A.P.)
2 Emergency Department, Emergency Clinical Municipal Hospital, 300079 Timisoara, Romania
3 Clinic of Anaesthesia and Intensive Care, "Pius Brinzeu" Emergency Clinical County Hospital, 300736 Timisoara, Romania
4 Department of Infectious Diseases, "Victor Babes" University of Medicine and Pharmacy, 300041 Timisoara, Romania; alexandra.mocanu@umft.ro
5 Department of Anesthesia and Intensive Care, Emergency County Hospital, 320210 Resita, Romania
6 Emergency Department, "Pius Brinzeu" Emergency Clinical County Hospital, 300736 Timisoara, Romania
* Correspondence: claudiu.barsac@umft.ro; Tel.: +40-728950041

Abstract: Synchronous electrical cardioversion is a relatively common procedure in the emergency department (ED), often performed for unstable supraventricular tachycardia (SVT) or unstable ventricular tachycardia (VT). However, it is also used for stable cases resistant to drug therapy, which carries a risk of deterioration. In addition to the inherent risks linked with procedural sedation, there is a possibility of malignant arrhythmias or bradycardia, which could potentially result in cardiac arrest following this procedure. Here, we present a case of complete heart block unresponsive to transcutaneous pacing and positive inotropic and chronotropic drugs for 90 min, resulting in multiple cardiac arrests. The repositioning of the transcutaneous cardio-stimulation electrodes, one of them placed in the left latero-sternal position and the other at the level of the apex, led to immediate stabilization of the patient. The extubation of the patient was performed the following day, with full recovery and discharge within 7 days after the insertion of a permanent pacemaker.

Keywords: supraventricular tachycardia; cardioversion; unstable patient; complete heart block; ineffective pacing; cardiac arrest; advanced life support

1. Introduction

Patients with symptomatic supraventricular arrhythmias commonly present in the emergency department (ED), necessitating urgent management. Sporadically, complications may arise, but there is a lack of comprehensive literature regarding post-cardioversion events for supraventricular tachycardia (SVT).

Traditionally, SVT encompasses all tachycardias except for ventricular tachycardias (VTs) and atrial fibrillation (AF), with atrial rates exceeding 100 beats per minute at rest [1]. Narrow QRS tachycardia is defined as a QRS duration of 120 ms or less, while sometimes, they may display a widened QRS complex exceeding 120 ms due to pre-existing conduction delays either related to heart rate or to bundle branch blocks [1–3].

In the general population, the prevalence of SVT is 2.25 per 1000 individuals, with an incidence of 35 per 100,000 person-years [1]; evidence from the United States indicates that they contribute to approximately 50,000 ED visits each year [4]. However, epidemiological studies on SVT populations are limited. Women face twice the risk of developing SVT compared to men, while individuals aged 65 years or older have over five times the risk compared to their younger counterparts [1]. Additionally, SVT is also frequent in patients with congenital heart disease [5].

The clinical presentations of SVT vary extensively, spanning from mild symptoms like palpitations and breathing disturbances to severe symptoms associated with hemodynamic instability and cardiogenic shock, which pose a risk to the patient's life [6,7]. The assessment and management of all arrhythmias consider both the patient's condition and the characteristics of the arrhythmia. The goal is to prevent cardiac arrest.

Therefore, the initial approach in the ABCDE assessment involves identifying the patient's adverse features, such as shock, syncope, acute heart failure, and myocardial ischemia. Additionally, it is essential to consistently monitor the heart rhythm and blood pressure and administer oxygen if SpO2 falls below 94%. Identifying and addressing reversible causes, such as electrolyte imbalances or hypovolemia, should be conducted in accordance with the 2021 European Resuscitation Council (ERC) Guidelines [8]. If these signs are absent in a patient with regular tachycardia, vagal maneuvers will be performed [9], with the inverted Valsalva maneuver demonstrated to be more efficient in adults [1]. In the ED, the standard protocol includes conducting a thorough history, physical examination, and a 12-lead ECG, supplemented by usual laboratory tests such as full blood counts, biochemistry profile, and thyroid function assessment. If feasible, transthoracic echocardiography should also be conducted.

If vagal maneuvers fail to resolve the issue, the initial drug of choice is adenosine (6–12–18 mg) [1,8]. A recently published study by Xiao et al. compared the efficiency of Valsalva maneuvers, adenosine, and their combination, but the results were inconclusive [10]. If adenosine proves ineffective, intravenous verapamil, diltiazem, or beta-blockers are the subsequent treatment options for narrow complex SVT, while intravenous procainamide or amiodarone are recommended for wide complex SVT. Given that atrioventricular node blockers are contraindicated for patients with pre-excited atrial fibrillation [11], the differential diagnosis should be meticulously performed before their administration. If these treatments are ineffective, synchronized cardioversion of up to three attempts is advised to terminate the tachycardia. Having a stable patient provides the advantage of granting the emergency physician the opportunity to seek expert advice for both the differential diagnosis of SVT and its treatment if initial measures prove unsuccessful.

For unstable patients exhibiting life-threatening features, synchronized cardioversion under sedation is the treatment of choice [12]. If unsuccessful, administering intravenous amiodarone at a dose of 300 mg over 10–20 min or intravenous procainamide at a dose of 10–15 mg/kg over 20 min is recommended, followed by repeating synchronized shocks, if necessary [1,8].

Here, we describe a case of a patient requiring electrical cardioversion for SVT. Following the synchronized shock, the patient experienced severe bradycardia, subsequently progressing to complete heart block unresponsive to medication and pacing, culminating in cardiorespiratory arrest.

2. Case Presentation

A 53-year-old male patient, a known smoker with no other comorbidities except for a right bundle branch block (RBBB), arrived at the ED via a physician-staffed ambulance. The patient presented with main complaints of palpitations and fatigue that started approximately 8 h before arrival, along with diaphoresis and dyspnea exacerbated by minimal efforts, particularly in the last hour.

Before reaching the hospital, a 12-lead ECG (Figure 1) and vital signs monitoring were conducted, revealing SVT with RBBB, a heart rate of 174 BPM, SpO2 at 98%, and blood pressure of 130/80 mmHg. Deeming the patient's condition stable, the emergency physician attempted vagal maneuvers, which had no effect on the heart rate. Adenosine was administered in three doses (6 mg, 12 mg, 18 mg), also with no impact on the patient's condition. After a 30 min period during which 10 mg of metoprolol was slowly intravenously administered without success, the decision was made to transfer the patient to the ED.

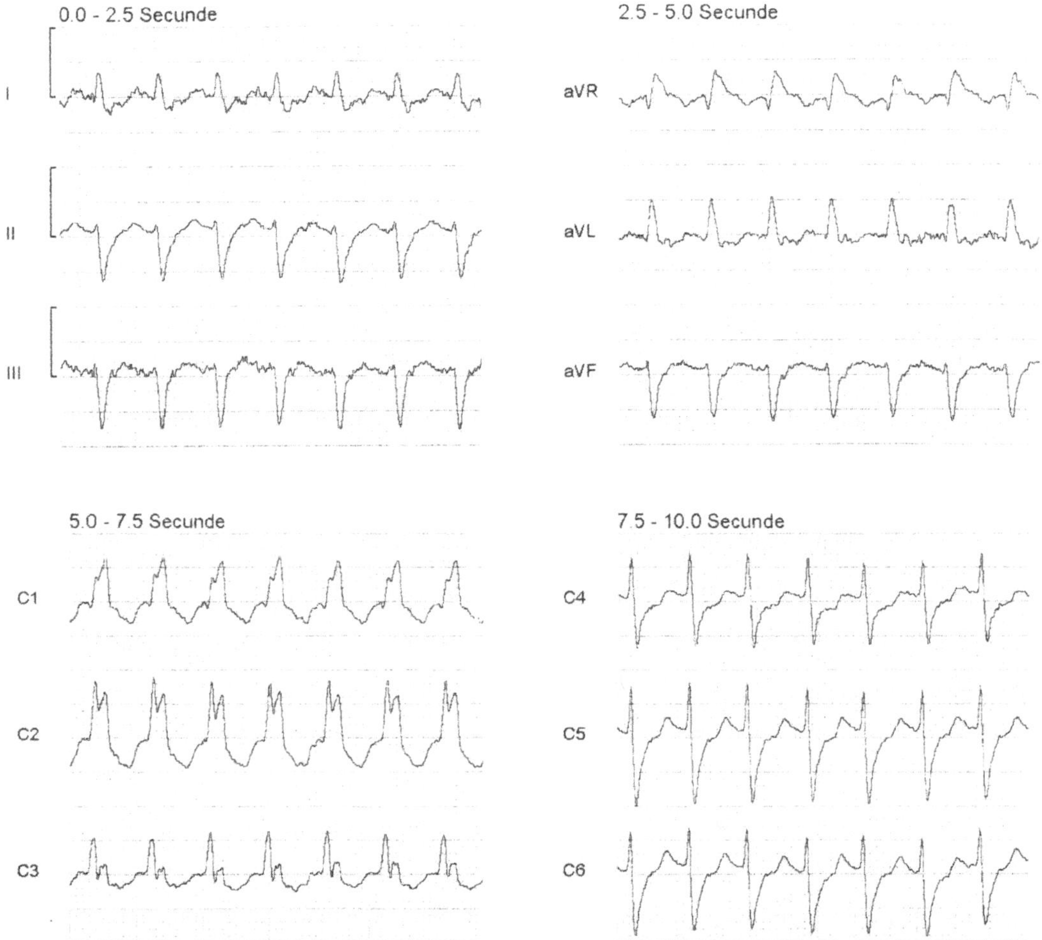

Figure 1. A 12 lead-ECG from the ambulance: regular rhythm tachycardia (heart rate 174 BPM) and wide QRS complexes of 0.14 s, with rSR′ pattern in V1 and V2; findings indicative of supraventricular tachycardia (SVT) with right bundle branch block (RBBB).

Upon arrival at the ED, the patient appeared conscious and cooperative, but he was pale, diaphoretic, and exhibited dyspnea at rest. Vital signs indicated a peripheral oxygen saturation of 93%, blood pressure at 90/60 mmHg, a heart rate of 174 BPM, a capillary refill time of 3 s, and a barely detectable radial pulse. The ECG showed SVT with RBBB, as seen in Figure 2.

The patient was administered supplemental oxygen at a rate of 3 L/min; blood work-up and arterial blood gas analysis were conducted (Table 1). After approximately 30 min, it was decided that synchronous cardioversion with 70 joules was the optimal course of action. The patient provided consent for the procedure and was sedated beforehand.

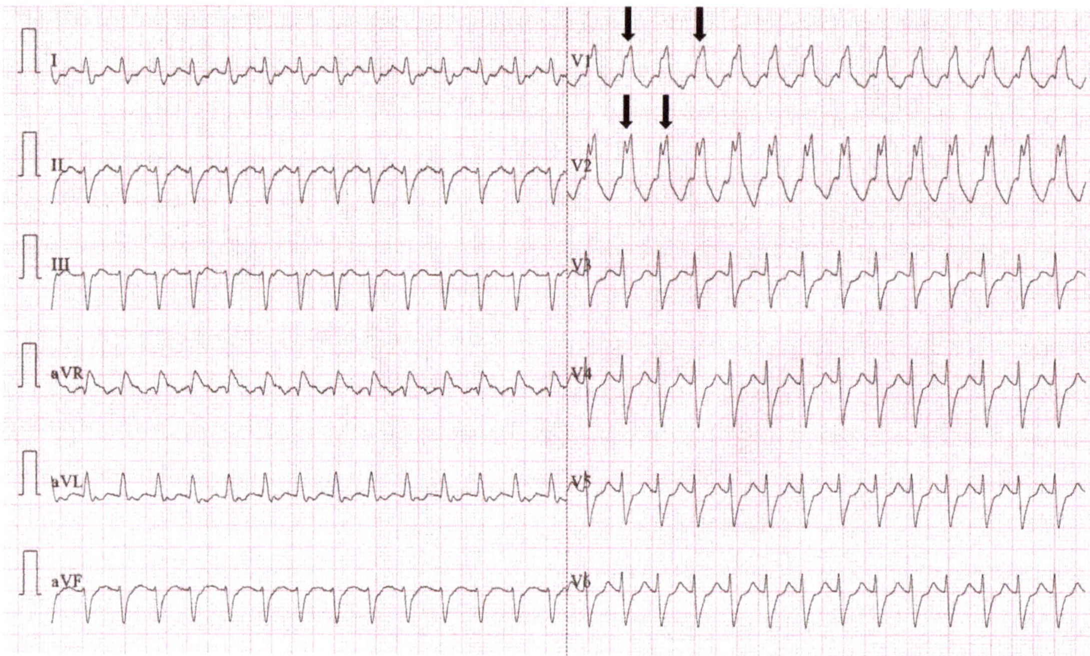

Figure 2. First 12-lead ECG (recorded at 25 mm/s, and a voltage of 10 mm/mV) from ED—regular rhythm tachycardia (heart rate 174 BPM), QRS duration of 0.14 s, rSR′ pattern in V1 and V2 (arrows), absent P waves, negative T waves in V1 and V2; findings suggestive for SVT with RBBB.

Table 1. Pathological values of the laboratory tests performed upon arrival in the ED.

Laboratory Test	Value	Reference Range Value	Conventional Units
Blood glucose	146	74–106	mg/dL
Creatinine	1.52	0.70–1.30	mg/dL
D-dimer	1.89	<0.68	mg/L
Lactate	2.52	0.36–0.75	mmol/L
NT-pro-BNP	10,217	<125	pg/mL
Troponin I	58.2	17–50	ng/L
White blood cells	11.1	4.0–10.0	$\times 10^9/\mu L$

Abbreviations: NT-pro-BNP, N-terminal pro-B-type natriuretic peptide.

Following the initial synchronous shock, the patient experienced severe bradycardia (Figure 3) for a few seconds, transitioning into asystole. Immediate resuscitation measures, including chest compressions and bag-mask ventilation, were initiated. After about 30 s, the patient exhibited spontaneous breathing and movement of limbs, opened his eyes, and responded to verbal stimuli.

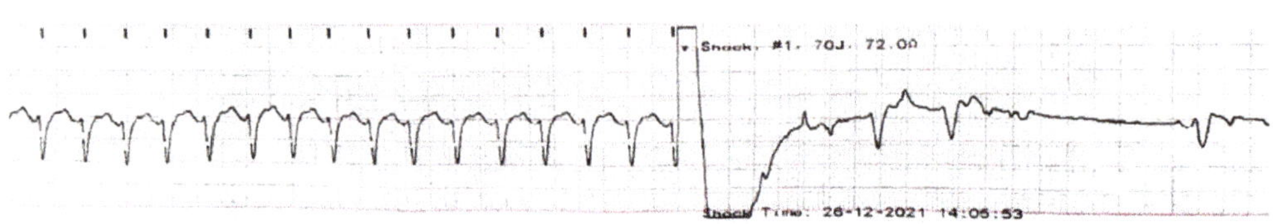

Figure 3. The defibrillator's rhythm recording during the electrical cardioversion shows irregular bradycardia after the synchronous shock for SVT.

A repeated ECG recording revealed a third-degree AV block (Figure 4), with a heart rate of 23 BPM, and the patient was hemodynamically unstable. Intravenous Atropine 0.5 mg was administered, followed by additional doses every 2 min, up to a maximum of 3 mg. Simultaneously, Adrenaline was administered via a syringe infusion pump with 2 mcg/min, with no improvement in the patient's condition. Transcutaneous pacing was initiated with a frequency set to "Demand" at 70 BPM, 80 mA intensity. Although the monitor indicated efficient capture, the femoral pulse was not concordant. Pacing parameters were adjusted to 70 BPM with an increase in intensity up to 160 mA and even 200 mA for short periods of time, yet the myocardium remained unresponsive to external pacing.

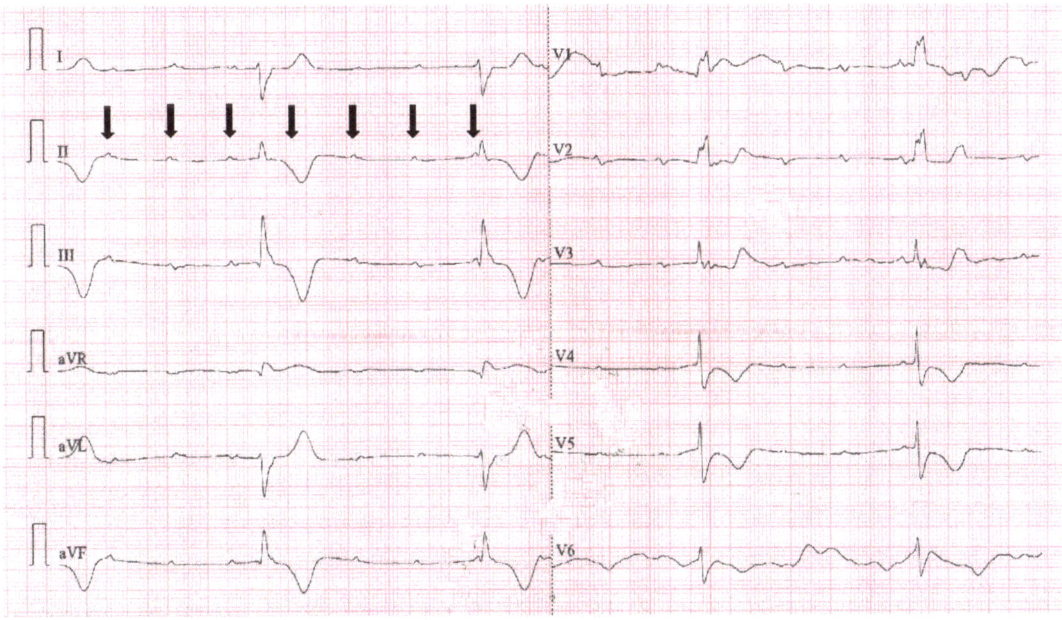

Figure 4. A 12-lead ECG (recorded at 25 mm/s, and a voltage of 10 mm/mV) after ROSC shows atrio-ventricular dissociation, with a ventricular heart rate of 27 BPM and QRS duration of 0.17 s, regular P waves (arrows), variable PR interval, right axis deviation, negative T waves in DII, DIII, aVF, V4–V6 and ST depression in the V3–V5 leads. The findings are consistent with a complete heart block and myocardial ischemia in the infero-lateral territory.

Despite efforts to improve hemodynamic stability, the transcutaneous pacing remained ineffective (Figure 5). The patient's thorax was shaved to enhance transcutaneous conduction, and the initial electrode position (right subclavian/cardiac apex) was changed to an antero-posterior and, later, to a latero-lateral position. The Adrenaline dose was increased from 2 mcg/min to 20 mcg/min. Additionally, alternative medications, including Aminophylline 24 mg over 10 min and Dopamine via a syringe infusion pump at 10 mcg/kg/min, were administered.

Throughout the patient's stay in the ED, he experienced cardiopulmonary arrest at least 10 times, manifesting as either asystole or pulseless electrical activity. Each time, the patient responded positively to external thoracic compressions, mechanical ventilation, and Adrenaline administration, achieving a return of spontaneous circulation in less than 2 min.

The on-call physician at the regional Institute for Cardiovascular Diseases was contacted and agreed to admit the patient once his condition was stable for transport. Despite exhausting all available treatment options in the ED (which lacked equipment for transvenous pacing), the patient continued to experience severe hypotension between cardiopulmonary arrest episodes due to the unresponsiveness to transthoracic cardio-stimulation. Considering the inefficacy of pacing, attributable to the patient's thoracic anatomy with a large anterior-to-posterior diameter, a decision was made to reposition the transthoracic pacing leads to subclavicular left (latero-sternal) and cardiac apex (replacing ECG lead V6) positions (Figure 6). Upon reassessment, the change in lead position resulted in successful pacing capture, confirmed by femoral artery pulse and an increase in blood pressure values.

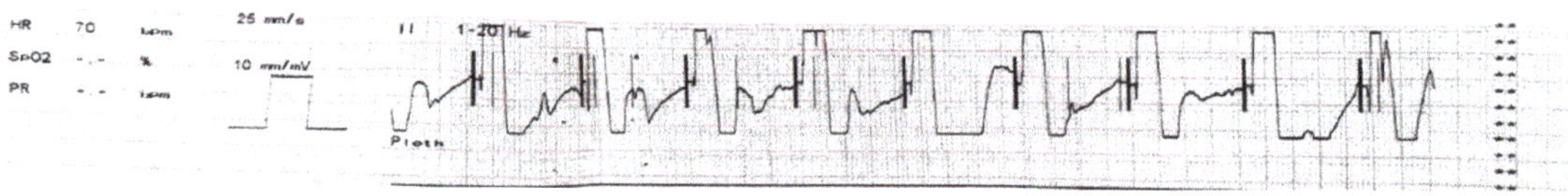

Figure 5. Transcutaneous pacing with ineffective capture and inconsistent femoral pulse. Pacing settings: mode—demand, frequency—70 BPM, intensity—160 mA.

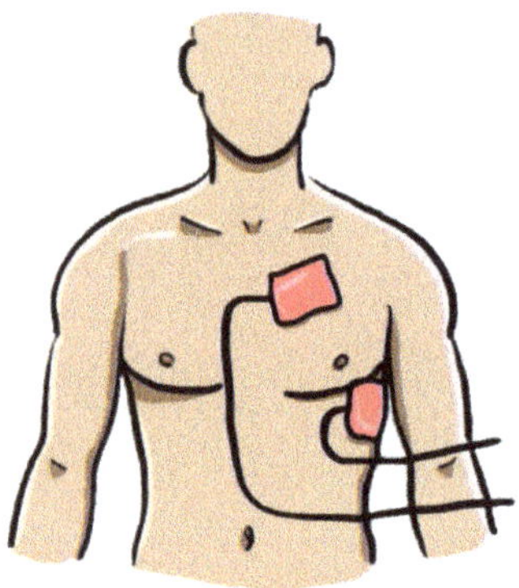

Figure 6. Placement of both transcutaneous stimulation electrodes on the left hemithorax: subclavicular left (latero-sternal) and cardiac apex (replacing ECG lead V6) positions.

Approximately 90 min after the initial cardioversion attempt, the patient's stability allowed for transportation to the regional Institute for Cardiovascular Diseases for transvenous pacing. The final evaluation indicated a blood pressure of 115/50 mmHg, heart rate of 70 BPM, consistent femoral pulse, GCS of 3 with the patient mechanically ventilated under continuous sedative medication and receiving inotropic and vasopressor medication (Adrenaline and Dopamine). Emergency transthoracic echocardiography showed a left ventricle of normal size with preserved systolic function, an ejection fraction of 50%, medio-basal hypokinesia of the lateral wall, concentric left ventricular hypertrophy, grade II mitral and tricuspid regurgitation, medium secondary pulmonary hypertension, dilated right ventricle, and a posterior pericardial fluid blade measuring below 1 cm.

Upon arrival at the regional Institute for Cardiovascular Diseases, the patient's condition improved with the placement of the transvenous pacing probe, later replaced with a permanent pacemaker implant. The following day, the patient was extubated, demonstrating complete hemodynamic and neurologic recovery, and was discharged from the hospital a week later.

3. Discussion

Synchronized cardioversion, a potentially life-saving procedure, is commonly utilized in the emergency department for hemodynamically unstable tachyarrhythmias. Emergency physicians should possess a thorough understanding of the indications and potential complications before recommending or performing this intervention. The effectiveness of frequently utilized anti-arrhythmic drugs is restricted in these situations, primarily due to concerns over side effects and their potential to induce arrhythmias, thereby limiting their usage [13].

When selecting the appropriate method for cardioversion, it is important to follow the current guidelines and carefully weigh the potential benefits and risks associated with each intervention. Sometimes, the patient is at the threshold of receiving either electrical or drug cardioversion and requires a prompt decision to distinguish between the two, given that both interventions carry inherent risks. Ventricular fibrillation (VF) as a complication of electrical cardioversion was documented in numerous studies, particularly when cardioversion takes place during the vulnerable period of repolarization, typically around the peak of the T wave on the ECG [14,15]. In 2004, Lyndon and Abdul described such a case, highlighting the significance of adjusting the lead configuration on the defibrillator monitor to prevent mistaking the high T wave for the R wave, thereby averting the induction of VF during the administration of synchronous external electric shock [15]. Kaufmann et al. described two cases of iatrogenic ventricular fibrillation after the cardioversion of pre-excited atrial fibrillation due to inadvertent T-wave synchronization [16].

In this scenario, the patient was presented with recent-onset palpitations lasting several hours, and appropriate drug therapy had already been administered in prehospital settings. Given the unavailability of intravenous verapamil or diltiazem in the region, the only remaining option for terminating the tachycardia was electrical cardioversion. Considering the patient's known history of right bundle branch block, the tachycardia was managed as SVT. Chronologically, the decision to proceed with electrical cardioversion was made over an hour after the last bolus of metoprolol, during which time no significant reduction in heart rate was observed.

Severe bradycardia, immediately followed by complete heart block and subsequent cardiac arrest with pulseless electrical activity, was an unexpected and rarely reported complication of synchronized cardioversion. Similar outcomes were described by Gallagher et al., who conducted a retrospective cohort study examining the relationship between shock energy and arrhythmic complications of electrical cardioversion. Sinus bradycardia or a slow junctional escape rhythm was observed in 22 cases, with 20 resolving within minutes after cardioversion. While two patients required permanent pacing before hospital discharge, neither needed rate support while awaiting pacemaker implantation. None of these patients experienced cardiac arrest. They also found that the incidence of ventricular fibrillation (VF) following shocks of <200 J was significantly higher compared to higher energy shocks (5 out of 2959 vs. 0 out of 3439 shocks, $p = 0.021$). Additionally, non-sustained broad complex tachycardia occurred in four cases, all lasting less than 10 s: two after shocks > 200 J and two after shocks less than 200 J. The induction of atrial fibrillation (AF) was significantly more common with shocks of <200 J (20 out of 930 shocks vs. 1 out of 313 shocks at ≥200 J, $p = 0.015$) [17].

The success of cardioversion relies on several factors, with time being the most crucial. In this case, the patient experienced symptoms for several hours, and the initial EKG recording, which revealed SVT with a heart rate of 174, was conducted more than three hours prior to arriving at the ED. Nevertheless, the patient initially declined to come to the hospital. The prolonged duration of the tachyarrhythmia could potentially lead to both post-repolarization and conduction delays due to global ischemia, as described in other studies, which reported VF as a complication following cardioversion for AF [18,19].

Furthermore, a proposed theory regarding the mechanism of complete heart block in this patient was the administration of intravenous metoprolol before cardioversion, given that beta blockers are known as drugs with sinoatrial and/or atrioventricular nodal-blocking properties [20]. In a retrospective and prospective study conducted by Osmonov et al. involving 108 patients treated with atrioventricular blockers and presenting symptomatic type II second- or third-degree AV block, 2:1 AV block, atrial fibrillation, and bradyarrhythmia, it was found that 36 patients treated with metoprolol experienced metoprolol-induced AV blocks that persisted or recurred in 24 patients [21].

However, the maximum therapeutic dose of 15 mg (recommended by ESC guidelines, American College of Cardiology/American Heart Association Task Force on Clinical Practice Guidelines, and the Heart Rhythm Society for stable SVT) [1,20] was not achieved in this case; only 10 mg was administered intravenously in 2.5 mg boluses, with no discernible effect on heart rate following the last bolus. This hypothesis was considered due to the lack of effectiveness of the transcutaneous pacing, assuming the patient had a stronger response to beta-blockers. Unfortunately, glucagon, the antidote for beta-blocker overdose, was unavailable at the time in any of the hospitals in the area, preventing the assessment of this hypothesis.

Also, myocardial ischemia or metabolic disturbances such as acidosis and hypoxia were described as factors that can elevate the pacing threshold and potentially prevent capture [22]. The patient experienced both metabolic acidosis and severe hypoxemia in the period following cardioversion, conditions that were rectified only after successful cardiac pacing.

Successful capture is typically identified by a widened QRS complex, succeeded by a clear ST segment and broad T wave. A pulse rate manually confirmed in the femoral artery or right carotid artery notably lower than the pacing rate displayed on the pacing unit monitor may suggest a lack of capture [22].

In this case, achieving efficient capture required placing the electrodes closer together. While we cannot definitively assert that this positional change was the sole factor stabilizing the patient, given the limited application to only one patient, it proved to be the sole measure in a unique and critical situation that yielded an immediate positive effect, leading to a sudden improvement in the patient's condition. Consequently, we cannot consistently advocate or recommend this procedure in routine practice. However, in similar situations where other well-known methods prove ineffective and the patient's condition continuously deteriorates, as exemplified in this case report, it may be considered a life-saving measure.

4. Conclusions

Cardiac arrest and complete heart block are uncommon complications following electrical cardioversion. Given the infrequency of capture failure cases with transcutaneous pacing, addressing each isolated case can provide significant benefits to both the ED and prehospital staff, particularly in the management of atypical situations.

Author Contributions: Conceptualization, A.M.M.; methodology, A.M.M. and C.B.; software, A.C.C.; validation, C.B., C.I.T. and A.P.; investigation, A.M.M., A.H. and C.I.T.; resources, A.M.M.; data curation, A.M.M.; writing—original draft preparation, A.M.M. and A.P.; writing—review and editing, A.M.M., D.S., C.B., A.C.C., A.H. and A.P.; visualization, D.S. and A.C.C.; supervision, A.P. All authors have read and agreed to the published version of the manuscript.

Funding: The APC was funded by "Victor Babes" University of Medicine and Pharmacy from Timisoara.

Institutional Review Board Statement: The study was conducted in accordance with the Declaration of Helsinki and approved by the Ethics Committee of Emergency Clinical Municipal Hospital from Timisoara, Romania (number 10050/12.04.2023).

Informed Consent Statement: Written informed consent has been obtained from the patient to publish this paper.

Data Availability Statement: The data presented in this study are available upon request from the corresponding author.

Conflicts of Interest: The authors declare no conflicts of interest.

References

1. Brugada, J.; Katritsis, D.G.; Arbelo, E.; Arribas, F.; Bax, J.J.; Blomström-Lundqvist, C.; Calkins, H.; Corrado, D.; Deftereos, S.G.; Diller, G.-P.; et al. 2019 ESC Guidelines for the Management of Patients with Supraventricular TachycardiaThe Task Force for the Management of Patients with Supraventricular Tachycardia of the European Society of Cardiology (ESC). *Eur. Heart J.* **2020**, *41*, 655–720. [CrossRef] [PubMed]
2. Bibas, L.; Levi, M.; Essebag, V. Diagnosis and Management of Supraventricular Tachycardias. *Can. Med Assoc. J.* **2016**, *188*, E466–E473. [CrossRef] [PubMed]
3. Ding, W.Y.; Mahida, S. Wide Complex Tachycardia: Differentiating Ventricular Tachycardia from Supraventricular Tachycardia. *Heart* **2021**, *107*, 1995–2003. [CrossRef] [PubMed]
4. Murman, D.H.; McDonald, A.J.; Pelletier, A.J.; Camargo, C.A. U.S. Emergency Department Visits for Supraventricular Tachycardia, 1993–2003. *Acad. Emerg. Med.* **2007**, *14*, 578–581. [CrossRef] [PubMed]
5. Wasmer, K.; Eckardt, L. Management of Supraventricular Arrhythmias in Adults with Congenital Heart Disease. *Heart* **2016**, *102*, 1614–1619. [CrossRef] [PubMed]
6. Patti, L.; Ashurst, J.V. *Supraventricular Tachycardia*; StatPearls Publishing: Treasure Island, FL, USA, 2024.
7. Shah, R.L.; Badhwar, N. Approach to Narrow Complex Tachycardia: Non-Invasive Guide to Interpretation and Management. *Heart* **2020**, *106*, 772–783. [CrossRef] [PubMed]
8. Current ERC Guidelines. Available online: https://cprguidelines.eu/ (accessed on 31 January 2024).
9. Prabakaran, S.; Slappy, R.; Merchant, F. Supraventricular Tachycardia. In *Handbook of Outpatient Cardiology*; Springer International Publishing: Cham, Switzerland, 2022; pp. 409–422.
10. Xiao, L.; Ou, X.; Liu, W.; Lin, X.; Peng, L.; Qiu, S.; Zhang, Q. Combined Modified Valsalva Maneuver with Adenosine Supraventricular Tachycardia: A Comparative Study. *Am. J. Emerg. Med.* **2024**, *78*, 157–162. [CrossRef] [PubMed]
11. Kotadia, I.D.; Williams, S.E.; O'Neill, M. Supraventricular Tachycardia: An Overview of Diagnosis and Management. *Clin. Med.* **2020**, *20*, 43–47. [CrossRef] [PubMed]
12. Littmann, L.; Olson, E.G.; Gibbs, M.A. Initial Evaluation and Management of Wide-Complex Tachycardia: A Simplified and Practical Approach. *Am. J. Emerg. Med.* **2019**, *37*, 1340–1345. [CrossRef] [PubMed]
13. Narasimhan, B.; Gandhi, K.; Moras, E.; Wu, L.; Da Wariboko, A.; Aronow, W. Experimental Drugs for Supraventricular Tachycardia: An Analysis of Early Phase Clinical Trials. *Expert Opin. Investig. Drugs* **2023**, *32*, 825–838. [CrossRef] [PubMed]
14. Ebrahimi, R.; Rubin, S.A. Electrical Cardioversion Resulting in Death from Synchronization Failure. *Am. J. Cardiol.* **1994**, *74*, 100–102. [CrossRef] [PubMed]
15. Xavier, L.C.; Memon, A. Synchronized Cardioversion of Unstable Supraventricular Tachycardia Resulting in Ventricular Fibrillation. *Ann. Emerg. Med.* **2004**, *44*, 178–180. [CrossRef] [PubMed]
16. Kaufmann, M.R.; McKillop, M.S.; Burkart, T.A.; Panna, M.; Conti, J.B.; Miles, W.M. Iatrogenic Ventricular Fibrillation after Direct-Current Cardioversion of Preexcited Atrial Fibrillation Caused by Inadvertent T-Wave Synchronization. *Tex. Heart Inst. J.* **2018**, *45*, 39–41. [CrossRef] [PubMed]
17. Gallagher, M.M.; Yap, Y.G.; Padula, M.; Ward, D.E.; Rowland, E.; Camm, A.J. Arrhythmic Complications of Electrical Cardioversion: Relationship to Shock Energy. *Int. J. Cardiol.* **2008**, *123*, 307–312. [CrossRef] [PubMed]
18. Sucu, M.; Davutoglu, V.; Ozer, O. Electrical Cardioversion. *Ann. Saudi Med.* **2009**, *29*, 201–206. [CrossRef] [PubMed]
19. SIMS, J.J.; MILLER, A.W.; UJHELYI, M.R. Regional Hyperkalemia Increases Ventricular Defibrillation Energy Requirements. *J. Cardiovasc. Electrophysiol* **2000**, *11*, 634–641. [CrossRef] [PubMed]
20. Page, R.L.; Joglar, J.A.; Caldwell, M.A.; Calkins, H.; Conti, J.B.; Deal, B.J.; Estes, N.A.M.; Field, M.E.; Goldberger, Z.D.; Hammill, S.C.; et al. 2015 ACC/AHA/HRS Guideline for the Management of Adult Patients With Supraventricular Tachycardia: Executive Summary. *Circulation* **2016**, *133*, e471–e505. [CrossRef] [PubMed]
21. Osmonov, D.; Erdinler, I.; Ozcan, K.S.; Altay, S.; Turkkan, C.; Yildirim, E.; Hasdemir, H.; Alper, A.T.; Cakmak, N.; Satilmis, S.; et al. Management of Patients with Drug-Induced Atrioventricular Block. *Pacing Clin. Electrophysiol.* **2012**, *35*, 804–810. [CrossRef] [PubMed]
22. Doukky, R.; Bargout, R.; Kelly, R.F.; Calvin, J.E. Using Transcutaneous Cardiac Pacing to Best Advantage: How to Ensure Successful Capture and Avoid Complications. *J. Crit. Illn.* **2003**, *18*, 219–225. [PubMed]

Journal of *Personalized Medicine*

MDPI

Article

Assessing the Impact of the Pandemic on Treatment Outcomes for Cardiac Arrest Patients Utilizing Mechanical CPR: A Nationwide Population-Based Observational Study in South Korea

Jae Hwan Kim, Young Taeck Oh and Chiwon Ahn *

Department of Emergency Medicine, College of Medicine, Chung-Ang University, Seoul 06974, Republic of Korea; thesult@cauhs.or.kr (J.H.K.); powerfreeze@cauhs.or.kr (Y.T.O.)
* Correspondence: cahn@cau.ac.kr; Tel.: +82-2-6299-2846

Abstract: Introduction: Cardiopulmonary resuscitation with mechanical devices (MCPR) was developed to provide high-quality cardiopulmonary resuscitation (CPR) for patients with cardiac arrest. However, the effect of this procedure on treatment outcomes remains controversial. Nevertheless, during the coronavirus disease-19 (COVID-19) pandemic, in-hospital MCPR gained attention, owing to its advantages such as saving medical staff and preventing infection. This study compared the treatment outcomes of in-hospital MCPR and manual CPR for out-of-hospital cardiac arrest (OHCA) patients during the COVID-19 pandemic. Materials and Methods: This retrospective nationwide population-based study was conducted in South Korea. Data were collected from the Out-of-Hospital Cardiac Arrest surveillance database managed by the Korea Disease Control and Prevention Agency. We included adult OHCA patients transported by emergency medical services from 2016 to 2021. The study compared outcomes during the COVID-19 pandemic years (2020–2021) with the preceding non-pandemic years (2018–2019). The primary outcome was survival to hospital discharge, and the secondary outcomes were good neurological outcome and sustained return of spontaneous circulation (ROSC). Results: The entire study included 72,050 patients with OHCA and, in the multivariable analyses, MCPR was associated with lower survival rates compared to manual CPR (AOR 0.63; 95% CI 0.51–0.77; $p < 0.001$). Interestingly, during the COVID-19 pandemic, while MCPR use increased, the survival rate did not differ significantly between the MCPR and manual-CPR groups. Conclusion: Our study findings suggest that while MCPR may offer potential benefits, such as decreased infection risk for healthcare workers, it did not demonstrate superior outcomes compared to manual CPR in our study population.

Keywords: cardiopulmonary resuscitation; cardiac arrest; mechanical device; mechanical CPR; COVID-19

1. Introduction

Sudden cardiac arrests remain an important public health concern [1]. Cardiopulmonary resuscitation (CPR) is a critical intervention for enhancing the survival of patients experiencing cardiac arrest [2]. Therefore, there have been continuous efforts to determine the proper chest-compression depth and rate to provide effective and high-quality CPR [3]. When CPR is performed with human-powered chest compressions (manual CPR), the quality of the chest compressions decreases over time, as the rescuer becomes fatigued [4,5]. In response, various mechanical CPR devices have been developed and used to provide automatic chest compressions [6,7]. However, in previous studies, the notion of whether these devices improve treatment outcomes in patients with cardiac arrest has been controversial [8,9]. Mechanical chest-compression devices provide external chest compressions in place of a human rescuer. In general, mechanical CPR devices can be divided into two categories. based on the mechanism by which they deliver chest compressions [10]. One is to press the thoracic cavity widely by a load-distributing band like AutoPulse™ (Revivant, Sunnyvale, CA, USA), and the other is to point and directly press the sternum by a piston device like LUCAS™ (LUCAS, Redmond, WA, USA) and Thumper™ (Michigan Instruments, Grand Rapids, MI, USA) [10]. Some animal studies have shown that mechanical chest compression can increase coronary perfusion pressure and myocardial blood flow, improving neurologically intact survival [11]. In a manikin study, MCPR resulted in better compliance with CPR guidelines compared to manual CPR. This was especially true during patient transport [12]. As such, while CPR with a mechanical device (MCPR) offers benefits such as supplementing the lacking manpower and ensuring constant chest compressions during CPR, evidence to date has not demonstrated its superiority over manual CPR [10]. Even the most recent CPR guidelines do not routinely recommend MCPR [13,14]. Consequently, MCPR is employed as a supplementary intervention, rather than as an alternative to manual CPR [13,14].

MCPR has disadvantages, such as mechanical trauma caused by the device and increased chest-compression hands-off time, due to device installation [15–17]. The pandemic has particularly highlighted the potential advantages of MCPR, including minimizing rescuer exposure to the virus and compensating for manpower shortages during peak periods of medical crisis. In particular, the need for MCPR has been highlighted during disasters such as the Coronavirus disease 2019 (COVID-19) pandemic [18,19]. Despite the risk of rescuers becoming infected with COVID-19 from the transmission generated during CPR, there are no immediate tests for COVID-19 in patients with out-of-hospital cardiac arrest (OHCA). The American Heart Association issued interim guidelines on resuscitation, suggesting that MCPR should be considered to reduce the number of rescuers [20].

This study endeavors to bridge this gap by leveraging recent nationwide data from South Korea to assess the impact of MCPR on the outcomes of patients experiencing OHCA. Particularly, it focuses on the COVID-19 pandemic period, during which the use of prehospital MCPR significantly increased to prevent infections and address understaffing issues, a trend that is likely to have extended to in-hospital MCPR, as well [19,21,22]. By comparing the survival rates to hospital discharge between patients treated with manual CPR and those receiving MCPR, and conducting an analysis to elucidate the pandemic's effect, this research aims to provide a timely and critical evaluation of MCPR's utility in contemporary emergency medicine. There have been previous studies that analyzed past data, but in this study, the analysis was carried out with updated information [23].

Our investigation aims to systematically assess the prognostic significance of MCPR during the COVID-19 pandemic, utilizing a comprehensive, nationwide dataset from South Korea. The main goal of our study is to evaluate the impact of MCPR on treatment outcomes for patients experiencing OHCA during the pandemic period. Additionally, we aim to shed light on the evolving emergency care practices during health crises, and offer critical insights into optimal CPR strategies. These insights are intended to support healthcare professionals in making well-informed decisions to improve patient care outcomes now and in the future. Furthermore, this study aims to establish a foundational basis for future guidelines on managing OHCA patients, especially in scenarios involving new infectious-disease outbreaks.

2. Materials and Methods

2.1. Study Design

This retrospective nationwide population-based observational study evaluated the characteristics of patients with OHCA and the prognostic factors associated with survival-to-hospital-discharge, good neurological outcomes, and the return of spontaneous circulation (ROSC) from January 2016 to December 2021, using the Out-of-Hospital Cardiac Arrest Surveillance (OHCAS) database (managed by the Korea Disease Control and Prevention Agency (KDCA)). The database includes all patients with acute OHCA transferred to medical institutions via the EMS (approximately 30,000 patients per year).

In South Korea, public EMSs are managed by the government (National Fire Agency, comprising 19 fire station headquarters), and are provided 24 h a day, 365 days a year [24]. Before visiting the hospital, the paramedics used an automated external defibrillator (AED) to perform CPR. CPR can be stopped, or advanced airway methods can be used, under the supervision of a doctor. However, advanced cardiac life-support drugs cannot be used. After the arrival of victims, each hospital has a policy for administering resuscitation treatments during hospitalization and after ROSC. The EMS data register and hospital medical records were used to obtain patient information from the OHCAS database. Medical-record investigators from the KCDA visited the medical facilities to review the patients' medical records and to verify several items, in accordance with the Utstein-style [25] and Resuscitation Outcomes Consortium Project [26].

2.2. Participants

This study included all adult patients with OHCA transported via the EMSs who were older than 18 years between January 2016 and December 2021. The intervention group comprised patients who underwent MCPR in the emergency department using various devices. The control group included patients who underwent manual CPR. We excluded patients younger than 18 years-old, cases with non-medical causes such as drowning, trauma, poisoning, or hanging, and cases in which CPR was not performed in the emergency department (patients with ROSC before arrival at the medical facility, death on arrival, patients with "do not resuscitate" orders, etc.). Of the total data, 2020 and 2021 were set as the COVID-19 pandemic period and the two previous years, 2018 and 2019, were set as the pre-pandemic period.

2.3. Outcome Measures

The primary outcome was survival-to-hospital-discharge, defined as normal discharge or transfer to another medical facility for long-term care after acute treatment. Secondary outcomes were good neurological outcomes and return of spontaneous circulation. Neurological outcomes were categorized using the Cerebral Performance Category (CPC) score, and good neurological outcomes were defined as CPC scores of 1 and 2.

2.4. Variables

The primary concern was the use of a mechanical resuscitation device during CPR in the emergency room for patients with OHCA. According to the Utstein style, several variables were collected, including age, sex, place of arrest (public and non-public), whether the arrest was witnessed, whether bystander CPR was performed, initial cardiac rhythm at scene (non-shockable vs. shockable), cause of arrest(cardiac origin; cause of cardiac arrest was due to failure of the heart itself vs. non-cardiac origin), whether defibrillation was performed, and whether advanced interventions were performed, such as percutaneous coronary intervention (PCI), target temperature management (TTM), pacemaker, and extracorporeal membrane oxygenation (ECMO).

2.5. Subgroup Analysis

Subgroup analyses were conducted according to the mechanical CPR devices (AutoPulse^{TM}, LUCAS^{TM} and Thumper^{TM}). This subgroup analysis utilized data from the entire study period (2016–2021) to ensure a sufficient sample size. The AutoPulse^{TM} compresses a wider area of chest by the load-distributing band. The Thumper^{TM} compresses the chest by a piston actuated by pneumatic pressure. These two devices are not capable of decompressing the chest. LUCAS^{TM} applies pointed compression to the chest by a cup-shaped piston, which adheres to the patient's chest surface to induce active decompression [10].

2.6. Statistical Analyses

Categorical variables were analyzed using Pearson's chi-square and Fisher's exact tests. Continuous variables were analyzed using an independent samples *t*-test for parametric data and the Mann–Whitney U test for non-parametric data. The Shapiro–Wilk test was used to assess data normality. Multivariable analysis using logistic regression with backward elimination was additionally performed using all statistically significant covariates from the univariate analysis. Following the stepwise elimination of factors in the regression, only the factors that optimized the model's coefficient of determination remained. Additionally, we performed the propensity score matching (PSM) for the pandemic population between the manual-CPR and mechanical-CPR groups. Propensity scores were computed to 10 decimal places. The closest non-exposure group members in each model were matched to patients in the mechanical-CPR group with a propensity score-difference threshold of less than 1×10^{-9}. No recurrence was observed in the manual-CPR group. For all data, a p-value of less than 0.05 was considered statistically significant. Data were analyzed using R (version 4.3.0; the R Foundation for Statistical Computing, Vienna, Austria).

2.7. Ethics Statement

The study protocol was approved by the Institutional Review Board of the Chung-Ang University Hospital, in May 2023 (IRB No. 2305-006-19469). The requirement for informed consent was waived because of the retrospective nature of the study and the use of anonymous clinical data. The Korea Disease Control and Prevention Agency approved the use of the data for this study.

3. Results

3.1. Patients' Characteristics

We identified 182,508 patients who had experienced OHCAs and assessed 77,350 patients for eligibility after excluding 105,158 patients with traumatic and unknown causes, CPR less than 20 min, do-not-resuscitate orders, ROSC before arrival at the hospital, and age < 18 years. Finally, 72,050 patients were included in our analysis, after excluding patients who were transferred. The patients were divided into two groups, based on the number of patients in each receiving manual or mechanical CPR. A total of 61,696 patients received manual CPR and 10,354 patients received mechanical CPR (Figure 1). Their mean age was 69.4 ± 14.8 years, and 56.5% of patients were male. There were some significant different prehospital factors between manual CPR and MCPR, such as bystander CPR (76.3% vs. 69.5%; $p < 0.001$), cardiac origin arrest (94.2% vs. 93.4%; $p = 0.003$), shockable EKG rhythm (14.9% vs. 13.3%; $p < 0.001$) and prehospital defibrillation (21.7% vs. 19.8%; $p < 0.001$), respectively. In-hospital factors between manual CPR and MCPR, such as TTM (3.5% vs. 4.8%; $p < 0.001$) and ECMO (1.5% vs. 2.9%; $p < 0.001$, respectively,) showed significant differences (Table 1).

Table 1. Comparison of patient characteristics for manual and mechanical CPR.

	Manual CPR (n = 61,696)	Mechanical CPR (n = 10,354)	Total (n = 72,050)	p Value
Male	39,617 (64.2%)	6775 (65.4%)	46,392 (64.4%)	0.017
Age, years	69.3 ± 14.8	69.5 ± 14.8	69.4 ± 14.8	0.277
Witnessed arrest	34,619 (58.3%)	5844 (58.1%)	40,463 (58.3%)	0.67
Bystander CPR	14,761 (23.9%)	3612 (34.9%)	18,373 (25.5%)	<0.001
Arrest in public place	9200 (18.5%)	1560 (18.1%)	10,760 (18.4%)	0.47
Cardiac origin	58,089 (94.2%)	9672 (93.4%)	67,761 (94.0%)	0.003
Shockable EKG rhythm	9138 (14.9%)	1370 (13.3%)	10,508 (14.7%)	<0.001
Prehospital defibrillation	13,352 (21.7%)	2044 (19.8%)	15,396 (21.4%)	<0.001
PCI	1571 (2.5%)	277 (2.7%)	1848 (2.6%)	0.46
TTM	2175 (3.5%)	494 (4.8%)	2669 (3.7%)	<0.001
Pacemaker	194 (0.3%)	34 (0.3%)	228 (0.3%)	0.89
ECMO	951 (1.5%)	303 (2.9%)	1254 (1.7%)	<0.001
ROSC	26,443 (42.9%)	4220 (40.8%)	30,663 (42.6%)	<0.001

Table 1. *Cont.*

	Manual CPR (n = 61,696)	Mechanical CPR (n = 10,354)	Total (n = 72,050)	p Value
Survival-to-hospital-discharge	2804 (4.5%)	382 (3.7%)	3186 (4.4%)	<0.001
Good neurologic outcome	1041 (1.7%)	113 (1.1%)	1154 (1.6%)	<0.001

Values are presented as the means ± standard deviations and frequency (proportion). CPR, cardiopulmonary resuscitation; PCI, percutaneous coronary intervention; TTM, targeted temperature management; ECMO, extracorporeal membrane oxygenation; ROSC, return of spontaneous circulation.

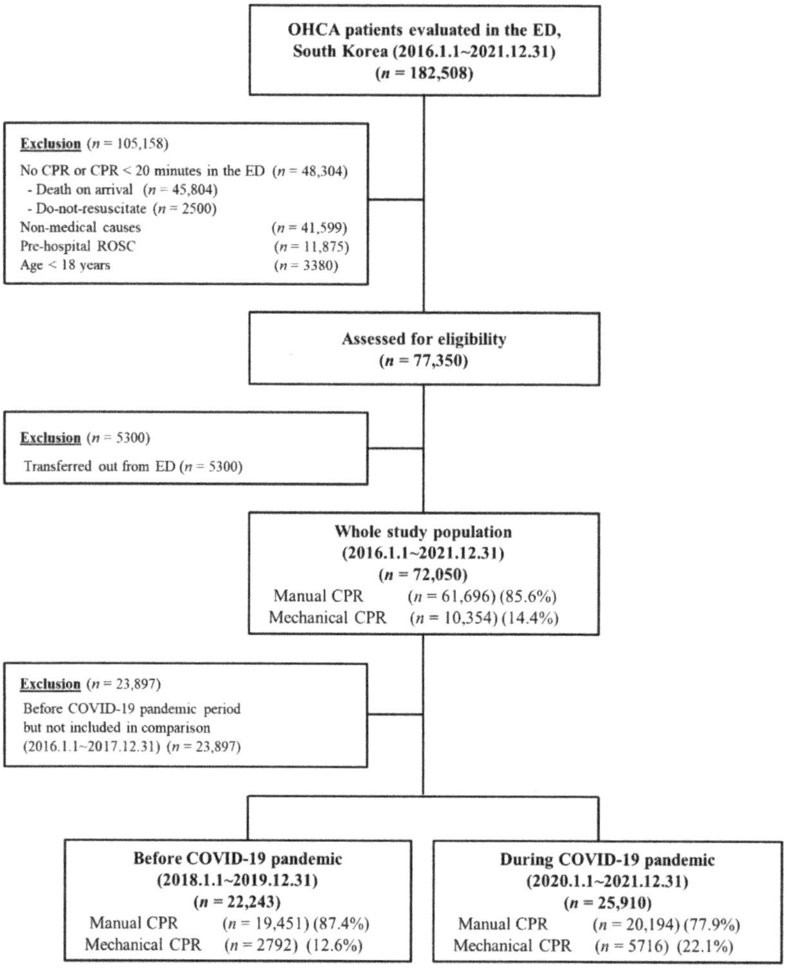

Figure 1. Comparison of patient characteristics in the manual-CPR and mechanical-CPR groups.

3.2. Outcomes: Whole Study Period

Survival-to-hospital-discharge (4.5% vs. 3.7%; $p < 0.001$), good neurological outcomes (1.7% vs. 1.1%; $p < 0.001$), and ROSC (42.9% vs. 40.8%; $p < 0.001$) rates were significantly lower in the MCPR group than in the manual-CPR group (Table 1). Multivariable logistic regression analysis revealed that age, witnessed arrest, arrest in a public place, shockable EKG rhythm, percutaneous coronary intervention, TTM, MCPR, and ECMO were independent risk factors for survival-to-hospital-discharge (Supplementary Table S1) and good neurological outcomes (Supplementary Table S2). Male, witnessed arrest, bystander

CPR, cardiac origin, shockable EKG rhythm, prehospital defibrillation, and MCPR were independently associated with ROSC (Supplementary Table S3). MCPR was significantly associated with lower survival-to-hospital-discharge (adjusted odds ratio (AOR) 0.63; 95% confidence interval (CI) 0.51–0.77; p <.001) (Figure 2A). Also, MCPR was significantly associated with poor neurologic outcome and ROSC (AOR 0.50; 95% CI 0.34–0.72; $p < 0.001$ and AOR 0.81, 95% CI 0.75–0.87; $p < 0.001$, respectively) (Figure 2B,C).

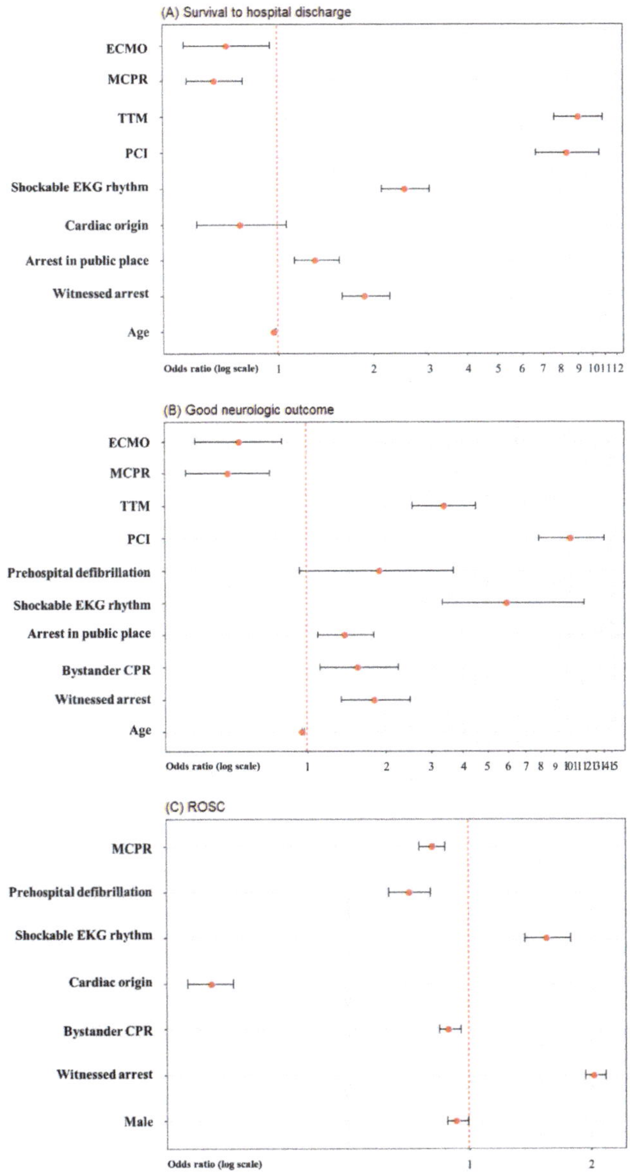

Figure 2. Forest plot depicting multivariable logistic regression analysis for mechanical CPR. **(A)** Survival-to-hospital-discharge. **(B)** Good neurologic outcome. **(C)** ROSC.

3.3. Outcomes: The COVID-19 Pandemic vs. Before the Pandemic

In an analysis comparing the pre-pandemic and pandemic periods, the frequency of MCPR was 12.6% (2792/22,243) before the pandemic and 22.1% (5716/25,910) during the pandemic ($p < 0.001$). In the pre-COVID-19-pandemic group, survival-to-hospital-discharge, good neurologic outcomes, and ROSC were all significantly reduced with MCPR, compared to manual CPR. In the COVID-19-pandemic group, good neurological outcomes were significantly reduced with MCPR, but ROSC and survival-to-hospital-discharge were not significantly different between the MCPR and manual-CPR groups (Table 2). In the COVID-19 group, MCPR was not significantly associated with survival-to-hospital-discharge (Figure 3A). However, MCPR was significantly associated with poor neurologic outcome (AOR 0.54; 95% CI 0.32–0.87; $p = 0.014$) (Figure 3B) in the COVID-19 pandemic. MCPR was not significantly associated with ROSC (Figure 3C).

Table 2. Comparison between manual CPR and mechanical CPR during the COVID-19 pandemic with before the pandemic.

Period	During COVID-19 Pandemic			Before COVID-19 Pandemic		
Chest-Compression Method	Manual CPR (n = 20,194)	Mechanical CPR (n = 5716)	p Value	Manual CPR (n = 19,451)	Mechanical CPR (n = 2792)	p Value
Male	12,883 (63.8%)	3719 (65.1%)	0.081	12,493 (64.2%)	1815 (65.0%)	0.434
Age, years	70.2 ± 14.7	70.1 ± 14.7	0.540	69.6 ± 14.9	69.3 ± 15.1	0.74
Witnessed arrest	11,615 (59.2%)	3302 (59.3%)	0.938	10,577 (56.6%)	1484 (55.0%)	0.125
Bystander CPR	5245 (26.0%)	2100 (36.7%)	<0.001	4810 (24.7%)	899 (32.2%)	<0.001
Arrest at public place	2718 (17.0%)	770 (16.4%)	0.351	2936 (19.5%)	459 (19.9%)	0.651
Cardiac origin	19,049 (94.3%)	5312 (92.9%)	<0.001	18,205 (93.6%)	2609 (93.4%)	0.796
Shockable EKG rhythm	2658 (13.3%)	703 (12.4%)	0.093	2907 (15.0%)	393 (14.1%)	0.218
Prehospital defibrillation	3937 (19.5%)	1064 (18.6%)	0.141	4174 (21.5%)	580 (20.8%)	0.410
PCI	505 (2.5%)	160 (2.8%)	0.225	560 (2.9%)	69 (2.5%)	0.248
TTM	722 (3.6%)	297 (5.2%)	<0.001	760 (3.9%)	114 (4.1%)	0.693
Pacemaker	54 (0.3%)	18 (0.3%)	0.646	54 (0.3%)	8 (0.3%)	1.000
ECMO	359 (1.8%)	156 (2.7%)	<0.001	319 (1.6%)	93 (3.3%)	<0.001
ROSC	8612 (42.6%)	2405 (42.1%)	0.449	8611 (44.3%)	1089 (39.0%)	<0.001
Survival-to-hospital-discharge	808 (4.0%)	210 (3.7%)	0.278	937 (4.8%)	101 (3.6%)	0.006
Good neurologic outcome	317 (1.6%)	66 (1.2%)	0.025	345 (1.8%)	26 (0.9%)	0.002

Values are presented as the means ± standard deviations and frequency (proportion). CPR, cardiopulmonary resuscitation; PCI, percutaneous coronary intervention; TTM, targeted temperature management; ECMO, extracorporeal membrane oxygenation; ROSC, return of spontaneous circulation.

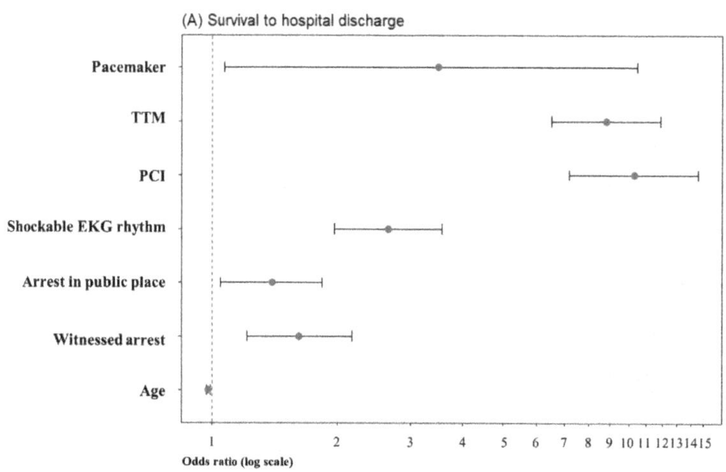

Figure 3. *Cont.*

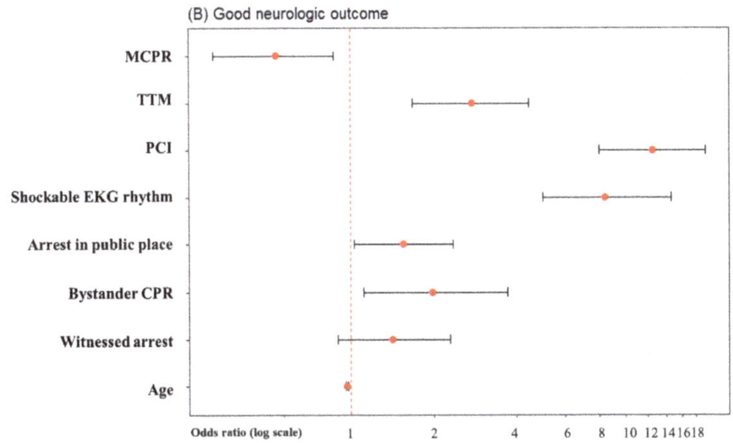

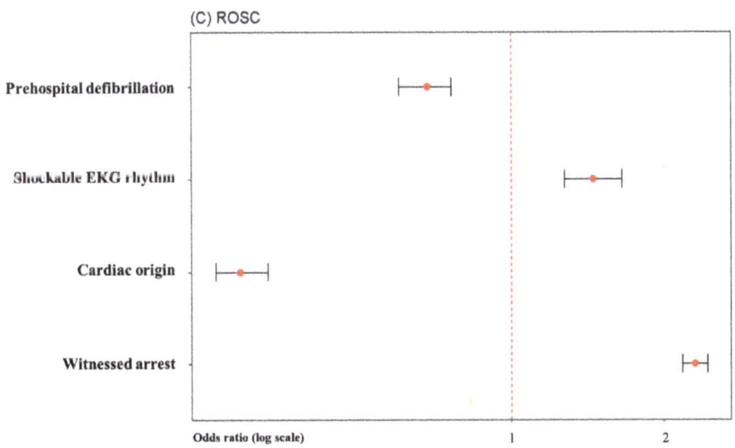

Figure 3. Forest plot depicting COVID-19 pandemic analysis of multivariate logistic regression analysis for mechanical CPR. (**A**) Survival-to-hospital-discharge. (**B**) Good neurologic outcome. (**C**) ROSC.

The PSM cohort extracted during the pandemic manual-CPR group was larger than the MCPR group. There were 5716 patients in the matching group. Both groups showed a well-balanced distribution of factors, except for PCI. In the PSM cohort, ROSC, survival, and neurological outcomes were significantly reduced with MCPR (Table 3).

Table 3. Comparison of patient characteristics and treatment outcomes in manual and mechanical CPR during the COVID-19 pandemic after the propensity score matching.

Chest-Compression Method	Manual CPR (n = 5716)	Mechanical CPR (n = 5716)	p Value
Male	3701 (64.7%)	3719 (65.1%)	0.739
Age, years	70.0 ± 14.5	70.1 ± 14.7	0.892
Witnessed arrest	3320 (57.8%)	3302 (59.3%)	0.747
Bystander CPR	2129 (37.2%)	2100 (36.7%)	0.588
Arrest at public place	778 (13.6%)	770 (13.5%)	0.848
Cardiac origin	5306 (92.8%)	5312 (92.9%)	0.856
Shockable EKG rhythm	707 (12.4%)	703 (12.3%)	0.932
Prehospital defibrillation	1030 (18.0%)	1064 (18.6%)	0.425

Table 3. *Cont.*

Chest-Compression Method	Manual CPR (n = 5716)	Mechanical CPR (n = 5716)	p Value
PCI	122 (2.1%)	160 (2.8%)	0.026
TTM	291 (5.1%)	297 (5.2%)	0.832
Pacemaker	10 (0.2%)	18 (0.3%)	0.185
ECMO	126 (2.2%)	156 (2.7%)	0.080
ROSC	2513 (44.0%)	2405 (42.1%)	0.043
Survival-to-hospital-discharge	267 (4.7%)	210 (3.7%)	0.009
Good neurologic outcome	106 (1.9%)	66 (1.2%)	0.003

Values are presented as the means ± standard deviations and frequency (proportion). CPR, cardiopulmonary resuscitation; PCI, percutaneous coronary intervention; TTM, targeted temperature management; ECMO, extracorporeal membrane oxygenation; ROSC, return of spontaneous circulation.

3.4. Subgroup Analysis: Types of Mechanical CPR Devices

Across all three mechanical CPR devices, the use of mechanical CPR devices did not appear to significantly affect survival-to-hospital-discharge, compared with manual CPR (4.0% vs. 3.3%; p = 0.598, 4.0% vs. 3.5%; p = 0.153, and 4.0% vs. 7.7%; p = 0.053) (Supplementary Tables S4–S6).

4. Discussion

The use of mechanical CPR devices is a subject of ongoing debate in the medical community, particularly regarding their effectiveness and impact on treatment outcomes. This study aimed to investigate the impact of in-hospital MCPR on the treatment outcomes of OHCA patients, comparing it with manual CPR, using nationwide population-based data from South Korea. During the COVID-19 pandemic, interim guidelines for the treatment of patients with OHCA were distributed by various organizations, and MCPR was recommended owing to staff shortages and to prevent infection. As a result, MCPR was used more frequently, and we hypothesized that the impact of MCPR on the prognosis of OHCA patients would differ. We compared the prognosis of MCPR with that of manual CPR before and after the COVID-19 pandemic. This was done to provide a basis for future guidelines for the treatment of OHCA patients in the event of a new infectious-disease outbreak.

An analysis of CPR data from OCHA in South Korea between 2016 and 2021 revealed that survival, neurological outcomes, and ROSC were poorer in patients who received MCPR during the hospital stage compared to those who received manual CPR. In multivariate analysis adjusting for various variables, age, witnessed status, occurrence of cardiac arrest in public places, and shockable rhythm were the major variables affecting survival rate. MCPR was significantly associated with a lower survival rate. In the analysis before the COVID-19 pandemic, the survival rate, neurological outcome, and ROSC all showed negative outcomes with MCPR, compared to manual CPR. During the COVID-19 pandemic, the survival rate did not differ significantly between the two groups. Although PSM analysis showed that the MCPR group had lower survival-to-hospital-discharge, in the multivariable logistic analysis, MCPR was not an influencing factor for survival-to-hospital-discharge during the COVID-19 pandemic. It is necessary to note that the impact of the MCPR during the pandemic showed differences from that prior to the pandemic. Based on the results of this study, it cannot be concluded whether or not the application of MCPR improved treatment outcomes.

Before the pandemic, the survival rate of MCPR was 3.8%, and during the pandemic, it was approximately 3.6%. However, with manual CPR, the survival rate was 4.9% before the pandemic and it decreased to approximately 4.0% during the pandemic. This indicates that manual CPR during the pandemic differed from that performed previously. During the COVID-19 pandemic, healthcare workers had been advised to wear personal protective equipment during in-hospital CPR for safety and to prevent the spread of the virus, and to perform resuscitations with fewer staff [27]. This placed an additional burden on the resuscitation efforts, which may have had a negative impact on factors affecting patient outcomes. This could explain why manual CPR did not show a significant difference in survival rate compared to MCPR during the pandemic period.

Additionally, before the pandemic, the MCPR rate was 12.6%, increasing significantly to 22.1% during the pandemic. Before the pandemic, manual CPR was primarily performed, and MCPR was used as an alternative when CPR was prolonged or rescuer fatigue was evident. In contrast, during the pandemic, MCPR was actively applied from the beginning, due to the overall shortage of medical resources and the need to protect medical staff from infection [19], and interim guidelines recommending its application had led to more widespread use of this technique [20,28,29]. As a characteristic of the pandemic, Lim et al. in Korea showed an increase in the use of MCPR in prehospital settings [21], which was the first study to confirm that MCPR was applied at a high frequency in patients admitted to the hospital with OHCA.

Although the findings from our study show reduced survival and neurological outcomes with MCPR, it is important to compare these results with findings from other studies. A meta-analysis of previous randomized controlled trials comparing MCPR with manual CPR found no statistically significant differences between MCPR and manual CPR in treatment outcomes, including ROSC, survival-to-hospital-discharge, and good neurological outcomes [30]. El-Menya et al. conducted an umbrella review of systematic reviews comparing MCPR and manual CPR, and concluded that they could not provide sufficient evidence that MCPR is superior to manual CPR [8] Other studies have indicated that MCPR might be useful in specific scenarios, such as prolonged resuscitation or during transport. However, our findings do not support these advantages in the context of the COVID-19 pandemic, where MCPR did not show a survival benefit.

Kim et al. found that, until 2016, AutoPulse™ was the most common mechanical CPR device used in South Korean hospitals [23]; however, more recently, LUCAS™ has been widely used (Supplementary Figure S1). However, when comparing each device with manual CPR in terms of survival, there was no significant difference, showing the same trend as that in previous studies. LUCAS™ differs from other devices, in that it can be performed according to CPR guidelines in terms of compression rate and depth [31]. The devices are also relatively simple to apply, and have a relative advantage in terms of side effects, which has made them preferred in recent years [32].

Previous studies have shown that in-hospital cardiac arrest (IHCA) cases tend to have specific characteristics and result in better clinical outcomes compared to OHCA cases [33,34]. It is important to note that our study only included patients who experienced OHCA and received CPR before hospital admission. Pure IHCA cases were not included in this analysis, due to the limitations of the OHCAS database. This database focuses exclusively on OHCA patients, and thus we could not investigate subgroup analyses between in-hospital and out-of-hospital CPR patients. As in-hospital cardiac arrest (IHCA) cases may benefit from immediate CPR and a systematic CPR team, the outcomes could differ significantly compared to OHCA cases. We acknowledge this as a limitation of the study, and future research, including both IHCA and OHCA data, is necessary to fully evaluate the effectiveness of mechanical CPR devices across different settings. This study has some limitations. First, the medical environment differs in each country and region, and it is difficult to generalize the results to all situations, as this study was conducted in South Korea. Especially in the analysis of the pandemic, South Korea has a relatively well-controlled COVID-19 situation; therefore, the results have been different in places with different patterns of COVID-19 prevalence. Second, this is a retrospective study, using the OHCAS database. We were unable to measure or adjust for certain factors that could potentially affect OHCA outcomes, such as EMS response times, socioeconomic status, patient history, and the quality of in-hospital CPR, due to the lack of these data in the database. Additionally, important clinical factors that could influence patient outcomes were not available in our database. Laboratory and clinical data could have provided further insights into the impact of these conditions on survival and neurological outcomes in cardiac arrest patients. The absence of such detailed clinical data limits the scope of our analysis, and future studies that incorporate these parameters are needed to better understand their effects on CPR outcomes. Third, the COVID-19 pandemic period included in the sub-analysis was limited to 2020–2021, which is the early- to mid-pandemic period, and is therefore not representative of the entire pandemic. In particular, South Korea experienced an increase in mortality among COVID-19 patients in the first half of 2022 during the early stages of the omicron variant, which was not reflected. This needs to be further analyzed once the raw data are released.

5. Conclusions

In conclusion, it is clear that MCPR did not demonstrate superior outcomes to manual CPR in our study population. Despite the potential benefits of MCPR during the COVID-19 pandemic, such as reduced infection risk for healthcare professionals, these might not outweigh the importance of patient outcomes. Our study highlights the importance of thoughtful decision-making when selecting MCPR or manual CPR. It is crucial to note that our findings do not definitively favor one method over the other in terms of patient survival and neurological outcomes. Further research is needed to explore safe and effective CPR methods that can also protect healthcare workers without compromising patient care.

Supplementary Materials: The following supporting information can be downloaded at: https://www.mdpi.com/article/10.3390/jpm14111072/s1.

Author Contributions: J.H.K.: conceptualization, writing—original draft, methodology, writing—review and editing, visualization; C.A.: conceptualization, writing—review and editing, project administration, validation, supervision; Y.T.O.: writing—review and editing, resource, data curation, software, investigation. All authors have read and agreed to the published version of the manuscript.

Funding: This research was supported by the Chung Ang University Research Grants in 2023 and a grant from the Korea Health Technology R&D Project through the Korea Health Industry Development Institute (KHIDI), funded by the Ministry of Health and Welfare, Republic of Korea (HI22C155300).

Institutional Review Board Statement: The study was conducted according to the guidelines of the Declaration of Helsinki, and it was approved by the Institutional Review Board (Institutional Review Board of the Chung-Ang University Hospital on 11 May 2023 (IRB No. 2305-006-19469).

Informed Consent Statement: Patient consent was waived due to the retrospective nature of the study.

Data Availability Statement: The datasets generated during the current study are available from the corresponding author on reasonable request.

Conflicts of Interest: The authors declare no conflicts of interest.

References

1. Nichol, G.; Thomas, E.; Callaway, C.W.; Hedges, J.; Powell, J.L.; Aufderheide, T.P.; Rea, T.; Lowe, R.; Brown, T.; Dreyer, J.; et al. Regional variation in out-of-hospital cardiac arrest incidence and outcome. *JAMA* **2008**, *300*, 1423–1431. [CrossRef] [PubMed]
2. Sasson, C.; Rogers, M.A.; Dahl, J.; Kellermann, A.L. Predictors of survival from out-of-hospital cardiac arrest: A systematic review and meta-analysis. *Circ. Cardiovasc. Qual. Outcomes* **2010**, *3*, 63–81. [CrossRef] [PubMed]
3. Cooper, J.A.; Cooper, J.D.; Cooper, J.M. Cardiopulmonary resuscitation: History, current practice, and future direction. *Circulation* **2006**, *114*, 2839–2849. [CrossRef]
4. Sugerman, N.T.; Edelson, D.P.; Leary, M.; Weidman, E.K.; Herzberg, D.L.; Vanden Hoek, T.L.; Becker, L.B.; Abella, B.S. Rescuer fatigue during actual in-hospital cardiopulmonary resuscitation with audiovisual feedback: A prospective multicenter study. *Resuscitation* **2009**, *80*, 981–984. [CrossRef]
5. Jo, C.H.; Cho, G.C.; Ahn, J.H.; Park, Y.S.; Lee, C.H. Rescuer-limited cardiopulmonary resuscitation as an alternative to 2-min switched CPR in the setting of inhospital cardiac arrest: A randomised cross-over study. *Emerg. Med. J.* **2015**, *32*, 539–543. [CrossRef] [PubMed]
6. Harrison-Paul, R. Resuscitation great. A history of mechanical devices for providing external chest compressions. *Resuscitation* **2007**, *73*, 330–336. [CrossRef] [PubMed]

7. Prinzing, A.; Eichhorn, S.; Deutsch, M.A.; Lange, R.; Krane, M. Cardiopulmonary resuscitation using electrically driven devices: A review. *J. Thorac. Dis.* **2015**, *7*, E459–E467. [CrossRef]
8. El-Menyar, A.; Naduvilekandy, M.; Rizoli, S.; Di Somma, S.; Cander, B.; Galwankar, S.; Lateef, F.; Rahman, M.A.A.; Nanayakkara, P.; Al-Thani, H. Mechanical versus manual cardiopulmonary resuscitation (CPR): An umbrella review of contemporary systematic reviews and more. *Crit. Care* **2024**, *28*, 259. [CrossRef]
9. Ji, C.; Lall, R.; Quinn, T.; Kaye, C.; Haywood, K.; Horton, J.; Gordon, V.; Deakin, C.; Pocock, H.; Carson, A.; et al. Post-admission outcomes of participants in the PARAMEDIC trial: A cluster randomised trial of mechanical or manual chest compressions. *Resuscitation* **2017**, *118*, 82–88. [CrossRef]
10. Poole, K.; Couper, K.; Smyth, M.A.; Yeung, J.; Perkins, G.D. Mechanical CPR: Who? When? How? *Crit. Care* **2018**, *22*, 140. [CrossRef]
11. Ikeno, F.; Kaneda, H.; Hongo, Y.; Sakanoue, Y.; Nolasco, C.; Emami, S.; Lyons, J.; Rezaee, M. Augmentation of tissue perfusion by a novel compression device increases neurologically intact survival in a porcine model of prolonged cardiac arrest. *Resuscitation* **2006**, *68*, 109–118. [CrossRef] [PubMed]
12. Sunde, K.; Wik, L.; Steen, P.A. Quality of mechanical, manual standard and active compression–decompression CPR on the arrest site and during transport in a manikin model. *Resuscitation* **1997**, *34*, 235–242. [CrossRef] [PubMed]
13. Panchal, A.R.; Bartos, J.A.; Cabanas, J.G.; Donnino, M.W.; Drennan, I.R.; Hirsch, K.G.; Kudenchuk, P.J.; Kurz, M.C.; Lavonas, E.J.; Morley, P.T.; et al. Part 3: Adult Basic and Advanced Life Support: 2020 American Heart Association Guidelines for Cardiopulmonary Resuscitation and Emergency Cardiovascular Care. *Circulation* **2020**, *142*, S366–S468. [CrossRef]
14. Soar, J.; Böttiger, B.W.; Carli, P.; Couper, K.; Deakin, C.D.; Djärv, T.; Lott, C.; Olasveengen, T.; Paal, P.; Pellis, T. European resuscitation council guidelines 2021: Adult advanced life support. *Resuscitation* **2021**, *161*, 115–151. [CrossRef]
15. Smekal, D.; Lindgren, E.; Sandler, H.; Johansson, J.; Rubertsson, S. CPR-related injuries after manual or mechanical chest compressions with the LUCAS device: A multicentre study of victims after unsuccessful resuscitation. *Resuscitation* **2014**, *85*, 1708–1712. [CrossRef]
16. Yost, D.; Phillips, R.H.; Gonzales, L.; Lick, C.J.; Satterlee, P.; Levy, M.; Barger, J.; Dodson, P.; Poggi, S.; Wojcik, K.; et al. As-sessment of CPR interruptions from transthoracic impedance during use of the LUCAS mechanical chest compression system. *Resuscitation* **2012**, *83*, 961–965. [CrossRef] [PubMed]
17. Esibov, A.; Banville, I.; Chapman, F.W.; Boomars, R.; Box, M.; Rubertsson, S. Mechanical chest compressions improved as-pects of CPR in the LINC trial. *Resuscitation* **2015**, *91*, 116–121. [CrossRef]
18. Baldi, E.; Sechi, G.M.; Mare, C.; Canevari, F.; Brancaglione, A.; Primi, R.; Palo, A.; Contri, E.; Ronchi, V.; Beretta, G. Treat-ment of out-of-hospital cardiac arrest in the COVID-19 era: A 100 days experience from the Lombardy region. *PLoS ONE* **2020**, *15*, e0241028. [CrossRef]
19. Ahn, J.Y.; Ryoo, H.W.; Cho, J.W.; Kim, J.H.; Lee, S.H.; Jang, T.C. Impact of the COVID-19 outbreak on adult out-of-hospital cardiac arrest outcomes in Daegu, South Korea: An observational study. *Clin. Exp. Emerg. Med.* **2021**, *8*, 137–144. [CrossRef]
20. Edelson, D.P.; Sasson, C.; Chan, P.S.; Atkins, D.L.; Aziz, K.; Becker, L.B.; Berg, R.A.; Bradley, S.M.; Brooks, S.C.; Cheng, A.; et al. Interim Guidance for Basic and Advanced Life Support in Adults, Children, and Neonates with Suspected or Confirmed COVID-19: From the Emergency Cardiovascular Care Committee and Get with The Guidelines-Resuscitation Adult and Pediatric Task Forces of the American Heart Association. *Circulation* **2020**, *141*, e933–e943. [CrossRef]
21. Lim, D.; Park, S.Y.; Choi, B.; Kim, S.H.; Ryu, J.H.; Kim, Y.H.; Sung, A.J.; Bae, B.K.; Kim, H.B. The comparison of emergency medical service responses to and outcomes of out-of-hospital cardiac arrest before and during the COVID-19 pandemic in an area of Korea. *J. Korean Med. Sci.* **2021**, *36*, e255. [CrossRef] [PubMed]
22. Kim, Y.S.; Lee, S.H.; Lim, H.J.; Hong, W.P. Impact of COVID-19 on Out-of-Hospital Cardiac Arrest in Korea. *J. Korean Med. Sci.* **2023**, *38*, e92. [CrossRef]
23. Kim, W.; Ahn, C.; Kim, I.Y.; Choi, H.Y.; Kim, J.G.; Kim, J.; Shin, H.; Moon, S.; Lee, J.; Lee, J.; et al. Prognostic Impact of In-Hospital Use of Mechanical Cardiopulmonary Resuscitation Devices Compared with Manual Cardiopulmonary Resuscitation: A Nationwide Population-Based Observational Study in South Korea. *Medicina* **2022**, *58*, 353. [CrossRef]
24. National Fire Agency. Organization of the National Fire Agency. Available online: https://www.nfa.go.kr/eng/agency/organization/organization (accessed on 1 December 2023).
25. Jacobs, I.; Nadkarni, V.; Bahr, J.; Berg, R.A.; Billi, J.E.; Bossaert, L.; Cassan, P.; Coovadia, A.; D'Este, K.; Finn, J.; et al. Car-diac arrest and cardiopulmonary resuscitation outcome reports: Update and simplification of the Utstein templates for resuscitation registries: A statement for healthcare professionals from a task force of the International Liaison Committee on Resuscitation (American Heart Association, European Resuscitation Council, Australian Resuscitation Council, New Zealand Resuscitation Council, Heart and Stroke Foundation of Canada, InterAmerican Heart Foundation, Resuscitation Councils of Southern Africa). *Circulation* **2004**, *110*, 3385–3397. [CrossRef] [PubMed]
26. Daya, M.R.; Schmicker, R.H.; Zive, D.M.; Rea, T.D.; Nichol, G.; Buick, J.E.; Brooks, S.; Christenson, J.; MacPhee, R.; Craig, A.; et al. Out-of-hospital cardiac arrest survival improving over time: Results from the Resuscitation Outcomes Consortium (ROC). *Resuscitation* **2015**, *91*, 108–115. [CrossRef] [PubMed]
27. Oh, H.S.; Choi, W.S.; Lim, Y.S.; Cho, J.-S.; Woo, J.-H.; Jang, J.H.; Choi, J.Y.; Choi, K.-K. The influence of changes in-hospital infection control protocols and cardiopulmonary resuscitation environment to treatment outcomes on out-of-hospital cardiac ar-rest due to the COVID-19 pandemic: A single center retrospective observational study. *J. Korean Soc. Emerg. Med.* **2023**, *34*, 1–9.

28. Perkins, G.D.; Morley, P.T.; Nolan, J.P.; Soar, J.; Berg, K.; Olasveengen, T.; Wyckoff, M.; Greif, R.; Singletary, N.; Castren, M.; et al. International Liaison Committee on Resuscitation: COVID-19 consensus on science, treatment recommendations and task force insights. *Resuscitation* **2020**, *151*, 145–147. [CrossRef]
29. Nolan, J.P.; Monsieurs, K.G.; Bossaert, L.; Bottiger, B.W.; Greif, R.; Lott, C.; Madar, J.; Olasveengen, T.M.; Roehr, C.C.; Semeraro, F.; et al. European Resuscitation Council COVID-19 guidelines executive summary. *Resuscitation* **2020**, *153*, 45–55. [CrossRef]
30. Chiang, C.-Y.; Lim, K.-C.; Lai, P.C.; Tsai, T.-Y.; Huang, Y.T.; Tsai, M.-J. Comparison between prehospital mechanical cardiopulmonary resuscitation (CPR) devices and manual CPR for out-of-hospital cardiac arrest: A systematic review, meta-analysis, and trial sequential analysis. *J. Clin. Med.* **2022**, *11*, 1448. [CrossRef]
31. Rubertsson, S.; Lindgren, E.; Smekal, D.; Ostlund, O.; Silfverstolpe, J.; Lichtveld, R.A.; Boomars, R.; Ahlstedt, B.; Skoog, G.; Kastberg, R.; et al. Mechanical chest compressions and simultaneous defibrillation vs. conventional cardiopulmonary resuscitation in out-of-hospital cardiac arrest: The LINC randomized trial. *JAMA* **2014**, *311*, 53–61. [CrossRef]
32. Koster, R.W.; Beenen, L.F.; van der Boom, E.B.; Spijkerboer, A.M.; Tepaske, R.; van der Wal, A.C.; Beesems, S.G.; Tijssen, J.G. Safety of mechanical chest compression devices AutoPulse and LUCAS in cardiac arrest: A randomized clinical trial for non-inferiority. *Eur. Heart J.* **2017**, *38*, 3006–3013. [CrossRef] [PubMed]
33. Høybye, M.; Stankovic, N.; Holmberg, M.; Christensen, H.C.; Granfeldt, A.; Andersen, L.W. In-Hospital vs. Out-of-Hospital Cardiac Arrest: Patient Characteristics and Survival. *Resuscitation* **2021**, *158*, 157–165. [CrossRef] [PubMed]
34. Fredriksson, M.; Aune, S.; Bång, A.; Thorén, A.-B.; Lindqvist, J.; Karlsson, T.; Herlitz, J. Cardiac arrest outside and inside hospital in a community: Mechanisms behind the differences in outcome and outcome in relation to time of arrest. *Am. Heart J.* **2010**, *159*, 749–756. [CrossRef] [PubMed]

Journal of
Personalized Medicine

MDPI

Article

Multi-Marker Approach in Patients with Acute Chest Pain in the Emergency Department

Andrea Piccioni [1,*,†], Silvia Baroni [2,†], Federica Manca [1], Francesca Sarlo [2], Gabriele Savioli [3], Marcello Candelli [1], Alessandra Bronzino [1], Marcello Covino [1], Antonio Gasbarrini [4] and Francesco Franceschi [1]

1 Department of Emergency, Anesthesiological and Reanimation Sciences, Fondazione Policlinico Universitario Agostino Gemelli-IRCCS, 00168 Roma, Italy; federica.manca@guest.policlinicogemelli.it (F.M.); marcello.candelli@policlinicogemelli.it (M.C.); alessandra.bronzino@policlinicogemelli.it (A.B.); marcello.covino@policlinicogemelli.it (M.C.); francesco.franceschi@policlinicogemelli.it (F.F.)

2 Unit of Chemistry, Biochemistry and Clinical Molecular Biology, Department of Laboratory and Hematological Sciences, Fondazione Policlinico Universitario Agostino Gemelli-IRCCS, Università Cattolica del Sacro Cuore, 00168 Roma, Italy; silvia.baroni@policlinicogemelli.it (S.B.); francesca.sarlo@guest.policlinicogemelli.it (F.S.)

3 Departement of Emergency, IRCCS Fondazione Policlinico San Matteo, 27100 Pavia, Italy; g.savioli@smatteo.pv.it

4 Medical and Surgical Science Department, Fondazione Policlinico Universitario Agostino Gemelli-IRCCS, Università Cattolica del Sacro Cuore, 00168 Roma, Italy; antonio.gasbarrini@policlinicogemelli.it

* Correspondence: andrea.piccioni@policlinicogemelli.it; Tel.: +39-333-3603442

† These authors contributed equally to this work.

Abstract: Background: Chest pain is a prevalent reason for emergency room referrals and presents diagnostic challenges. The physician must carefully differentiate between cardiac and noncardiac causes, including various vascular and extracardiovascular conditions. However, it is crucial not to overlook serious conditions such as acute coronary syndrome (ACS). Diagnosis of acute myocardial infarction (AMI) and early discharge management become difficult when traditional clinical criteria, ECG, and troponin values are insufficient. Recently, the focus has shifted to a "multi-marker" approach to improve diagnostic accuracy and prognosis in patients with chest pain. Methods: This observational, prospective, single-center study involved, with informed consent, 360 patients presenting to the emergency department with typical chest pain and included a control group of 120 healthy subjects. In addition to routine examinations, including tests for hsTnI (Siemens TNIH kit), according to the 0–1 h algorithm, biochemical markers sST2 (tumorigenicity suppression-2) and suPAR (soluble urokinase plasminogen activator receptor) were also evaluated for each patient. A 12-month follow-up was conducted to monitor outcomes and adverse events. Results: We identified two groups of patients: a positive one (112 patients) with high levels of hsTnI, sST2 > 24.19 ng/mL, and suPAR > 2.9 ng/mL, diagnosed with ACS; and a negative one (136 patients) with low levels of hsTnI, suPAR < 2.9 ng/mL, and sST2 < 24.19 ng/mL. During the 12-month follow-up, no adverse events were observed in the negative group. In the intermediate group, patients with hsTnI between 6 ng/L and the ischemic limit, sST2 > 29.1 ng/mL and suPAR > 2.9 ng/mL, showed the highest probability of adverse events during follow-up, while those with sST2 < 24.19 ng/mL and suPAR < 2.9 ng/mL had a better outcome with no adverse events at 12 months. Conclusion: Our data suggest that sST2 and suPAR, together with hsTnI, may be useful in the prognosis of cardiovascular patients with ACS, providing additional information on endothelial damage. These biomarkers could guide the clinical decision on further diagnostic investigations. In addition, suPAR and sST2 emerge as promising for event prediction in patients with chest pain. Their integration into the standard approach in PS could facilitate more efficient patient management, allowing safe release or timely admission based on individual risk.

Keywords: multi-marker approach; suPAR; sST2; chest pain; hsTnI; acute coronary syndrome (ACS); emergency department (ED); early risk stratification

1. Introduction

Chest pain is a frequent cause of admission to the ER [1–4] and can result from multiple origins, both cardiac and extracardiac [3–5]. It is crucial to quickly begin management of patients with life-threatening conditions such as acute coronary syndrome (ACS), aortic dissection, and pulmonary embolism, as well as other serious nonvascular conditions. Subsequently, targeted therapy must be given to those with less critical diseases. Although there are several life-threatening causes, chest pain often reflects more benign conditions [5].

Guidelines recommend an ECG within 10 min of arrival in the emergency department for patients with suspected acute myocardial infarction (AMI) [5–7]. High-sensitivity cardiac troponins are critical in identifying cardiac damage but do not specify the cause [7,8]. They may indeed be elevated in conditions such as acute heart failure, pericarditis, myocarditis, or arrhythmias [8]. However, a significant increase in cardiac troponins is an indicator of high risk for ACS [7–9].

The emergency physician must then stratify the patient's risk for ACS or MACE in the short term. Prognostic tools such as HEART, GRACE, and TIMI scores are used to evaluate patients for whom ECG and troponin tests are not diagnostic [7–14]. According to these scores, patients with cardiac chest pain, non-elevated hsTnI, and a negative ECG for ACS, but with risk factors such as diabetes, hypertension, hypercholesterolemia, or smoking, are considered to be at intermediate risk and need further diagnostic tests. These may include stress testing, exercise imaging, CCTA, or ICA, which often prolong hospital stays [7].

Our goal is to propose a safe and efficient clinical pathway for intermediate-risk patients, allowing the clinician to safely discharge those who do not need further attention and focus on those at higher risk of ACS or MACE in the short term, using a multi-marker approach based on suPAR and sST2 values.

2. Biomarkers

Cardiac biomarkers are an essential component of the criteria used to establish the diagnosis of an acute myocardial infarction. Troponin is the biomarker of first choice for the detection of myocardial damage and has a class I indication for the diagnosis of myocardial infarction according to the most recent ESC guidelines [15].

The current limitation, but at the same time the strength, of high-sensitivity troponin assay methods is the possibility of detecting "biochemical positivity" that cannot always be ascribed to a context of myocardial ischemia but also of myocardial injury.

The high sensitivity of the troponin kits allows for the evaluation of a wide range of clinical conditions that are non-ischemic, both acute and chronic, cardiac and extracardiac, such as pericarditis, myocarditis, Takotsubo syndrome, tachyarrhythmias, heart failure, pulmonary embolism, stroke, and sepsis [8]. Thus, hs-troponins have a high specificity for "myocardial damage" with a high negative predictive value. In addition, their values should be interpreted as a quantitative marker of myocardial damage, as there is a direct proportionality between the troponin level and the extent of injury.

SST2 has recently emerged as a promising biomarker in the field of acute cardiovascular disease. ST2 is a protein that belongs to the interleukin-1 receptor family (IL-1 RL-1) and exists in two isoforms, one transmembrane (ST2L) and one soluble (sST2). The natural ligand of ST2 is IL-33, a member of the IL-1 family, which plays an anti-inflammatory, anti-hypertrophic, and anti-fibrotic role in the myocardium [16] and is produced by different cell types, such as endothelial cells.

sST2, the soluble variant of ST2, on the other hand, is over-expressed under specific pathological conditions of myocardial stress or damage and is associated with inflammation and immune response; it is a decoy receptor that reduces the cardioprotective effect of the IL-33/ST2L pathway by binding free IL-33, which will no longer be available to the ST2L receptor [17].

In fact, sST2 is released by myocardial cells in response to myocardial infarction [18].

Although sST2 does not add elements to the initial diagnosis of AMI, its prognostic role has become conspicuous: early levels of sST2 during AMI seem to reflect the extent of myocardial necrosis [19]. Indeed, although sST2 cannot replace natriuretic peptides (NPs) in the diagnosis of AHF, its baseline increase has been shown to be superior to NT-pro BNP as a prognostic marker of mortality at 1 year and 4 years [19].

The role of ST2 in the pathophysiology of CAD and the clinical value of this biomarker in acute ST-segment elevation myocardial infarction (STEMI) have broadly expanded. Several studies suggest an important prognostic value of sST2 [20–22], both in chronic heart failure [23], in which it predicts the outcome of patients in addition to the N-terminal pro-B type natriuretic peptide (NT-proBNP) and the highly sensitive troponin T [24], and in acute heart failure [25], where it is useful in monitoring and guiding therapeutic decisions in patients with acute decompensated heart failure and acute myocardial infarction [26]. As a biomarker related to inflammation and fibrosis, sST2 has important clinical value in CAD, which may guide prognosis prediction and treatment [25,27,28].

In clinical practice, sST2 can be used in the prognostic stratification of patients and for the identification of patients at high risk of mortality and re-hospitalization in patients diagnosed with heart failure [29], providing unique prognostic information as well as complementary to that provided by the natriuretic peptides BNP and NT-proBNP, from which it is independent [30].

Although sST2 does not add elements to the initial diagnosis of AMI, its prognostic role has become conspicuous. Early levels of sST2 in AMI appear to reflect the extent of myocardial necrosis [19]. Starting from these data, sST2 could be recognized as a marker of early and late post-infarction remodeling [26–31].

SuPAR is the soluble form of uPAR, the membrane receptor of urine-type plasminogen activator or urokinase (uPA), and is released from the plasma membrane upon cleavage from the GPI anchor in response to inflammatory stimuli, regardless of the underlying cause [32].

Serum levels of suPAR are thus closely related to immune and inflammatory activation, and in the context of cardiovascular disease, suPAR has emerged as a very promising biomarker as a prognostic indicator for early prediction of events in chest pain emergency patients [33].

In fact, although its non-cardiac-specific nature limits its diagnostic value for heart disease, when used in conjunction with imaging studies and clinical rating scales in a multi-marker approach, it has been shown to ameliorate the clinical capacity to identify patients at risk for adverse cardiovascular events, morbidity, and mortality [34]. In the setting of an ACS, suPAR is associated with long-term all-cause death, heart failure, and MACE and provides incremental prognostic value beyond traditional risk factors [35].

3. Endpoint

The study sought to investigate a multi-marker approach in patients presenting to the emergency department (ED) with chest pain suggestive of acute coronary syndrome (ACS), using sST2 and suPAR, in addition to hsTnI, in the diagnostic workup and early risk stratification, to assess whether this approach improves diagnostic or prognostic accuracy, especially in those patients without a clear diagnosis. In addition, the effectiveness and validity of the multi-marker approach were evaluated through a follow-up of our patients at 12 months after ED admission.

4. Methods

4.1. Study Design

We performed a monocentric and prospective study evaluating a multi-marker approach for patients presenting cardiac pain in the Emergency Department. This study was conducted and developed in close cooperation with the High Automation Corelab and the Emergency Medicine Department of the A. Gemelli University Polyclinic Foundation, IRCCS of Rome. We prospectively and consecutively enrolled a total of 360 patients who presented to the ED of our polyclinic with chest pain or other typical symptoms. The inclusion criteria for the patient group were: (1) age $\geq$ 18 years; (2) chest pain or suggestive symptoms suspecting ACS; and (3) ability to give informed consent. Patients only presenting with dyspnoea or palpitations were not included in our study. All enrolled patients underwent standard diagnostic and therapeutic procedures according to the updated guidelines and good clinical practices. There were no alterations to the approved ACS protocol by our Polyclinic Foundation.

High-sensitivity troponins were determined following the European Society of Cardiology's (ESC) 0/1-h protocol.

Baseline demographic and clinical data (age, gender, cardiovascular risk factors, blood pressure, heart rate, electrocardiogram, respiratory rate, arterial oxygen saturation) as well as information on medications were collected and recorded on standardized data collection forms (see Table 1).

Table 1. Baseline characteristics of the studied population (N = 360 patients).

Characteristics	%
N pts	360
Sex (M:F)	57.6% 42.4%
Age (aa)	56.7 aa (33–86) M 215 (33–86) F 145 (36–77)
Risk factors	
Hypertension	52.8% M 58.3% F 45.2%
Diabetes	16.8% M 20.8% F 11.3%
Dyslipidemia	36.4% M 36.1% F 36.8%
Familiarity with cardiovascular disease	22.4% M 22.9% F 21.7%
Smoke	16.4% M 22.2% F 8%
Vasculopathy	10.4% M 14.6% F 4.7%

Plus, multi-markers' measurements (sST2 and suPAR) were performed for each patient enrolled, using the same blood sample provided by the clinical care pathway for chest pain approved in our hospital. Blood samples were immediately stored in the High Automation CoreLab of our hospital; plasma and serum were aliquoted in Eppendorf tubes and frozen at −80 °C until sST2 and suPAR analysis. The levels of all biomarkers were also examined in a control group of 120 healthy subjects with homogeneous characteristics regarding sex and age [35–37].

In our study, we did not utilize the GRACE or TIMI score, as we aimed to enhance prognostic value with actual measurements rather than clinical management tools.

4.2. Biomarker Measurements

Biomarker measurements were performed in the High Automation CoreLab of the A. Gemelli University Polyclinic Foundation, IRCCS Rome", by an Atellica Solution analyzer (Siemens Healthineers, Malvern, PA, USA).

- hs-troponin was measured by the TnIH kit (Siemens Healthcare Diagnostics, USA) using the CLIA method. The limit of detection (LOD) is 2.5 ng/L; the 99th percentile cut-off is 57 ng/L for males and 37 ng/L for females, with 10% CV at 6 ng/L. The TNIH assay-specific cut-off level (6 ng/L) within the 0 h/1 h protocol was derived from pre-defined criteria for sensitivity and specificity for ASC, as reported in ESC guidelines 2023 [15].
- sST2 was measured by the Sequent-IA kit, Critical Diagnostics USA, using the turbidimetric method applied to Atellica CH Siemens [38]. The LOD is 8 ng/mL, the measuring range is from 8 to 360 ng/mL, and the cut-off value for heart failure risk is 35 ng/mL.

- suPAR was measured by the turbidimetric method with the SUPARNOSTIC kit (Virogates DK) applied to Atellica CH Siemens. The LOD is 1.7 ng/mL, and the range is from 1.7 to 26.5 ng/mL; the cut-off is 3.0 ng/mL.

4.3. *Follow-Up*

Follow-up data were retrieved from digital and written patients' records, including discharge letters, revascularization reports, and any other relevant documentation. The 12-month clinical follow-up data were obtained from all patients included in the study by phone interview to assess clinical outcome (symptoms such as chest pain), hospital re-admission (myocardial infarction, revascularization), coronary angiography, and death.

4.4. *Ethics Statements*

The study protocol did not alter the diagnostic workup or therapeutic management of enrolled patients in any way. The study was approved by the A. Gemelli University Polyclinic Foundation, IRCCS, Ethics Review Board (protocol n° 4896/22). All patients provided written informed consent for their participation in the study.

4.5. *Statistical Analysis*

Statistical analysis was conducted using MedCalc®Statistical version 19.5.6 (MedCalc Software Ltd., Ostend, Belgium; https://www.medcalc.org (accessed on 16 May 2024); 2020) (version 15.0) software. Continuous variables were expressed as mean values ± standard deviation or as median (range), and categorical variables were expressed as frequencies. The data distribution was assessed by the Kolmogorov–Smirnov test or the Shapiro–Wilk test in order to verify the population distribution. The most appropriate statistical parametric and non-parametric tests (the Student's *t*-test or Mann–Whitney and chi-squared or Fisher) were used based on the data distribution. The Youden Index was used to choose the optimal cut-off points for biomarkers' diagnostic and prognostic effectiveness. The correlation analysis between variables was carried out using the Spearman coefficient. We calculated odds ratios (ORs) with their respective 95% confidence intervals (95% CI). A p value < 0.05 was considered statistically significant.

5. Results

Table 2 reports baseline values of hsTnI, sST2, and suPAR in all patients (N = 360).

Table 2. Baseline biomarker levels in the patients enrolled (N = 360).

	Min	Max	Mean	Median	SD	25–75 P
Age (y)	23.0	90.0	64.47	66.0	15.3	55.0 to 76.0
hsTnI ng/L	2.5	87,239.0	850.64	6.0	7353.5	3.0 to 21.0
sST2 ng/mL	12.0	501.6	34.48	24.8	48.6	19.1 to 37.5
su-PAR ng/mL	1.70	26.5	4.07	3.5	2.8	2.7 to 4.3

Then, we identified our study population in 2 groups:

- The "healthy control" group, composed of 120 subjects with hsTnI < 2.5 ng/L, in which levels of sST2 and suPAR were ≤ 2 4.19 ng/mL and ≤ 2.9 ng/mL, respectively;
- The "true positives" group, composed of 112 patients with hs-cTn concentration at presentation at least moderately elevated above the ischemic cut-off level (57 ng/L for males and 47 ng/L for females) or with a significant rise within the first hour (1 hΔ) of hsTnI levels.

The ACS diagnosis was confirmed, and all patients in this group had sST2 levels above 24.19 ng/mL and suPAR levels above 2.9 ng/mL.

We identified that sST2 and suPAR levels were significantly different in true positives versus the healthy group ($p < 0.001$); ST2 levels above 24.19 ng/mL had 100% specificity and

100% sensitivity for ACS, while suPAR levels above 2.9 ng/mL had 100% sensitivity and 85.7% specificity (see Figures 1 and 2). These cut-offs were calculated with Youden's index.

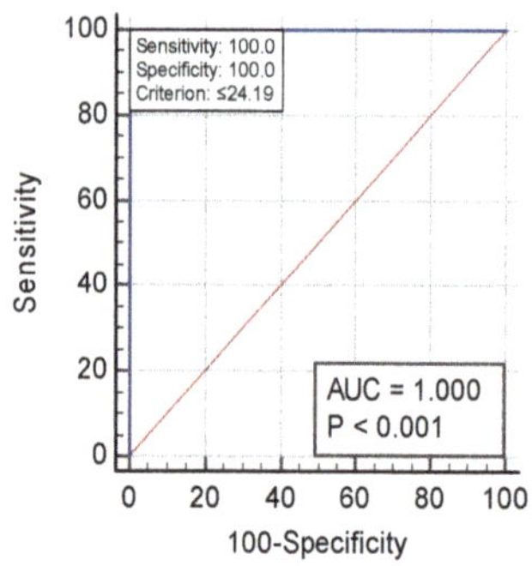

Figure 1. ROC for sST2.

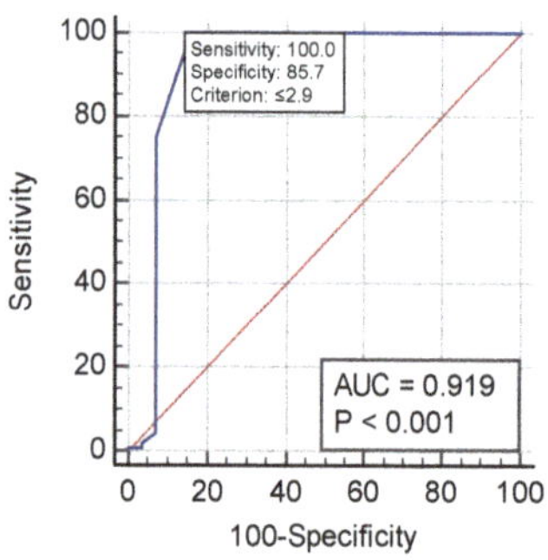

Figure 2. ROC for suPAR.

Figures 1 and 2 display the ROC for sST2 (Figure 1) and suPAR (Figure 2) in the *true positives* vs. *healthy group* (cut-off of 24.19 ng/mL for sST2 and 2.9 ng/mL for suPAR).

Then, we divided the patients according to hsTnI levels into a *"negative"* group composed of 136 patients with hsTnI below 6 ng/L and an *"intermediate"* group composed of 112 patients with troponin levels > 6 ng/L but below the ACS diagnostic cut-off for hsTnI (< 47 /57 ng/L F/M).

According to the suPAR normal cut-off, we observed that in the *"negative"* group, patients with suPAR $\leq$ 2.9 ng/mL (n 59) showed all sST2 levels $\leq$ 24.19 ng/mL, while patients with suPAR > 2.9 ng/mL (n 77) showed sST2 > 29.1 ng/mL in 65% of the cases. In the *"intermediate"* group, patients with suPAR $\leq$ 2.9 ng/mL (n 52) had sST2 $\leq$ 24.19 ng/mL, while all patients with suPAR > 2.9 ng/mL had sST2 > 29.1 ng/mL.

After 12 months from ED admission, it was possible to obtain information about the patients' follow-up through a telephone interview; we considered any event reported that we defined as MACE to be a negative outcome, regardless of the score (presence of single or multiple events).

sST2 and suPAR's cut-offs, previously calculated with ROC curves, were related to the presence or absence of adverse events of cardiac origin at the one-year follow-up through the chi-square "χ^2" hypothesis test and the relative risk.

We observed that in the *negative* and *intermediate groups*, none with suPAR $\leq$ 2.9 ng/mL and sST2 < 24.19 ng/mL reported adverse events in the follow-up (specificity 100%); these patients seem like healthy subjects.

While in the *negative* group, patients with suPAR > 2.9 ng/mL and sST2 > 29.1 ng/mL reported events in 70% of the cases.

In the *intermediate group*, almost all of the patients (84%) with sST2 > 29.1 ng/mL had adverse events at 1 year, while none showed events if sST2 was lower than 24.19 ng/mL.

The ROC curve AUC of sST2 for the excluding of events was 0.974 at the optimal threshold of 24.19 ng/mL, with a sensitivity of 100% and a specificity of 87.5% (Figure 3). The ROC curve AUC of sST2 for the prediction of events was 0.852 at the optimal threshold of 29.1 ng/mL, with a sensitivity of 85.7% and a specificity of 81.8% (Figure 4).

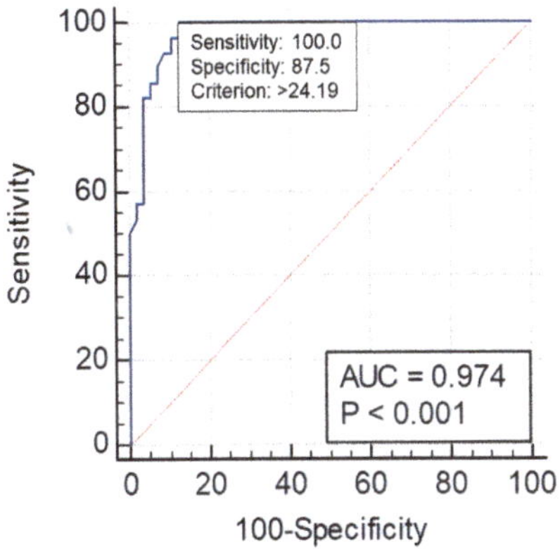

Figure 3. The *intermediate group* sST2 cut-off for the excluding of events (24.19 ng/mL).

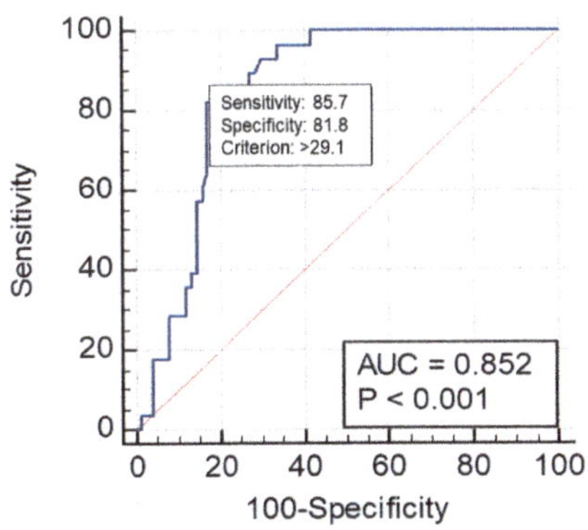

Figure 4. The *intermediate group* with a high risk of adverse events for the sST2 cut-off of 29.1 ng/mL.

In the *intermediate group*, according to the suPAR 2.9 ng/mL cut-off, the sensitivity was 86% and the specificity was 95.7% for identifying patients at risk or not for adverse events at 1 year. In fact, 80% of patients with values higher than 2.9 ng/mL showed adverse events at 1 year, while only 2% of patients with values lower than 2.9 ng/mL had adverse events in the follow-up.

sST2 was highly sensitive and specific (100% sensitivity, 90.9% specificity, positive predictive value 83.8%, negative predictive value 100%) for adverse events during follow-up; values above the cut-off of 29.1 ng/mL were therefore indicative of myocardial distress and associated with patients with a positive outcome.

suPAR was specific and highly sensitive (98.02% sensitivity, 74.5% specificity, positive predictive value 80%, negative predictive value 97.6%) for adverse events during follow-up with values above the cut-off of 2.9 ng/mL.

We also verified the significance of the association of sST2 and suPAR levels with outcome using the "χ^2" chi-square hypothesis test, which showed high statistical significance (p value < 0.001). We calculated the relative risk of an adverse event at one year in the case of sST2 higher than the cut-off of 29.1 ng/mL ($\chi^2 = 70.66$, RR = 51.11, 95% CI 7.28–358.87, p-value < 0.001) and in the case of suPAR higher than the cut-off of 2.9 ng/mL ($\chi^2 = 63.28$, RR = 3.86, 95% CI 2.45–6.07, p-value < 0.001).

6. Discussion

Patients presenting to the ED with acute chest pain are a challenge for emergency physicians and acute medicine departments, as a wide spectrum of diagnoses may cause the pain, ranging from acute myocardial infarction (AMI) and pulmonary embolism to harmless muscular tension belonging to the group of chest wall syndromes, as well as gastrointestinal causes such as gastroesophageal reflux disease. Noncardiac causes are very common, but it is important not to overlook serious conditions.

The decision to admit or discharge a patient can be difficult for the physician, especially in an acute setting such as the ED, which requires making this decision within hours. Currently, the evaluation of patients consists of a clinical investigation concerning medical history, a physical examination, followed by a 12-channel electrocardiogram (ECG), and further focused diagnostics, including cardiac biomarkers.

Despite the development of improved cardiac biomarkers and the validation of clinical scoring systems, medical decisions about hospital admission or discharge do not always come promptly. The introduction of highly sensitive cardiac troponin (hs-cTn) has significantly improved the diagnostic accuracy of acute coronary syndrome, both in the rule-in phase (with anticipation of the diagnosis) and in the rule-out phase, with the possibility of excluding acute injury with a 1-hour blood sample. On the other hand, hsTnI can highlight any kind of myocardiocyte suffering, not only that due to an ischemic cause, thus adding doubts to the decision-making process in which the physician must choose between hospital admission, 24-h observation, or a safe discharge. Recently, the standardization and validation of new diagnostic methods have increased clinicians' confidence in the use of circulating biomarkers to improve diagnostic accuracy, assess individual risk of developing cardiovascular disease, and monitor associated adverse events.

sST2 has been studied in patients with heart failure and has recently been introduced as an additional prognostic marker for natriuretic factors in heart failure, as it increases when myocardial tissue remodels in fibrosis. Plus, because of sST2's increase in different pathophysiological cardiac pathways, other studies have highlighted that sST2 has a complementary role in the prognostic stratification of cardiac ischemic patients. While hsTnI's increase represents miocardiocyte suffering, the sST2 plasma level may reflect endothelial damage.

Recently, many studies have taken into consideration suPAR as a cardiovascular marker, as it is related to immune activation, inflammation, and endothelial damage. suPAR has been proposed as a biomarker for risk stratification and for monitoring the therapeutic response in patients with heart disease.

Our research is based on a multi-marker approach for patients who are admitted to the ED with acute chest pain. We enrolled 360 consecutive patients in whom ACS was suspected. We measured hsTnI 0–1 h and the other biomarkers with the same blood sample. The aim of our research was to evaluate whether the combination of different biomarkers could help the clinician find an accurate diagnosis, explain the origin of the patients' symptoms, and improve risk stratification and prognosis. From our statistical analysis, we noticed that the distribution of values was very heterogeneous, considering the multiple clinical features that can be responsible for acute chest pain.

HsTnI was the only biomarker able to vary between time 0 and time 1, as its immediate release was an expression of an acute event; the other biomarkers did not show significant variation between the two measurements.

Our findings confirmed that troponin has a diagnostic role and highlighted that suPAR and sST2 could help the clinician better understand and personalize each patient's cardiovascular risk.

According to troponin levels, we divided the patients into different groups.

To evaluate the reliability of a multi-marker approach in these patients, we divided the *negative* subjects on the suPAR level: suPAR $\leq$ 2.9 ng/mL and sST2 $\leq$ 24.19 ng/mL showed high accuracy for excluding ACS, while suPAR > 2.9 ng/mL and sST2 > 29.1 ng/mL could discriminate patients with ACS.

The group of patients with "*intermediate*" troponin is the group that usually creates the biggest problems for the clinician. Patients with sST2 > 29.1 ng/mL or suPAR > 2.9 ng/mL presented a high risk of ACS. On the other hand, patients with sST2 $\leq$ 24.19% and suPAR $\leq$ 2.9 ng/mL were found to be healthy, non-ACS patients.

Among patients with *negative* or *intermediate* troponin, sST2 and suPAR appear to be able to separate those who could be discharged safely from the ED from those who may need more attention.

For follow-up, we relied mainly on objective data such as re-hospitalization, treatment changes, and new visits to the PS, rather than exclusively on the limited value of the 12-month telephone analysis. This is because patients' re-presentation of symptoms often lacks accuracy and timeliness. Follow-up showed that ST2 > 29.1 ng/mL was highly specific for adverse events and thus associated with patients with adverse outcomes, and suPAR > 2.9 ng/mL was specific and highly sensitive for adverse events.

For the first time in the evaluation of patients with acute chest pain, our study suggests the use of a multi-marker approach with sST2 and suPAR in association with troponin. Troponin, sST2, and suPAR explore totally distinct pathways that can each independently contribute to the genesis of cardiovascular pathology, despite being able to coexist without a causal relationship in some cases. Furthermore, sST2 and suPAR must also be considered indicators of endothelial health, as they are strongly influenced by conditions such as inflammatory states, autoimmune diseases, neoplasms, and non-ischemic heart conditions. SuPAR and sST2 are promising biomarkers for early prediction of events in chest pain emergency patients. Our data are preliminary and require an expansion of patients to be enrolled. However, since clinicians increasingly ask the laboratories for support in guiding their diagnostic choices using an evidence-based, biomarker-based approach, our findings appear interesting and deserve to be carefully considered and evaluated so as to manage patients more efficiently in a difficult setting such as the emergency department.

7. Limitations

There are some limitations to our study that are worth taking into consideration. First, the study is limited by a small sample size, which may influence our findings. However, our research should be viewed as a starting point for a multi-center study with a larger sample size. Plus, multi-center studies are needed to determine the potential role of this multi-marker approach in the diagnostic work-up as well as in patient stratification for rule-in and rule-out. Second, we lacked serial measurement of biomarkers in our study; the plasma levels of sST2 and suPAR were only detected at the time of admission to the ED. Temporal variation in biomarker measurements from admission to discharge in the ED could be an important finding. However, despite these limitations, it is important to underline our great findings regarding this multi-marker approach in patients with chest pain. The follow-up is still in progress.

8. Conclusions

Our data suggest that hsTnI remains the biomarker of choice for acute cardiological evaluations, considering its peculiar cardio-specificity and its rapid increase in acute ischemic settings; on the other hand, it is known that numerous different pathophysiological elements can influence each other and associate, determining multiple clinical pictures in patients. SST2 may play a complementary role to troponin in the prognostic stratification of ischemic patients. SuPAR, as a marker of endothelial damage and involvement in various pathophysiological pathways, can guide clinicians in determining the need for further diagnostic investigations. Our data suggest that a future integration of these biomarkers into the routine approach to the patient with acute chest pain in the ED might allow better patient stratification and proper patient management, helping the clinician to make an early safe discharge or a timely admission for those who deserve in-depth diagnostic and therapeutic investigations.

Author Contributions: Conceptualization, A.P. and F.F.; methodology, S.B.; validation, A.G. and F.F.; formal analysis, F.S. and M.C. (Marcello Covino); investigation, M.C. (Marcello Candelli); data curation, S.B., G.S., and A.B.; writing—original draft preparation, A.P. and F.M.; writing—review and editing, A.P., S.B., and A.B.; supervision, A.G. and F.F. All authors have read and agreed to the published version of the manuscript.

Funding: This research received no external funding.

Institutional Review Board Statement: Not applicable.

Informed Consent Statement: Not applicable.

Data Availability Statement: The original contributions presented in the study are included in the article, further inquiries can be directed to the corresponding author.

Conflicts of Interest: The authors declare no conflicts of interest.

References

1. McDevitt-Petrovic, O.; Kirby, K.; Shevlin, M. The prevalence of non-cardiac chest pain (NCCP) using emergency department (ED) data: A Northern Ireland based study. *BMC Health Serv. Res.* **2017**, *17*, 549. [CrossRef] [PubMed] [PubMed Central]
2. Pitts, S.R.; Niska, R.W.; Xu, J.; Burt, C.W. National Hospital Ambulatory Medical Care Survey: 2006 emergency department summary. *Natl. Health Stat. Rep.* **2008**, *6*, 1–38. [PubMed]
3. Fass, R.; Navarro-Rodriguez, T. Noncardiac chest pain. *J. Clin. Gastroenterol.* **2008**, *42*, 636–646. [CrossRef] [PubMed]
4. Eslick, G.D. Classification, natural history, epidemiology, and risk factors of noncardiac chest pain. *Dis. Mon.* **2008**, *54*, 593–603. [CrossRef] [PubMed]
5. Cayley, W.E., Jr. Diagnosing the cause of chest pain. *Am. Fam. Physician* **2005**, *72*, 2012–2021. [PubMed]
6. Diercks, D.B.; Peacock, W.F.; Hiestand, B.C.; Chen, A.Y.; Pollack, C.V., Jr.; Kirk, J.D.; Smith, S.C., Jr.; Gibler, W.B.; Ohman, E.M.; Blomkalns, A.L.; et al. Frequency and consequences of recording an electrocardiogram > 10 minutes after arrival in an emergency room in non-ST-segment elevation acute coronary syndromes (from the CRUSADE Initiative). *Am. J. Cardiol.* **2006**, *97*, 437–442. [CrossRef] [PubMed]
7. Gulati, M.; Levy, P.D.; Mukherjee, D.; Amsterdam, E.; Bhatt, D.L.; Birtcher, K.K.; Blankstein, R.; Boyd, J.; Bullock-Palmer, R.P.; Conejo, T.; et al. 2021 AHA/ACC/ASE/CHEST/SAEM/SCCT/SCMR Guideline for the Evaluation and Diagnosis of Chest Pain: A Report of the American College of Cardiology/American Heart Association Joint Committee on Clinical Practice Guidelines. *Circulation* **2021**, *144*, e368–e454, Erratum in *Circulation* **2021**, *144*, e455. [CrossRef] [PubMed]
8. Agewall, S.; Giannitsis, E.; Jernberg, T.; Katus, H. Troponin elevation in coronary vs. non-coronary disease. *Eur. Heart J.* **2011**, *32*, 404–411. [CrossRef] [PubMed]
9. Daubert, M.A.; Jeremias, A. The utility of troponin measurement to detect myocardial infarction: Review of the current findings. *Vasc. Health Risk Manag.* **2010**, *6*, 691–699. [CrossRef] [PubMed] [PubMed Central]
10. Six, A.J.; Backus, B.E.; Kelder, J.C. Chest pain in the emergency room: Value of the HEART score. *Neth. Heart J.* **2008**, *16*, 191–196. [CrossRef] [PubMed] [PubMed Central]
11. Eagle, K.A.; Lim, M.J.; Dabbous, O.H.; Pieper, K.S.; Goldberg, R.J.; Van de Werf, F.; Goodman, S.G.; Granger, C.B.; Steg, P.G.; Gore, J.M.; et al. A validated prediction model for all forms of acute coronary syndrome: Estimating the risk of 6-month postdischarge death in an international registry. *JAMA* **2004**, *291*, 2727–2733. [CrossRef] [PubMed]
12. Antman, E.M.; Cohen, M.; Bernink, P.J.; McCabe, C.H.; Horacek, T.; Papuchis, G.; Mautner, B.; Corbalan, R.; Radley, D.; Braunwald, E. The TIMI risk score for unstable angina/non-ST elevation MI: A method for prognostication and therapeutic decision making. *JAMA* **2000**, *284*, 835–842. [CrossRef] [PubMed]
13. Pollack, C.V., Jr.; Sites, F.D.; Shofer, F.S.; Sease, K.L.; Hollander, J.E. Application of the TIMI risk score for unstable angina and non-ST elevation acute coronary syndrome to an unselected emergency department chest pain population. *Acad. Emerg. Med.* **2006**, *13*, 13–18. [CrossRef] [PubMed]
14. Poldervaart, J.M.; Langedijk, M.; Backus, B.E.; Dekker, I.M.C.; Six, A.J.; Doevendans, P.A.; Hoes, A.W.; Reitsma, J.B. Comparison of the GRACE, HEART and TIMI score to predict major adverse cardiac events in chest pain patients at the emergency department. *Int. J. Cardiol.* **2017**, *227*, 656–661. [CrossRef] [PubMed]
15. Byrne, R.A.; Rossello, X.; Coughlan, J.J.; Barbato, E.; Berry, C.; Chieffo, A.; Claeys, M.J.; Dan, G.A.; Dweck, M.R.; Galbraith, M.; et al. 2023 ESC Guidelines for the management of acute coronary syndromes: Developed by the task force on the management of acute coronary syndromes of the European Society of Cardiology (ESC). *Eur. Heart J.* **2023**, *44*, 3720–3826. [CrossRef] [PubMed]
16. Miller, A.M.; Xu, D.; Asquith, D.L.; Denby, L.; Li, Y.; Sattar, N.; Baker, A.H.; McInnes, I.B.; Liew, F.Y. IL-33 reduces the development of atherosclerosis. *J. Exp. Med.* **2008**, *205*, 339–346. [CrossRef] [PubMed]

17. Schmitz, J.; Owyang, A.; Oldham, E.; Song, Y.; Murphy, E.; McClanahan, T.K.; Zurawski, G.; Moshrefi, M.; Qin, J.; Li, X.; et al. IL-33, an interleukin- 1-like cytokine that signals via the IL-1 receptor-related protein ST2 and induces T helper type 2-associated cytokines. *Immunity* **2005**, *23*, 479–490. [CrossRef] [PubMed]
18. Weinberg, E.O.; Shimpo, M.; De Keulenaer, G.W.; MacGillivray, C.; Tominaga, S.; Solomon, S.D.; Rouleau, J.L.; Lee, R.T. Expression and regulation of ST2, an interleukin-1 receptor family member, in cardiomyocytes and myocardial infarction. *Circulation* **2002**, *106*, 2961–2966. [CrossRef] [PubMed]
19. Altara, R.; Ghali, R.; Mallat, Z.; Cataliotti, A.; Booz, G.W.; Zouein, F.A. Conflicting vascular and metabolic impact of the IL-33/sST2 axis. *Cardiovasc. Res.* **2018**, *114*, 1578–1594. [CrossRef]
20. Pascual-Figal, D.A.; Lax, A.; Perez-Martinez, M.T.; del Carmen Asensio-Lopez, M.; Sanchez-Mas, J. Clinical Relevance of sST2 in cardiac diseases. *De Gruyter* **2016**, *54*, 29–35. [CrossRef]
21. Gül, İ.; Yücel, O.; Zararsız, A.; Demirpençe, Ö.; Yücel, H.; Zorlu, A.; Yılmaz MBGül, İ.; Yücel, O.; Zararsız, A.; Demirpençe, Ö.; et al. Prognostic role of soluble suppression of tumorigenicity-2 on cardiovascular mortality in outpatients with heart failure. *Anatol. J. Cardiol.* **2017**, *18*, 200. [CrossRef] [PubMed]
22. Mueller, T.; Gegenhuber, A.; Leitner, I.; Poelz, W.; Haltmayer, M.; Dieplinger, B. Diagnostic and prognostic accuracy of galectin-3 and soluble ST2 for acute heart failure. *Clin. Chim. Acta* **2016**, *463*, 158–164. [CrossRef] [PubMed]
23. Ahmad, T.; Fiuzat, M.; Neely, B.; Neely, M.L.; Pencina, M.J.; Kraus, W.E.; Zannad, F.; Whellan, D.J.; Donahue, M.P.; Piña, I.L.; et al. Biomarkers of myocardial stress and fibrosis as predictors of mode of death in patients with chronic heart failure. *JACC Heart Fail.* **2014**, *2*, 260–268. [CrossRef]
24. Emdin, M.; Aimo, A.; Vergaro, G.; Bayes-Genis, A.; Lupón, J.; Latini, R.; Meessen, J.; Anand, I.S.; Cohn, J.N.; Gravning, J.; et al. sST2 Predicts Outcome in Chronic Heart Failure Beyond NT−proBNP and High-Sensitivity Troponin T. *J. Am. Coll. Cardiol.* **2018**, *72*, 2309–2320. [CrossRef]
25. Aimo, A.; Vergaro, G.; Ripoli, A.; Bayes-Genis, A.; Pascual Figal, D.A.; de Boer, R.A.; Lassus, J.; Mebazaa, A.; Gayat, E.; Breidthardt, T.; et al. Meta-Analysis of Soluble Suppression of Tumorigenicity-2 and Prognosis in Acute Heart Failure. *JACC Hear. Fail.* **2017**, *5*, 287–296. [CrossRef] [PubMed]
26. Maisel, A.S.; Filippatos, G.S. *Algorithms in Heart Failure. Jaypee*; The Health Sciences Publisher: New Delhi, India, 2016.
27. Aleksova, A.; Paldino, A.; Beltrami, A.P.; Padoan, L.; Iacoviello, M.; Sinagra, G.; Emdin, M.; Maisel, A.S. Cardiac Biomarkers in the Emergency Department. *J. Clin. Med.* **2019**, *8*, 270. [CrossRef]
28. Januzzi, J.L., Jr.; Rehman, S.; Mueller, T.; Van Kimmenade, R.R.; Lloyd-Jones, D.M. Importance of biomarkers for long-term mortality prediction in acutely dyspneic patients. *Clin. Chen* **2010**, *56*, 1814–1821. [CrossRef]
29. Bayes-Genis, A.; Pascual-Figal, D.; Januzzi, J.L.; Maisel, A.; Casas, T.; Valdés Chávarri, M.; Ordóñez-Llanos, J. Soluble ST2 monitoring provides additional risk stratification for outpatients with decompensated heart failure. *Rev. Esp. Cardiol.* **2010**, *63*, 1171–1178. [CrossRef] [PubMed]
30. Sabatine, M.S.; Morrow, D.A.; Higgins, L.J.; MacGillivray, C.; Guo, W.; Bode, C.; Rifai, N.; Cannon, C.P.; Gerszten, R.E.; Lee, R.T. Complementary roles for biomarkers of biomechanical strain ST2 and N-terminal prohormone B-type natriuretic peptide in patients with ST-elevation myocardial infarction. *Circulation* **2008**, *117*, 1936–1944. [CrossRef]
31. Jenkins, W.S.; Roger, V.L.; Jaffe, A.S.; Weston, S.A.; AbouEzzeddine, O.F.; Jiang, R.; Manemann, S.M.; Enriquez-Sarano, M. Prognostic Value of Soluble ST2 After Myocardial Infarction: A Community Perspective. *Am. J. Med.* 2017; 130, 1112.e9–1112.e15.
32. Pope, J.H.; Aufderheide, T.P.; Ruthazer, R.; Woolard, R.H.; Feldman, J.A.; Beshansky, J.R.; Griffith, J.L.; Selker, H.P. Missed Diagnoses of Acute Cardiac Ischemia in the Emergency Department. *N. Engl. J. Med.* **2000**, *342*, 1163–1170. [CrossRef]
33. Lyngbæk, S.; Andersson, C.; Marott, J.L.; Møller, D.V.; Christiansen, M.; Iversen, K.K.; Clemmensen, P.; Eugen-Olsen, J.; Hansen, P.R.; Jeppesen, J.L. Soluble urokinase plasminogen activator receptor for risk prediction in patients admitted with acute chest pain. *Clin. Chem.* **2013**, *59*, 1621–1629. [CrossRef] [PubMed]
34. Velissaris, D.; Zareifopoulos, N.; Koniari, I.; Karamouzos, V.; Bousis, D.; Gerakaris, A.; Platanaki, C.; Kounis, N. Soluble Urokinase Plasminogen Activator Receptor as a Diagnostic and Prognostic Biomarker in Cardiac Disease. *J. Clin. Med. Res.* **2021**, *13*, 133–142. [CrossRef] [PubMed] [PubMed Central]
35. Chenevier-Gobeaux, C.; Lemarechal, H.; Doumenc, B.; Peschanski, N.; Claessens, Y.E.; Borderie, D.; Ray, P. Prognostic value of soluble urokinase plasminogen activator receptor in patients presenting to the emergency department with chest pain suggestive of acute coronary syndrome. *Clin. Biochem.* **2021**, *92*, 19–24. [CrossRef] [PubMed]
36. Ren, Y.; Hou, M.; Ren, Y.; Zhang, L. Diagnostic efficacy of serum ST2 in patients with ASC. *J. Clin. Lab. Anal.* **2022**, *36*, e24511. [CrossRef] [PubMed] [PubMed Central]
37. Peiró, Ó.M.; Cediel, G.; Bonet, G.; Rojas, S.; Quintern, V.; Carrasquer, A.; González-Del-Hoyo, M.; Sanz, E.; Bardají, A. Soluble urokinase plasminogen activator receptor as a long-term prognostic biomarker in acute coronary syndromes. *Biomarkers* **2020**, *25*, 402–409. [CrossRef] [PubMed]
38. Sarlo, F.; De Luca, C.; Moretti, G.; Urbani, A.; Baroni, S. Analytical performance evaluation of the new sST2 turbidimetric assay implemented in laboratory automation systems. *Clin. Chem. Lab. Med.* **2021**, *60*, e54–e56. [CrossRef] [PubMed]

Journal of
Personalized Medicine

MDPI

Review

Pregnancy-Related Thromboembolism—Current Challenges at the Emergency Department

Ștefan-Ionuț Moroi [1], Emma Weiss [2,3], Silviu Stanciu [2,4], Elisabeta Bădilă [2,5], Adriana Mihaela Ilieșiu [2,6] and Ana-Maria Balahura [2,6,*]

1 Department of Cardiology, Emergency Institute for Cardiovascular Diseases "Prof. Dr. C.C. Iliescu", 022328 Bucharest, Romania; stefan-ionut.moroi@rez.umfcd.ro
2 "Carol Davila" University of Medicine and Pharmacy, 050474 Bucharest, Romania; emma.weiss@umfcd.ro (E.W.); silviu.stanciu@umfcd.ro (S.S.); elisabeta.badila@umfcd.ro (E.B.); adriana.iliesiu@umfcd.ro (A.M.I.)
3 Internal Medicine Department, Bucharest Clinical Emergency Hospital, 014461 Bucharest, Romania
4 Dr. Carol Davila University Central Military Emergency Hospital, Calea Plevnei 134, 010825 Bucharest, Romania
5 Department of Cardiology, Colentina Hospital, 020125 Bucharest, Romania
6 Department of Cardiology, "Prof. Dr. Theodor Burghele" Clinical Hospital, 061344 Bucharest, Romania
* Correspondence: ana-maria.balahura@umfcd.ro; Tel.: +40-0742092269

Abstract: Thrombotic events during pregnancy are burdened by an increased risk of morbidity and mortality, despite innovations in their diagnosis and treatment. Given their multifactorial etiology, it is important to understand all the pathophysiological mechanisms but especially to achieve correct and timely diagnosis. Pulmonary embolism (PE) during pregnancy represents a rare event, with an incidence of 1 per 1000 pregnancies, but it is also one of the leading causes of death during pregnancy. Managing PE in the acute setting is even more challenging and complex due to the attempt to maintain a balance between hemorrhagic and thrombotic complications while ensuring an optimal outcome for both the mother and the baby. In this review, our aim is to analyze the most significant challenges of acute PE during pregnancy and identify suitable management approaches for specific situations in order to improve the prognosis of pregnant women.

Keywords: pregnancy; pulmonary embolism; emergency department

1. Introduction

Venous thromboembolism (VTE) is an important cause of morbidity and mortality during pregnancy and the peripartum period, with an incidence of 1 per 1000 pregnancies [1]. Despite advances in the diagnosis and management of VTE, it remains a leading cause of maternal mortality worldwide. Pregnancy-related VTE can have both serious short- and long-term complications, including post-thrombotic syndrome, which can alter the quality of life of the mother [2].

Thromboembolic events are often generated by pregnancy-related risk factors, most of them being preventable [3]. Therefore, it is crucial to diagnose, prevent, and manage VTE, including its complications. However, this population comes with the physiological alterations associated with pregnancy and the potential risks that the imaging techniques present to the fetus, which makes an accurate diagnosis highly challenging.

Therapeutic interventions must take into consideration the balance of the possible advantages and drawbacks of each approach to the mother and fetus [4]. In this regard, although it is a rare but deadly event, high-risk PE is the primary indication for thrombolysis, a challenging situation due to its high risk of bleeding complications.

However, data from a systematic review point out that thrombolysis in patients with high-risk PE has good maternal and fetal survival rates [5,6].

The aim of this review is to examine the key challenges of acute PE during pregnancy and to identify appropriate management strategies for different scenarios, with the goal of improving outcomes for pregnant women.

2. Epidemiology

Pregnant and postpartum women have a six-time higher risk of VTE, compared with non-pregnant women. This risk also increases with gestational age. It is widely agreed that the greatest risk occurs during the postpartum period, with the incidence reaching its peak in the first six weeks after childbirth [6].

A meta-analysis that included 93 million pregnant and postpartum women revealed that the incidence of VTE was 1.2 per 1000 deliveries [7]. The global application of computer tomographic pulmonary angiography (CTPA) in pregnant and postpartum women has increased the rates of diagnosed PE during delivery admissions and during postpartum hospitalizations [8]. The incidence varies based on several risk factors and populations, with a higher incidence in women with a history of VTE or thrombophilia or those with diabetes or hypertension [9].

There are data that suggest racial differences in the occurrence of VTE during pregnancy and the postpartum period, with Black women being the most impacted. A potential explanation is the fact that Black women have a higher prevalence of certain risk factors, such as hypertension and sickle cell disease [10].

3. Pathophysiology of VTE in Pregnancy

Virchow's triad, which consists of endothelial trauma, venous stasis, and hypercoagulability, all of which are increased during pregnancy, contributes to a higher risk of thrombus formation. These alterations in the coagulation and fibrinolytic systems are intended to minimize intrapartum blood loss but also increase the risk of thromboembolism [9]. Venous stasis of the lower limbs occurs due to changes in venous capacitance related to pregnancy and compression of the inferior vena cava or iliac veins by the gravid uterus. This augmentation of stasis in the lower limb venous system can occur even before the uterus has a marked increase in size [11]. There are also immunological changes, with a sudden increase in cytokines and vascular endothelial dysfunction that can lead to VTE [12].

Pregnancy and the postpartum period are also associated with a hypercoagulable state, with a physiologic increase in certain coagulation factors, such as factors II, VII, VIII, IX, and X. Conversely, there is also a reduction in the production of protein S and a decrease in the activation of the fibrinolysis inhibitors PAI-I and PAI-2 [13].

4. Risk Factors

Pregnancy itself is an important risk factor for VTE, but apart from it, other risk factors for thromboembolic events can be classified into maternal-specific, obstetric-specific, and new onset and transient risk factors [6]. Of note, traditional pre-existing risk factors are less prevalent in pregnant women compared with non-pregnant women who present with VTE [14].

Maternal-specific risk factors for venous thrombotic events in pregnancy include previous VTE, acquired or heritable thrombophilia, extensive varicose veins, body mass index > 30 kg/m^2, maternal age > 35 years, parity of more than 2, smoking, pre-existing comorbidities, such as hypertension, gestational diabetes, heart failure, inflammatory bowel disease [15], or cancer [11]. Women who present with a history of both provoked and unprovoked VTE or with first-degree relatives diagnosed with inherited thrombophilia should be evaluated with a thrombophilia panel, including tests for antiphospholipid syndrome, factor V Leiden, and the prothrombin G20210A gene variant, as well as for deficiencies in antithrombin III, protein C, and protein S [15].

Obstetric-specific risk factors are current pre-eclampsia, multiple pregnancy, prolonged labor (>24 h), preterm birth, stillbirth, postpartum hemorrhage (blood loss exceeding 1 L or blood loss that requires transfusion), and Caesarean section [16].

Newly acquired or transient risk factors, which can be potentially reversible, may emerge later in pregnancy than when the initial risk assessment was conducted. Therefore, it is of utmost importance to carefully monitor the individual risk. These risk factors encompass hyperemesis gravidorum, ovarian hyperstimulation syndrome, fertility treatments including in vitro fertilization, postpartum sterilization, hospital admission or immobility, bone fracture, any surgical procedure during pregnancy or the postpartum period, existing systemic illness, and long distance travel exceeding 4 h [11].

5. Risk Assessment of Pregnancy-Related VTE

Considering that VTE is a leading cause of mortality, it is essential to assess the risk of developing VTE in all pregnant women as early as possible. Most women may exhibit one or more thrombotic risk factors during pregnancy. Conducting an initial risk assessment and implementing preventive strategies are essential in reducing the incidence of VTE in pregnant women [11]. Special attention should be given to women with a previous history of VTE, those with known thrombophilia, and those with a family history of VTE [17]. Those identified as having a high risk for VTE should receive both an antepartum and postpartum prophylactic or intermediate dose of low-molecular-weight heparin (LMWH) or unfractioned heparin (UFH) [18].

The risk scoring approach should evaluate the necessity of thromboprophylaxis during pregnancy and the postpartum period. Based on the associated risk factors, all women will be categorized into various risk levels, and the appropriate thromboprophylaxis regimen will be chosen. This approach can include observation alone, mechanical methods or LMWH, and the choice should be tailored based on each patient's specific risk factors [19]. A scoring system to assess the risk of VTE in pregnant women would be highly beneficial, but unfortunately, no validated score currently exists for this purpose.

If pharmacological thromboprophylaxis is chosen as the appropriate regimen during pregnancy and the postpartum period, the risk of VTE must outweigh the risk of severe bleeding complications due to anticoagulation treatment. Recent guidelines and expert panels have taken this into consideration and suggested that pharmacologic prophylaxis should be considered only if the absolute risk of VTE exceeds 1 to 5%, with the prioritization of the woman's preferences [20].

6. Clinical Presentation

Clinical suspicion of deep vein thrombosis (DVT) is essential to ensure optimal diagnosis and treatment, because, without treatment, it may advance to PE, which can be life-threatening for both the mother and the fetus. DVT is significantly more prevalent in pregnant women compared to those who are not pregnant. In contrast to the general population, where thrombosis typically starts in the distal veins of the calf and progresses proximally, in pregnant women, it often originates in the proximal veins of the lower limb (primarily from iliac or femoral veins) due to compression by the pregnant uterus [4].

VTE during pregnancy can manifest as various forms, ranging from asymptomatic cases to severe and life-threatening conditions, such as hemodynamic unstable PE. Symptoms that suggest VTE in non-pregnant women include tachycardia, dyspnea, tachypnea, and lower limb edema and pain. However, these symptoms are non-specific and frequently encountered in various conditions, often imitating standard symptoms of pregnancy [9].

For DVT during pregnancy, the most frequent symptoms are pain and predominantly unilateral edema. These symptoms can be associated with warmth, erythema, or lower limb tenderness. Almost 80% of pregnant women with DVT exhibit these symptoms, yet the diagnosis is often overlooked [21]. In symptomatic pregnant women, DVT is more commonly diagnosed in the left lower limb, involving the proximal and iliac veins (70 to 90%) [22]. A possible explanation for this phenomenon is the dual compression of the left iliac vein, first by the normal anatomical crossing of the right iliac artery above the left iliac vein and second by the compression of the gravid uterus [4]. Although there are several scoring systems to evaluate the pre-test probability of VTE in non-pregnant women (such as Well's criteria and the modified Geneva score), it is important to recognize that the studies validating these scoring systems did not include pregnant or postpartum women; therefore, their applicability to this population may be limited [4]. Chan et al. proposed a clinical prediction tool to aid in the diagnosis of DVT in pregnant women during the first trimester, which includes the following: (1) left lower limb symptoms; (2) more than 2 cm difference in calf circumference; (3) presentation during the first trimester of pregnancy. These three components are together referred to as the LEFt rule. If none of these factors is identified, the negative predictive value is 100%. The LEFt rule should, however, not be used as the only test to rule out DVT in pregnancy but rather as one component of a diagnostic approach, including other tests, such as D-dimer measurements and lower extremity duplex ultrasound (DUS) [23,24].

D-dimer levels increase during pregnancy compared with non-pregnant women, limiting the diagnostic value when evaluating the probability of VTE. However, normal D-dimer levels are a low-cost, non-invasive, simple test to rule out VTE during pregnancy in cases with low-to-intermediate clinical pretest probability [25]; conversely, a high D-dimer level necessitates an additional investigation, similar to the approach used for non-pregnant women [26]. Being widely available and without the risk of radiation to the fetus, DUS is the first-line diagnostic tool for symptomatic DVT. If DVT is found via DUS and PE is clinically suspected, additional chest imaging is not required, since the management approach would remain the same. Nevertheless, if PE is suspected clinically and DUS does not reveal DVT, a CT pulmonary angiogram (CTPA) or lung perfusion scintigraphy (V/Q scan) is required [27]. The detection of DVT in iliofemoral veins via compression ultrasonography (CUS) is often inadequate, due to the veins' incompressibility from pregnancy-related changes in blood flow mechanics, their increased compressibility in the proximal veins, and their location within the pelvis. In this setting, adjunctive DUS parameters should be used, such as the venous flow changes with respiration and with the Valsalva maneuver in order to identify downstream occlusive thrombosis [28]. In pregnant women who are suspected of having iliac vein thrombosis, the diagnostic approach can be continued via magnetic resonance imaging (MRI) venography if the initial compressive ultrasound is negative. Also, if the CUS is negative but the clinical suspicion of DVT is high, reassessment with highly sensitive D-dimer testing on days 3 and 7 and/or repeat CUS should be performed. In cases of suspected pelvic DVT, CT venography can be considered; however, MRI venography is a valid option with excellent diagnostic precision, without exposing the mother and fetus to radiation [29]. Protocols without gadolinium should be taken into consideration, as fetal exposure to high doses of gadolinium is associated with developmental anomalies in small animals models [30], while evidence in humans is very limited [31]. It should be noted that MRI venography for DVT diagnosis is infrequent due to its restricted accessibility at the point of care.

The most frequent symptoms of PE, which are shortness of breath, tachycardia, and chest pain, are nonspecific and may also occur as normal physiological alterations during pregnancy, making the diagnostic management particularly challenging [32]. Varrias et al. demonstrated that sinus tachycardia is primarily regarded as a normal physiological aspect of pregnancy, but it is linked to adverse outcomes [33]. Therefore, a thorough assessment of the medical history, physical examination, laboratory evaluation, and diagnostic imaging are essential for the precise and prompt diagnosis of PE in pregnant women. The PERC (PE rule-out criteria) rule, used in the overall population to exclude PE in cases with a low pre-test probability, is insufficient during pregnancy [34]. Neglecting or missing a PE diagnosis can be fatal for both the mother and the child, whereas the careless use of imaging tests can expose both the mother and fetus to radiation [35]. A few rules of pre-test probability assessment have been proposed for pregnant patients with a working diagnosis of PE (Table 1).

Table 1. Clinical pre-test assessment of DVT and PE. CTPA—computer tomography pulmonary angiography, DVT—deep vein thrombosis, I—intermediate, L—low, LL-DUS—lower limb Doppler ultrasound, pts.—patients, PE—pulmonary embolism, V/Q scan—ventilation/perfusion scan, Sb—sensibility, Sp—specificity, VTE—venous thromboembolism.

Clinical Pre-Test Probability Assessment	Components and Interpretation	Efficiency	Studies Evaluating Pregnancy-Adapted Algorithms for the Diagnosis of PE Including the Specified PTP Scores
LEFt rule (for DVT in pregnancy) [24]	Left lower limb symptoms A difference in calf circumference exceeding 2 cm Presentation in the first trimester LEFt rule score interpretation • If all factors are absent, the negative predictive value of DVT is 100%	Sb 100% Sp 50%	NA
Revised Geneva score(for PE) [36]	Age ≥ 65 years—1p Previous DVT or PE—3p Surgery or fracture within 1 month—2p Active cancer—2p Unilateral lower limb pain—3p Hemoptysis—2p Heart rate 75 to 94 bpm—3p Heart rate 95 or more bpm—5p Pain on deep palpation of the lower limb accompanied by unilateral swelling—4p Revised Geneva score interpretation • Low probability of PE < 4p • Intermediate probability of PE 4–10p • High probability of PE > 10p	Sb 70% Sp 52%	**CT-PE pregnancy study** Multicenter, multinational, prospective **Algorithm**: - L or I pretest probability + negative D-dimer = rule-out PE otherwise LL-CUS - Negative LL-CUS, CTPA was performed. A V/Q scan was done if CTPA inconclusive. **Results**: Rate of symptomatic VTE 0.0% (95% CI, 0.0% to 1.0%) among untreated pts. [26]

Table 1. *Cont.*

Clinical Pre-Test Probability Assessment	Components and Interpretation	Efficiency	Studies Evaluating Pregnancy-Adapted Algorithms for the Diagnosis of PE Including the Specified PTP Scores
The Pregnancy-Adapted Geneva (PAG) score (for PE in pregnancy) [37]	Age 40 years or over—1p Previous DVT or PE—3p Surgery or lower limb fracture within 1 month—2p Unilateral lower limb pain—3p Hemoptysis—2p Heart rate > 110 bpm—5p Pain on deep palpation of the lower limb accompanied by unilateral swelling—4p Revised Geneva score interpretation • Low probability of PE 0–1 p • Intermediate probability of PE 2–6 p • High probability of PE ≥ 7p	Reported AUC	Needs further external validation
YEARS	YEARS Items • Clinical signs of DVT • Hemoptysis • PE most likely diagnosis YEARS rule score interpretation • 0 YEARS items and D-dimer < 1000 ng/mL − PE excluded • 0 YEARS items and D-dimer ≥ 1000 ng/mL − Order CTPA • ≥1 YEARS items and D-dimer < 500 ng/mL − PE excluded • ≥1 YEARS items and D-dimer ≥ 500 ng/mL − Order CTPA	Sb 90% Sp 65%	**1. ARTEMIS** Prospective, multicenter, international study **Algorithm**: Adaptation of YEARS algorithm by including LL-DUS in pts with symptoms of DVT. - DVT present—patient received AC, no CTPA - DVT negative and all other pts. in which PE was not ruled out—underwent CTPA **Results**: From the ruled-out PE pts, 1 patient was diagnosed with VTE during follow-up (0.21%; 95% CI, 0.04 to 1.2) CTPA (thus radiation) was avoided in 32–65% of pts. [38] **2. The YEARS algorithm in the CT-PE population.** Post-hoc analysis of outcomes from a prospective study on PE diagnosis in pregnant women **Algorithm**: 371 pregnant patients from the original CT-PE study—retrospective application of the YEARS algorithm. **Results**: Failure rate of YEARS algorithm 0 out of 77 pts (95% CI, 0.0–3.9) [39]

YEARS is an algorithm that can help in the treatment decision, which uses three clinical parameters: (1) clinical signs of DVT; (2) hemoptysis; (3) PE being the most probable diagnosis, in conjunction with the D-dimer levels. With this algorithm, PE can be excluded if all three criteria are absent and the D-dimer level is less than 1000 ng/mL, or if one or more of the three elements are present and the D-dimer level is <500 ng/mL. If PE cannot be ruled out by the YEARS criteria, further investigations need to be pursued [40]. Pregnant women with suspected PE and criteria for hemodynamic instability face a high risk of mortality in the initial hours and days. Therefore, it is recommended to start heparin anticoagulation without delay in those cases with a high or intermediate clinical probability of PE, even prior to confirming the diagnosis, while diagnostic tests are ongoing [27].

7. Risk Stratification of Pregnancy-Associated Pulmonary Embolism

Risk stratification is crucial to adjust the best possible treatment of acute PE. It should take into consideration the impact of the elevated right ventricular (RV) afterload on RV performance, because the main cause of mortality in acute PE is circulatory failure [41].

The current European guidelines propose a two-step risk assessment approach [27]. High-risk PE is defined by the presence of hemodynamic instability or cardiac arrest, where reperfusion therapy is of utmost importance (systemic thrombolysis) because of the significant risk of mortality in the acute phase. Current criteria, aside from cardiac arrest, include obstructive shock with associated inadequate end-organ perfusion or persistent hypotension, defined as a systolic blood pressure (BP) < 90 mmHg or a fall in the systolic BP $\geq$ 40 mmHg without an alternative etiology. Intermediate-risk PE identifies hemodynamically stable patients, in which the presence of RV dilatation, increased troponin or increased B-type natriuretic peptide (BNP), or N-terminal-proBNP (NTproBNP) should emphasize careful hemodynamic monitoring due to the enhanced risk of short-term clinical deterioration. The reminder of PE patients are classified as low risk.

There is no research study that proves that this risk stratification applies to pregnancy-associated PE, but indirect evidence encourages that the physiological changes in pregnancy should not alter the current clinical assessment approach of hemodynamic compromise employed to identify high-risk PE [41].

Cardiac output increases by 50% during pregnancy to satisfy the metabolic demands of both the mother and the fetus. The heart rate rises, cardiac preload is elevated based on the increased blood volume, and cardiac afterload is decreased through a drop in systemic vascular resistance. This hyperdynamic state is associated with left ventricular eccentric remodeling [42]. Shortly after delivery, the hemodynamic parameters revert to pre-pregnancy levels. Because of this, the 90 mmHg threshold used to define high-risk PE is suitable in the context of pregnancy [41].

The biomarker criteria that indicate an intermediate risk of PE can also be applied during pregnancy. Troponin and NT proBNP fluctuate mildly during pregnancy and the postpartum period, and the 95th percentile stays under the non-gravid threshold levels of 14 ng/L and 300 ng/L, respectively [43]. Concerning RV dilatation, all heart chambers enlarge during pregnancy, including right heart dimensions [42]. Because the change in volume in left and right cavities is similar, it is not expected that the physiological RV/LV ratio will be altered in pregnancy [41].

Fetal distress can also indicate end-organ hypoperfusion. It is therefore proposed that, in late pregnancy, an obstetrical assessment of the fetal status using ultrasound and cardiotocogram should be performed, for the risk stratification of severe pregnancy-associated PE [41].

8. Diagnosis

Ongoing discussions in clinical practice focus on determining the most appropriate imaging modality for ruling out or diagnosing PE during pregnancy. The challenges associated with various modalities will be briefly discussed to aid in clinical decision-making [44].

A chest X-ray should be conducted to exclude other conditions, such as pneumonia or pneumothorax, that present with similar symptoms to those of PE. It should be noted that in up to 50% of cases, the thoracic X-ray can appear normal. The most frequent radiological findings in PE are pleural fluid accumulation, pulmonary edema, basal atelectasis, and localized opacities [45].

The electrocardiogram may suggest and strengthen the diagnosis of PE, with changes, such as sinus tachycardia, right bundle branch block, rightward axis deviation, or the S1Q3T3 pattern. It is important to highlight that these changes may not be present even in cases of a massive embolism [46].

Lung ultrasound (LUS) could potentially help in excluding or confirming some of the alternative diagnoses of PE, such as pleural effusion, pneumothorax, or interstitial syndrome, including pulmonary edema [47]. Moreover, the A profile in the BLUE protocol for LUS in conjunction with a positive DUS scan has 81% sensitivity, 99% specificity, and 98% negative predictive value for PE in non-pregnant patients [48]. Currently, there are no available protocols for LUS in pregnancy except for COVID-19 disease management [49]. However, a combination of POCUS (point of care ultrasound) with LUS, transthoracic echocardiography, and DUS could potentially improve the diagnostic accuracy, in addition to reducing the time to diagnosis of PE with a lower radiation-associated risk for the mother and fetus.

In patients with hemodynamic instability, a transthoracic echocardiography (TTE) should be conducted, as it can rapidly detect acute RV dysfunction if acute PE is the cause of the hemodynamic deterioration [27]. When no imaging signs of RV dysfunction are identified, other causes of hemodynamic instability, such as acute coronary or aortic syndromes, pericardial tamponade, and acute valvular conditions, can be evaluated by TTE as well [32]. If PE is indirectly confirmed, all PE patients with hemodynamic compromise are considered for a rescue thrombolytic treatment, in the absence of contraindications. However, if a contraindication exists, alternative treatment options should be reviewed, such as percutaneous thrombectomy. Nonetheless, cardio-pulmonary resuscitation is necessary in patients with hemodynamic collapse and concomitant cardiac arrest, due to the very limited treatment options. Even though pregnancy is considered a relative contraindication for systemic thrombolytic treatment, current guidelines still suggest considering thrombolysis or surgical embolectomy as the primary reperfusion strategies in these patients [32]. A recent analysis of a contemporary cohort shows that 1 in 3 pregnant women with PE and hemodynamic instability underwent systemic thrombolysis [50].

In women with suspected PE, the key components of the diagnostic algorithm are the assessment of pre-test clinical probability, combined with high-sensitivity D-dimer testing and bilateral lower limb CUS (Figure 1). If a high or intermediate pre-test probability exists, therapeutic anticoagulation should be started before waiting for the confirmation or ruling out the diagnosis [51]. In the presence of signs or symptoms of DVT, CUS needs to be carried out. If DVT is identified, the diagnosis of PE is indirectly confirmed. If proximal DVT is not identified or the CUS is not conclusive, thoracic X-ray and then ventilation/perfusion scintigraphy (V/Q scan) or CTPA are the recommended imaging modalities to rule out suspected PE. However, due to a low prevalence of confirmed PE in pregnant women (2 to 7%), several diagnostic challenges emerge, which translate in the different algorithms proposed for the confirmation of PE in pregnancy by the current guidelines [32,52]. Recently, a multicenter prospective study validated a diagnostic approach for pregnant women with suspected PE. This strategy combined a pre-test clinical probability assessment using the Geneva score, with high-sensitivity D-dimer tests, CTPA, and CUS (see Table 1). In cases with low or intermediate pre-test clinical probability combined with a negative D-dimer test result, PE was ruled out. All remaining patients underwent lower limb CUS; if this was negative, CTPA was performed. The study included 395 women, with PE confirmed in 28 (7.1%) and excluded in 367 (92.9%). Among untreated women with excluded PE, the rate of symptomatic VTE events was 0.0%. Thus, this diagnostic algorithm effectively rules out PE in pregnancy [26]. However, it is important to note that normal D-dimer values have been observed in patients with confirmed PE [53] further emphasizing the need for a systematic and individualized approach to the pregnant patient with suspected VTE.

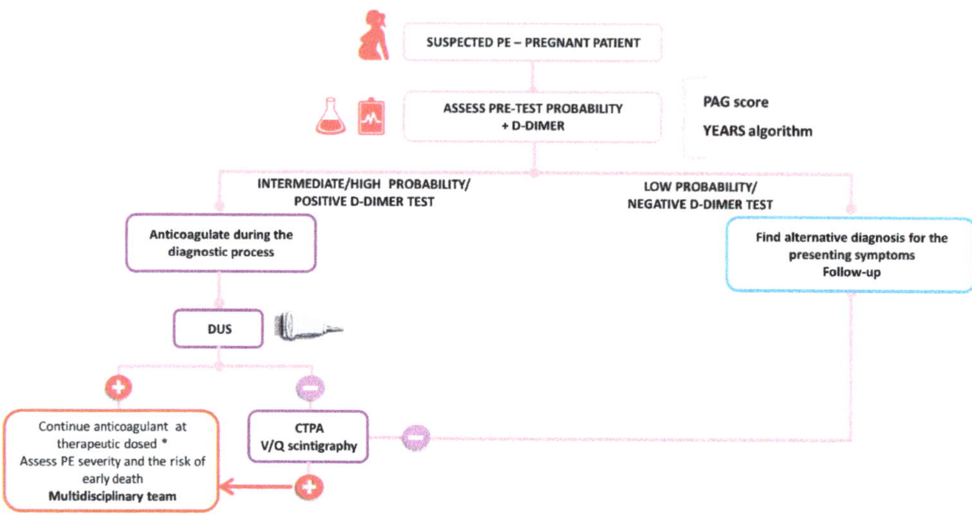

Figure 1. Proposed algorithm for the diagnosis of pulmonary embolism in pregnancy. CTPA—computer tomography pulmonary angiography, DUS—Doppler ultrasound, PAG—pregnancy-adapted Geneva score, V/Q—ventilation-perfusion; * See Tables 2 and 3.

Table 2. Anticoagulant options for VTE during pregnancy. APTT—activated partial thromboplastin time; DOAC—direct oral anticoagulant; INR—international normalized ratio; LMWH—low molecular weight heparin; UFH—unfractioned heparin; VKA—vitamin K antagonist; VTE—venous thromboembolism; kg—kilogram; i.v.—intravenous. & Based on the early pregnancy weight (8–12 weeks). * Fondaparinux can be used exceptionally in pregnancy in patients with heparin-induced thrombocytopenia [17,22,50].

Anticoagulant	Prophylactic Dose	Therapeutic Dose &	Recommended during Pregnancy	Recommended during Breastfeeding	Crossing of the Placental Barrier
UFH	3 × 5000 Units/day 2 × 7500 Units/day	80 Units bolus i.v., followed by 18 Units/kg/h i.v. Target APTT: 1.5–2 × baseline	Yes	Yes	No
LMWH			Yes	Yes	No
- Dalteparin	1 × 5000 Units/day	1 × 200 Units/kg/day 2 × 100 Units/kg/day			
- Enoxaparin	1 × 4000 Units/day	2 × 100 Units/kg/day 1 × 150 Units/kg/day			
- Nadroparin	1 × 2850 Units/day	2 × 85 Units/kg/day			
- Tinzaparin	1 × 4500 Units/day	1 × 175 Units/kg/day			

Table 2. *Cont.*

Anticoagulant	Prophylactic Dose	Therapeutic Dose [&]	Recommended during Pregnancy	Recommended during Breastfeeding	Crossing of the Placental Barrier
FONDAPARINUX	1 × 2.5 mg/day	<50 kg: 1 × 5 mg/day 50–100 kg: 1 × 7.5 mg/day >100 kg: 1 × 10 mg/day	No *	Yes	Yes
VKA	-	INR between 2–3 Preferably <5 mg/day	No past 6 weeks gestation. First trimester embriopathy Can be taken into consideration in women with mechanical heart valves	Yes	Yes
DOAC	-	-	No	No	Yes

The current ESC guidelines suggest that in pregnant women with suspected PE, an X-ray should be first performed. If the X-ray results are normal, a V/Q scan is recommended due to its low radiation exposure to both the fetus and the mother. If the X-ray reveals abnormalities, such as pulmonary opacities or infiltrates, a CTPA should be conducted directly [27]. Unfortunately, a V/Q scan at the point of care has a low availability, even more so outside working hours, which makes CTPA a frequent first choice as a diagnostic tool for PE suspicion [30].

9. Differential Diagnosis

The differential diagnosis of DVT in pregnant women is similar to that outside pregnancy. Several disorders presenting with warmth, erythema, edema, and pain in the lower limb, flank, pelvis, or back should be excluded. Such conditions can be superficial thrombophlebitis, cellulitis, lymphatic oedema, chronic venous disease, aneurysm of the popliteal vein or artery, Baker's cyst, lymphadenopathy, hematoma, or muscle tears [11].

The clinical presentation of DVT in pregnancy can also resemble normal manifestations in pregnancy, such as cramps and lower limb swelling.

Symptoms of PE in pregnancy can range from mild dyspnea to severe shock. Other conditions that can mimic PE are pneumothorax, heart failure, peripartum cardiomyopathy, pneumonia, and acute aortic syndrome. It is crucial to recognize that PE can occur in conjunction with other disorders [11].

10. Treatment

10.1. Management of VTE in Pregnancy

The primary treatment for acute VTE during pregnancy and the post-partum period is anticoagulation (Table 2). The selection of the anticoagulant agent is determined by a few factors, including the anatomical location, extension and severity of the thrombosis, the gestational age, and the possible risks to the fetus.

Heparin, preferably LMWH, is to be used, although UFH can be used as well, since neither agent crosses the placental barrier [54]. This differs from anti-vitamin K oral anticoagulant (AVK) warfarin that can cross the placenta and has the potential to cause severe complications, such as stillbirth, miscarriage, teratogenicity, pregnancy loss, neurodevelopmental deficits, and excessive bleeding. Nonetheless, warfarin can be used during breastfeeding.

The direct oral anticoagulants (DOACs) pass through the placenta and are not recommended in pregnancy [54]. Moreover, LMWH is preferred as a first-line treatment for preventing and treating VTE in pregnancy instead of UFH because it exhibits a lower risk of adverse effects, such as hemorrhage, osteoporosis, heparin-induced thrombocytopenia and allergic reactions [55]. The initial dose of UFH is established according to the patient's weight and then changed based on to the activated partial tromboplastin time (aPTT). Conversely, the dose of LMWH is based on the patient's early pregnancy body weight (8–12 weeks of gestation) and administered twice daily, mostly without monitoring. However, monitoring the anti-activated coagulation factor X can be taken into account in patients with extreme body weights, significant renal impairment, or recurrent thromboembolic events [27].

Fondaparinux is another indirect factor Xa inhibitor, but its use during pregnancy is not routinely indicated as there is little evidence regarding efficacy and safety and a minor transplacental passage has been shown [56]. Therefore, it is not considered a first-line anticoagulant; however, it can be used with caution as an alternative choice for patients with heparin-induced thrombocytopenia [27].

The anticoagulant treatment duration in VTE and PE associated with pregnancy ranges from 3 to 6 months, including up to six weeks after delivery [9]. AVK and LMWH are recommended after delivery, while DOACs should neither be used during pregnancy nor during lactation. Extended anticoagulation is reserved for women with a history of VTE and two or more thrombophilias or for women with history of recurrent thrombotic events and any thrombophilia or women diagnosed with antiphospholipid antibody syndrome [57].

Several clinical situations require the careful assessment of risk versus benefit of anticoagulation for VTE in pregnancy, such as active bleeding or high-risk of bleeding: obstetrical risk factors, like placenta praevia, a low platelet count (bellow 75×109) or acquired coagulopathy, severe liver disease (with increased prothrombin time), a history of allergy, stroke in the past 28 days, or inadequately controlled hypertension (BP more than 200 mmHg systolic or 120 mmHg diastolic) [16].

Pregnant women with VTE need careful monitoring to evaluate their response to treatment, prevent recurrent VTE, and address potential complications. The nature and complexity of monitoring depends on a number of variables, including VTE severity, the type of anticoagulant administered, and the gestational age of the fetus [54]. Other important aspects to consider during follow-up are the coagulation parameters, as well as routine periodic fetal surveillance to evaluate fetal growth and welfare.

Non-pharmacological treatment is also important in managing VTE symptoms in pregnancy. Compression stockings may assist in reducing the risk of post-thrombotic syndrome and alleviating symptoms, such as leg swelling or pain [58].

Additionally, pregnant women with VTE should be provided with information regarding the clinical aspects of recurrent VTE and be instructed to request medical assistance in the case of new or worsening symptoms [59].

10.2. Management of PE in Pregnancy

The management of acute PE in pregnancy requires a comprehensive clinical assessment and risk evaluation, incorporating the hemodynamic status, RV function and size, imaging, biomarkers, and validated scoring systems for PE severity stratification [27]. A multidisciplinary approach consisting of cardiology, obstetrics, pulmonology, vascular medicine, hematology, anesthesiology/intensive care, cardiothoracic surgery, and interventional radiology is essential for decision making (Figure 2) [6].

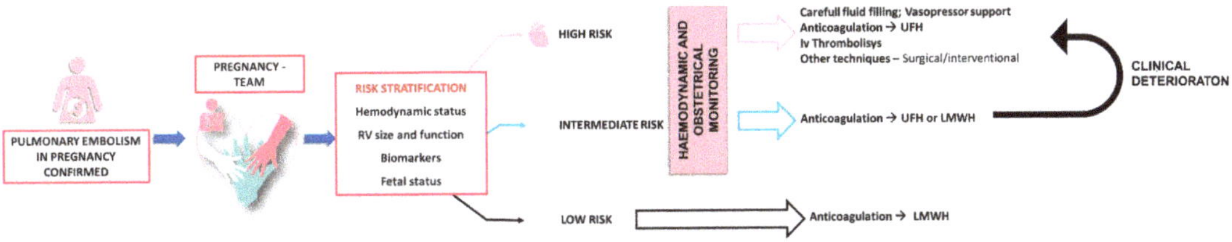

Figure 2. Proposed therapeutic management according to the pulmonary embolism severity. LMWH—low molecular weight heparin, UFH—unfractioned heparin.

Patients with acute low-risk PE, characterized by stable hemodynamics, normal RV function, and no end-organ damage, can be managed with LMWH or with UFH as an alternative option. These patients could potentially be managed on an outpatient basis [54].

Patients with hemodynamic stability but exhibiting RV strain on echocardiography or those with clinically severe PE—including oxygen saturation < 90%, tachycardia, tachypnea, numerous risk factors, or concurrent disease, such as old age, cancer, heart failure, or chronic pulmonary disease—are classified as intermediate risk. If troponin is elevated and RV dilatation/dysfunction is present, patients are additionally stratified into intermediate-high-risk groups as opposed to intermediate-low-risk groups in which troponin levels are normal. Sole anticoagulation is the mainstay treatment for intermediate-low-risk groups, while intensive monitoring is necessary for patients in intermediate-high-risk groups due to the potential for clinical worsening [27].

High-risk PE in pregnancy can be severe, with a case-fatality rate reaching as high as 37% [50]. If hemodynamic instability is present, UFH is administered as the primary treatment. Thrombolytic agents may be used if the hemodynamic status deteriorates. Immediate thrombolytic therapy is advised, provided there are no absolute contraindications to systemic thrombolysis [27].

Other treatment options of high-risk PE should be taken into account, such as surgical or percutaneous thrombectomy. If necessary, extracorporeal membrane oxygenation (ECMO) should be considered for depressurizing the RV and lung circulation [5]. Even though pregnancy is listed as a relative contraindication for thrombolysis, in women with circulatory collapse accompanied by cardiac arrest and the need for cardiopulmonary resuscitation, there are no alternative treatment possibilities [32]. Recent data demonstrated that as much as a third of high-risk PE women undergo systemic thrombolytic treatment. Nonetheless, thrombolysis seems to be associated with a favorable outcome, with 94% maternal survival and 88% fetal survival. Frequent side effects following thrombolytic treatment are bleeding complications, with a reported frequency of 18% during pregnancy up to 58% of cases in the post-partum period [5].

The peripartum period, along with spinal and epidural anesthesia, carries a high risk of bleeding; thus, thrombolysis should be performed peripartum only in a life-threatening situation [32]. Fibrinolytic drugs do not cross the placental barrier, so the fetal risk is low [60]. However, the lack of studies rule out conclusions regarding the safety profile and efficacy of thrombolysis in pregnancy high-risk PE. Therefore, important maternal or fetal adverse reactions cannot be extrapolated on for the use of a thrombolytic agent only [32].

If absolute contraindications are present, other treatment strategies need to be provided, such as percutaneous low-dose thrombolysis (CDT), surgical embolectomy, or thrombectomy [61]. Several small studies confirmed that CDT, in intermediate- and high-risk PE, is associated with better outcomes concerning bleeding complications compared to systemic thrombolysis [62]. In the post-partum period, surgical pulmonary embolectomy and percutaneous thrombectomy can be considered suitable treatment options to mitigate the hemorrhagic risks associated with systemic thrombolytic therapy. Nonetheless, these methods are usually not readily available and are used only in a life-threatening situation as a bailout therapeutic strategy [5].

In cases with hemodynamic instability where reperfusion therapy is not available or effective, recent data suggest that a bridging therapy with the transit use of mechanical circulatory support via ECMO can improve outcomes until mechanical thrombolysis or embolectomy is available [63]. ECMO has not been widely used in patients with acute high-risk PE and pregnancy. Limited date from a systematic review of 21 pregnant women with PE report a maternal survival rate of 76%, and a fetal survival rate of 63% with the use of ECMO [41]. Table 3 describes the current options for the treatment of high-risk PE with hemodynamic instability.

Table 3. Treatment for high-risk PE with hemodynamic instability. LMWH—low-molecular-weight heparin; UFH—unfractioned heparin; PE—pulmonary embolism.

Technique	Description
Anticoagulation	UFH is a first-line anticoagulation therapy in a patient with hemodynamic instability. Since they do not penetrate the placental barrier, they are safe during pregnancy and breastfeeding [53]. Can be given both intravenously or subcutaneously [44].
Thrombolytic treatment	Systemic thrombolysis is recommended only for high-risk patients with hemodynamic instability [27]. In patients with massive PE, favorable maternal outcomes were observed. The rate of maternal survival is approximatively 92% [5]. Lethal complications, including cardiac arrest or severe maternal hemorrhage, may arise [44]. Alteplase is given at a dose of 100 mg administered over two hours [41].
Catheter-directed therapy (CDT)	In high-risk patients where thrombolysis and anticoagulation have failed or are contraindicated, CDT can be beneficial [64]. The incidence of major hemorrhage is infrequent, about 18% [65]. The devices use mechanical fragmentation, aspiration, or thrombolytic infusion [44]. Should be conducted only in experienced centers [41].
Surgical thrombectomy	It is particularly taken into account for treating PE during pregnancy when anticoagulation is insufficient or the patient has hemodynamic instability [66]. Surgical thrombectomy with cardiopulmonary bypass is typically carried out without cardioplegia involving the removal of pulmonary clots through surgical openings in the two primary pulmonary arteries. Maternal survival occurred in about 86% of patients [5].
Extracorporeal membrane oxygenation (ECMO)	In patients with high-risk PE, it is regarded as a lifesaving intervention [67]. Venous and arterial cannulas are inserted into the inferior vena cava and the common femoral artery [44]. To improve outcomes, it can be combined with fibrinolysis or embolectomy [68]. The most suitable indication for ECMO is unresponsive cardiac arrest resulting from PE [44].

Inferior vena cava (IVC) filters can be taken into consideration in gravid women when an absolute contraindication to anticoagulation is present or when recurrent PE occurs despite optimal anticoagulant treatment in order to prevent further embolic events in the pulmonary circulation. However, data on this approach are limited. In the RIETE registry, recruiting between the years 2001 and 2019, a cohort of women with VTE, either pregnant or in the postpartum period, only one patient from the 34 receiving an IVC filter had a complication (vein tear during filter recovery) [14]. In a systematic review analyzing

124 pregnant women with DVT who underwent an IVC filter implantation, no fatal PE occurred after device placement, and the complication rates from retrieval were similar with those observed in the general population. The most common adverse events are migration, perforation, fracture, or death [69]. However, despite the authors' conclusion that IVC filters can be used effectively in pregnant women to prevent PE, more studies are needed to suggest that they can be used routinely [70].

In general, the evidence supporting advanced therapeutic options in pregnant women with high-risk PE is lacking. Due to the complexity of diagnosis and treatment, optimal treatment strategies should be individualized and based on a multidisciplinary team approach with expertise in managing PE during pregnancy [27].

11. Conclusions

It is widely acknowledged that pregnancy involves physiological changes that increase the risk of thromboembolic events. VTE, as well as its complications, is an important cause of morbidity and mortality in the mother and the fetus. Hence, it is crucial to promptly and accurately identify women for whom preventive anticoagulation would be beneficial. PE is a rare event, but with a high-risk of mortality, especially during pregnancy. The diagnosis of acute PE in pregnant women can be difficult due to significant overlap between symptoms due to embolism and symptoms secondary to the inherent anatomical and physiological changes in pregnancy; a tailored diagnostic algorithm should be implemented based on currently available pre-test probability assessment tools along with D-dimer testing, DUS, CTPA, and V/Q scans. However, PE with hemodynamic instability is a major emergency, and this diagnosis needs to be established as soon as possible, utilizing the appropriate diagnostic tools in order to implement a prompt and immediate reperfusion strategy. Although pregnancy is regarded as a relative contraindication for thrombolysis, it should still be considered for pregnant women with high-risk PE, alongside other therapeutic approaches, including low-dose CDT, surgical embolectomy, or percutaneous thrombectomy. Overall, decision-making should be supported by a multidisciplinary approach, informed by guideline recommendations and currently available data, with careful consideration of the benefits and risks of the mother, as well as the fetus, available resources, and the level of expertise.

Author Contributions: Conceptualization: Ș.-I.M., S.S., E.W., A.M.I., E.B. and A.-M.B.; writing—original draft preparation, Ș.-I.M., A.M.I., E.B. and A.-M.B.; writing—review and editing, Ș.-I.M., S.S., E.W. and A.-M.B.; supervision: E.B. and A.-M.B. All authors have read and agreed to the published version of the manuscript.

Funding: Publication of this paper was supported by the "Carol Davila" University of Medicine and Pharmacy Bucharest, Romania, through the institutional program "Publish not Perish".

Institutional Review Board Statement: Not applicable.

Informed Consent Statement: No potentially identifiable human images or data are presented in this study. According to national legislation and institutional requirements, this study did not require informed consent for participation.

Data Availability Statement: The data presented in this study are available upon request from the corresponding author.

Conflicts of Interest: The authors declare no conflicts of interest.

References

1. Bourjeily, G.; Paidas, M.; Khalil, H.; Rosene-Montella, K.; Rodger, M. Pulmonary embolism in pregnancy. *Lancet* **2010**, *375*, 500–512. [CrossRef]
2. Wik, H.S.; Jacobsen, A.F.; Sandvik, L.; Sandset, P.M. Prevalence and predictors for post-thrombotic syndrome 3 to 16years after pregnancy-related venous thrombosis: A population-based, cross-sectional, case-control study. *J. Thromb. Haemost.* **2012**, *10*, 840–847. [CrossRef] [PubMed]

3. Testa, S.; Passamonti, S.M.; Paoletti, O.; Bucciarelli, P.; Ronca, E.; Riccardi, A.; Rigolli, A.; Zimmermann, A.; Martinelli, I. The "Pregnancy Health-care Program" for the prevention of venous thromboembolism in pregnancy. *Intern. Emerg. Med.* **2015**, *10*, 129–134. [CrossRef] [PubMed]
4. Kalaitzopoulos, D.R.; Panagopoulos, A.; Samant, S.; Ghalib, N.; Kadillari, J.; Daniilidis, A.; Samartzis, N.; Makadia, J.; Palaiodimos, L.; Kokkinidis, D.G.; et al. Management of venous thromboembolism in pregnancy. *Thromb. Res.* **2022**, *211*, 106–113. [CrossRef] [PubMed]
5. Martillotti, G.; Boehlen, F.; Robert-Ebadi, H.; Jastrow, N.; Righini, M.; Blondon, M. Treatment options for severe pulmonary embolism during pregnancy and the postpartum period: A systematic review. *J. Thromb. Haemost.* **2017**, *15*, 1942–1950. [CrossRef]
6. Bukhari, S.; Fatima, S.; Barakat, A.F.; Fogerty, A.E.; Weinberg, I.; Elgendy, I.Y. Venous thromboembolism during pregnancy and postpartum period. *Eur. J. Intern. Med.* **2022**, *97*, 8–17. [CrossRef]
7. Kourlaba, G.; Relakis, J.; Kontodimas, S.; Holm, M.V.; Maniadakis, N. A systematic review and meta-analysis of the epidemiology and burden of venous thromboembolism among pregnant women. *Int. J. Gynecol. Obstet.* **2016**, *132*, 4–10. [CrossRef]
8. Callaghan, W.M.; Creanga, A.A.; Kuklina, E.V. Severe maternal morbidity among delivery and postpartum hospitalizations in the United States. *Obstet. Gynecol.* **2012**, *120*, 1029–1036. [CrossRef]
9. Varrias, D.; Spanos, M.; Kokkinidis, D.G.; Zoumpourlis, P.; Kalaitzopoulos, D.R. Venous Thromboembolism in Pregnancy: Challenges and Solutions. *Vasc. Health Risk Manag.* **2023**, *19*, 469–484. [CrossRef]
10. Karlsson, O.; Sporrong, T.; Hillarp, A.; Jeppsson, A.; Hellgren, M. Prospective longitudinal study of thromboelastography and standard hemostatic laboratory tests in healthy women during normal pregnancy. *Anesth. Analg.* **2012**, *115*, 890–898. [CrossRef]
11. Kearsley, R.; Stocks, G. Venous thromboembolism in pregnancy—Diagnosis, management, and treatment. *BJA Educ.* **2021**, *21*, 117–123. [CrossRef] [PubMed]
12. Van Pampus, M.G.; Dekker, G.A.; Wolf, H.; Huijgens, P.C.; Koopman, M.M.; von Blomberg, B.M.; Büller, H.R. High prevalence of hemostatic abnormalities in women with a history of severe preeclampsia. *Am. J. Obstet. Gynecol.* **1999**, *180*, 1146–1150. [CrossRef] [PubMed]
13. Khan, K.S.; Wojdyla, D.; Say, L.; Gülmezoglu, A.M.; Van Look, P.F. WHO analysis of causes of maternal death: A systematic review. *Lancet* **2006**, *367*, 1066–1074. [CrossRef] [PubMed]
14. Elgendy, I.Y.; Fogerty, A.; Blanco-Molina, Á.; Rosa, V.; Schellong, S.; Skride, A.; Portillo, J.; Lopez-Miguel, P.; Monreal, M.; Weinberg, I. Clinical Characteristics and Outcomes of Women Presenting with Venous Thromboembolism during Pregnancy and Postpartum Period: Findings from the RIETE Registry. *Thromb. Haemost.* **2020**, *120*, 1454–1462. [CrossRef]
15. Kim, Y.H.; Pfaller, B.; Marson, A.; Yim, H.W.; Huang, V.; Ito, S. The risk of venous thromboembolism in women with inflammatory bowel disease during pregnancy and the postpartum period: A systematic review and meta-analysis. *Medicine* **2019**, *98*, e17309. [CrossRef]
16. Royal College of Obstetricians and Gynaecologists (RCOG). Reducing the Risk of Venous Thromboembolism during Pregnancy and the Puerperium Green-Top Guideline No. 37a. 2015. Available online: https://www.rcog.org.uk/globalassets/documents/guidelines/gtg-37a.png (accessed on 14 April 2024).
17. Hoffman, R.; Brenner, B. Can we program VTE prevention in pregnancy? *Intern. Emerg. Med.* **2015**, *10*, 123–124. [CrossRef]
18. ACOG. American College of Obstetricians and Gynecologists—ACOG Practice Bulletin No. 196: Thromboembolism in Pregnancy. *Am. Coll. Obstet. Gynecol.* **2018**, *132*, e1-17. [CrossRef]
19. Hart, C.; Bauersachs, R.; Scholz, U.; Zotz, R.; Bergmann, F.; Rott, H.; Linnemann, B. Prevention of Venous Thromboembolism during Pregnancy and the Puerperium with a Special Focus on Women with Hereditary Thrombophilia or Prior VTE-Position Paper of the Working Group in Women's Health of the Society of Thrombosis and Haemostasis (GTH). *Hamostaseologie* **2020**, *40*, 572–590. [CrossRef]
20. Abdelhafez, M.M.; Ahmed, K.A.; Daud, M.N.; Eldiasty, A.M.; Amri, M.F.; Jeffree, M.S.; Kadir, F.B.; Baharuddin, D.M.; Rahim, S.S.; Than, W.W.; et al. Venous thromboembolism and pregnancy: A review of the literature. *Afr. J. Reprod. Health* **2023**, *27*, 81–94.
21. James, A.H.; Tapson, V.F.; Goldhaber, S.Z. Thrombosis during pregnancy and the postpartum period. *Am. J. Obstet. Gynecol.* **2005**, *193*, 216–219. [CrossRef]
22. Chan, W.S.; Spencer, F.A.; Ginsberg, J.S. Anatomic distribution of deep vein thrombosis in pregnancy. *Can. Med. Assoc. J.* **2010**, *182*, 657–660. [CrossRef] [PubMed]
23. Righini, M.; Jobic, C.; Boehlen, F.; Broussaud, J.; Becker, F.; Jaffrelot, M.; Blondon, M.; Guias, B.; Le Gal, G.; EDVIGE Study Group. Predicting deep venous thrombosis in pregnancy: External validation of the LEFT clinical prediction rule. *Haematologica* **2013**, *98*, 545–548. [CrossRef] [PubMed]
24. Field, L.; Chan, W.; Lee, A.; Spencer, F.A.; Crowther, M.; Rodger, M. Annals of Internal Medicine Article Predicting Deep Venous Thrombosis in Pregnancy: Out in. *Ann. Intern. Med.* **2009**, *151*, 85–92.
25. Bellesini, M.; Robert-Ebadi, H.; Combescure, C.; Dedionigi, C.; Le Gal, G.; Righini, M. D-dimer to rule out venous thromboembolism during pregnancy: A systematic review and meta-analysis. *J. Thromb. Haemost.* **2021**, *19*, 2454–2467. [CrossRef]
26. Righini, M.; Robert-Ebadi, H.; Elias, A.; Sanchez, O.; Le Moigne, E.; Schmidt, J.; Le Gall, C.; Cornuz, J.; Aujesky, D.; Roy, P.M.; et al. Diagnosis of pulmonary embolism during pregnancy a multicenter prospective management outcome study. *Ann. Intern. Med.* **2018**, *169*, 766–773. [CrossRef]

27. Konstantinides, S.V.; Meyer, G.; Becattini, C.; Bueno, H.; Geersing, G.J.; Harjola, V.P.; Huisman, M.V.; Humbert, M.; Jennings, C.S.; Jiménez, D.; et al. 2019 ESC Guidelines for the diagnosis and management of acute pulmonary embolism developed in collaboration with the European Respiratory Society (ERS). *Eur. Respir. J.* **2019**, *54*, 1901647. [CrossRef] [PubMed]
28. Chan, W.S.; Spencer, F.A.; Lee, A.Y.; Chunilal, S.; Douketis, J.D.; Rodger, M.; Ginsberg, J.S. Serial Compression Ultrasound and Iliac Vein Imaging. *Can. Med. Assoc.* **2013**, *185*, 194–200. [CrossRef]
29. Torkzad, M.R.; Bremme, K.; Hellgren, M.; Eriksson, M.J.; Hagman, A.; Jörgensen, T.; Lund, K.; Sandgren, G.; Blomqvist, L.; Kälebo, P. Magnetic resonance imaging and ultrasonography in diagnosis of pelvic vein thrombosis during pregnancy. *Thromb. Res.* **2010**, *126*, 107–112. [CrossRef]
30. Nguyen, E.T.; Hague, C.; Manos, D.; Memauri, B.; Souza, C.; Taylor, J.; Dennie, C. Canadian Society of Thoracic Radiology/Canadian Association of Radiologists Best Practice Guidance for Investigation of Acute Pulmonary Embolism, Part 1: Acquisition and Safety Considerations. *Can. Assoc. Radiol. J.* **2022**, *73*, 203–213. [CrossRef]
31. Cohen, S.L.; Feizullayeva, C.; McCandlish, J.A.; Sanelli, P.C.; McGinn, T.; Brenner, B.; Spyropoulos, A.C. Comparison of international societal guidelines for the diagnosis of suspected pulmonary embolism during pregnancy. *Lancet Haematol.* **2020**, *7*, e247–e258. [CrossRef]
32. Hobohm, L.; Farmakis, I.T.; Münzel, T.; Konstantinides, S.; Keller, K. Pulmonary Embolism and Pregnancy—Challenges in Diagnostic and Therapeutic Decisions in High-Risk Patients. *Front. Cardiovasc. Med.* **2022**, *9*, 856594. [CrossRef]
33. Varrias, D.; Sharma, N.; Hentz, R.; Ma, R.; Gurciullo, D.; Kleiman, J.; Kossack, A.; Wolf, E.; Lam, B.; Bimal, T.; et al. Clinical significance of unexplained persistent sinus tachycardia in women with structurally normal heart during the peripartum period. *BMC Pregnancy Childbirth* **2022**, *22*, 677. [CrossRef] [PubMed]
34. Kline, J.A.; Slattery, D.; O'Neil, B.J.; Thompson, J.R.; Miller, C.D.; Schreiber, D.; Briese, B.A.; Pollack, C.V. Clinical features of patients with pulmonary embolism and a negative PERC rule result. *Ann. Emerg. Med.* **2013**, *61*, 122–124. [CrossRef] [PubMed]
35. Perisinakis, K.; Seimenis, I.; Tzedakis, A.; Damilakis, J. Perfusion scintigraphy versus 256-slice CT angiography in pregnant patients suspected of pulmonary embolism: Comparison of radiation risks. *J. Nucl. Med.* **2014**, *55*, 1273–1280. [CrossRef]
36. Le Gal, G.; Righini, M.; Pierre-Marie, R.; Sanchez, O.; Aujesky, D.; Bounameaux, H. Prediction of Pulmonary Embolism in the Emergency Department. *Ann. Intern. Med.* **2006**, *144*, 165–171. [CrossRef] [PubMed]
37. Robert-Ebadi, H.; Elias, A.; Sanchez, O.; Le Moigne, E.; Schmidt, J.; Le Gall, C., Aujesky, D., Roy, P.M.; Moumneh, T.; Chauleur, C.; et al. Assessing the clinical probability of pulmonary embolism during pregnancy: The Pregnancy-Adapted Geneva (PAG) score. *J. Thromb. Haemost.* **2021**, *19*, 3044–3050. [CrossRef] [PubMed]
38. Roth, C.K. Pregnancy-Adapted years algorithm for diagnosis of suspected pulmonary embolism. *MCN Am. J. Matern. Nurs.* **2019**, *44*, 302A.
39. Langlois, E.; Cusson-Dufour, C.; Moumneh, T.; Elias, A.; Meyer, G.; Lacut, K.; Schmidt, J.; Le Gall, C.; Chauleur, C.; Glauser, F.; et al. Could the YEARS algorithm be used to exclude pulmonary embolism during pregnancy? Data from the CT-PE-pregnancy study. *J. Thromb. Haemost.* **2019**, *17*, 1329–1334. [CrossRef]
40. Singh, C.; Jain, A.; Tandon, R.; Malhotra, P. Management of thromboembolic disorders during pregnancy in resource-constrained settings: An Indian perspective. *Indian J. Med. Res.* **2023**, *157*, 533–542.
41. Blondon, M.; Martinez de Tejada, B.; Glauser, F.; Righini, M.; Robert-Ebadi, H. Management of high-risk pulmonary embolism in pregnancy. *Thromb. Res.* **2021**, *204*, 57–65. [CrossRef]
42. Melchiorre, K.; Sharma, R.; Khalil, A.; Thilaganathan, B. Maternal cardiovascular function in normal pregnancy: Evidence of maladaptation to chronic volume overload. *Hypertension* **2016**, *67*, 754–762. [CrossRef]
43. Furenäs, E.; Eriksson, P.; Wennerholm, U.B.; Dellborg, M. Pregnancy in a healthy population: Dynamics of NTproBNP and hs-cTroponin T. *Open Heart* **2020**, *7*, e001293. [CrossRef] [PubMed]
44. Makowska, A.; Treumann, T.; Venturini, S.; Christ, M. Pulmonary Embolism in Pregnancy: A Review for Clinical Practitioners. *J. Clin. Med.* **2024**, *13*, 2863. [CrossRef]
45. Urriago-Osorio, G.A.; Melo-Burbano, L.Á.; Van Den Berghe, J.L.; Muñoz-Córdoba, A.M.; Daza-Arana, J.E.; Contreras-Zúñiga, E. Pulmonary Thromboembolism in Pregnancy: A Case Report and Literature Review. *Open Access Emerg. Med.* **2023**, *15*, 217–225. [CrossRef] [PubMed]
46. Thomson, D.; Kourounis, G.; Trenear, R.; Messow, C.M.; Hrobar, P.; Mackay, A.; Isles, C. ECG in suspected pulmonary embolism. *Postgrad. Med. J.* **2019**, *95*, 12–17. [CrossRef]
47. Demi, L.; Wolfram, F.; Klersy, C.; De Silvestri, A.; Ferretti, V.V.; Muller, M.; Miller, D.; Feletti, F.; Wełnicki, M.; Buda, N.; et al. New International Guidelines and Consensus on the Use of Lung Ultrasound. *J. Ultrasound Med.* **2023**, *42*, 309–344. [CrossRef]
48. Lichtenstein, D.A. BLUE-Protocol and FALLS-Protocol: Two applications of lung ultrasound in the critically ill. *Chest* **2015**, *147*, 1659–1670. [CrossRef] [PubMed]
49. Moro, F.; Buonsenso, D.; Moruzzi, M.C.; Inchingolo, R.; Smargiassi, A.; Demi, L.; Larici, A.R.; Scambia, G.; Lanzone, A.; Testa, A.C. How to perform lung ultrasound in pregnant women with suspected COVID-19. *Ultrasound Obstet. Gynecol.* **2020**, *55*, 593–598. [CrossRef]
50. Hobohm, L.; Keller, K.; Valerio, L.; Ni Ainle, F.; Klok, F.A.; Münzel, T.; Kucher, N.; Lankeit, M.; Konstantinides, S.V.; Barco, S. Fatality rates and use of systemic thrombolysis in pregnant women with pulmonary embolism. *ESC Heart Fail.* **2020**, *7*, 2365–2372. [CrossRef]

51. Simcox, L.E.; Ormesher, L.; Tower, C.; Greer, I.A. Pulmonary thrombo-embolism in pregnancy: Diagnosis and management. *Breathe* **2015**, *11*, 282–289. [CrossRef]
52. Wan, T.; Skeith, L.; Karovitch, A.; Rodger, M.; Le Gal, G. Guidance for the diagnosis of pulmonary embolism during pregnancy: Consensus and controversies. *Thromb. Res.* **2017**, *157*, 23–28. [CrossRef]
53. Greer, I.A. Pregnancy Complicated by Venous Thrombosis. *N. Engl. J. Med.* **2015**, *373*, 540–547. [CrossRef]
54. Bates, S.M.; Rajasekhar, A.; Middeldorp, S.; McLintock, C.; Rodger, M.A.; James, A.H.; Vazquez, S.R.; Greer, I.A.; Riva, J.J.; Bhatt, M.; et al. American Society of Hematology 2018 guidelines for management of venous thromboembolism: Venous thromboembolism in the context of pregnancy. *Blood Adv.* **2018**, *2*, 3317–3359. [CrossRef]
55. Greer, I.A.; Nelson-Piercy, C. Low-molecular-weight heparins for thromboprophylaxis and treatment of venous thromboembolism in pregnancy: A systematic review of safety and efficacy. *Blood* **2005**, *106*, 401–407. [CrossRef]
56. Dempfle, C.-E.H. Minor Transplacental Passage of Fondaparinux in Vivo. *N. Engl. J. Med.* **2004**, *350*, 1914–1915. [CrossRef]
57. Schulman, S.; Granqvist, S.; Holmström, M.; Carlsson, A.; Lindmarker, P.; Nicol, P.; Eklund, S.G.; Nordlander, S.; Lärfars, G.; Leijd, B.; et al. The duration of oral anticoagulant therapy after a second episode of venous thromboembolism. *Pneumologie* **1997**, *51*, 996. [CrossRef] [PubMed]
58. Middleton, P.; Shepherd, E.; Gomersall, J.C. Venous thromboembolism prophylaxis for women at risk during pregnancy and the early postnatal period. *Cochrane Database Syst. Rev.* **2021**, *2021*, CD001689.
59. Gris, J.C. Venous thromboembolism during pregnancy and puerperium. *Hematologie* **2018**, *24*, 145–155. [CrossRef]
60. Leonhardt, G.; Gaul, C.; Nietsch, H.H.; Buerke, M.; Schleussner, E. Thrombolytic therapy in pregnancy. *J. Thromb. Thrombolysis* **2006**, *21*, 271–276. [CrossRef] [PubMed]
61. Hobohm, L.; Keller, K.; Münzel, T.; Gori, T.; Konstantinides, S.V. EkoSonic® endovascular system and other catheter-directed treatment reperfusion strategies for acute pulmonary embolism: Overview of efficacy and safety outcomes. *Expert Rev. Med. Devices* **2020**, *17*, 739–749. [CrossRef]
62. Hobohm, L.; Schmidt, F.P.; Gori, T.; Schmidtmann, I.; Barco, S.; Münzel, T.; Lankeit, M.; Konstantinides, S.V.; Keller, K. In-hospital outcomes of catheter-directed thrombolysis in patients with pulmonary embolism. *Eur. Heart J. Acute Cardiovasc. Care* **2021**, *10*, 258–264. [CrossRef]
63. Hobohm, L.; Sagoschen, I.; Habertheuer, A.; Barco, S.; Valerio, L.; Wild, J.; Schmidt, F.P.; Gori, T.; Münzel, T.; Konstantinides, S.; et al. Clinical use and outcome of extracorporeal membrane oxygenation in patients with pulmonary embolism. *Resuscitation* **2022**, *170*, 285–292. [CrossRef] [PubMed]
64. Pruszczyk, P.; Klok, F.A.; Kucher, N.; Roik, M.; Meneveau, N.; Sharp, A.S.; Nielsen-Kudsk, J.E.; Obradović, S.; Barco, S.; Giannini, F.; et al. Percutaneous treatment options for acute pulmonary embolism: A clinical consensus statement by the ESC Working Group on Pulmonary Circulation and Right Ventricular Function and the European Association of Percutaneous Cardiovascular Interventions. *EuroIntervention* **2022**, *18*, E623. [CrossRef] [PubMed]
65. Rodriguez, D.; Jerjes-Sanchez, C.; Fonseca, S.; Garcia-Toto, R.; Martinez-Alvarado, J.; Panneflek, J.; Ortiz-Ledesma, C.; Nevarez, F. Thrombolysis in massive and submassive pulmonary embolism during pregnancy and the puerperium: A systematic review. *J. Thromb. Thrombolysis* **2020**, *50*, 929–941. [CrossRef] [PubMed]
66. Taenaka, H.; Ootaki, C.; Matsuda, C.; Fujino, Y. Successful pulmonary embolectomy for massive pulmonary embolism during pregnancy: A case report. *JA Clin. Rep.* **2017**, *3*, 2–5. [CrossRef]
67. Agerstrand, C.; Abrams, D.; Biscotti, M.; Moroz, L.; Rosenzweig, E.B.; D'Alton, M.; Brodie, D.; Bacchetta, M. Extracorporeal Membrane Oxygenation for Cardiopulmonary Failure During Pregnancy and Postpartum. *Ann. Thorac. Surg.* **2016**, *102*, 774–779. [CrossRef]
68. Meneveau, N.; Guillon, B.; Planquette, B.; Piton, G.; Kimmoun, A.; Gaide-Chevronnay, L.; Aissaoui, N.; Neuschwander, A.; Zogheib, E.; Dupont, H.; et al. Outcomes after extracorporeal membrane oxygenation for the treatment of high-risk pulmonary embolism: A multicentre series of 52 cases. *Eur. Heart J.* **2018**, *39*, 4196–4204. [CrossRef]
69. Harris, S.A.; Velineni, R.; Davies, A.H. Inferior Vena Cava Filters in Pregnancy: A Systematic Review. *J. Vasc. Interv. Radiol.* **2016**, *27*, 354–360.e8. [CrossRef]
70. Bikdeli, B.; Chatterjee, S.; Desai, N.R.; Kirtane, A.J.; Desai, M.M.; Bracken, M.B.; Spencer, F.A.; Monreal, M.; Goldhaber, S.Z.; Krumholz, H.M. Inferior Vena Cava Filters to Prevent Pulmonary Embolism: Systematic Review and Meta-Analysis. *J. Am. Coll. Cardiol.* **2017**, *70*, 1587–1597. [CrossRef]

Journal of *Personalized Medicine*

MDPI

Article

The Absence of Typical Stroke Symptoms and Risk Factors Represents the Greatest Risk of an Incorrect Diagnosis in Stroke Patients

Rakesh Jalali [1,*], Aleksandra Bieniecka [2], Marek Jankowski [2], Patryk Stanisław Michel [2], Marta Popielarczyk [3], Mariusz Krzysztof Majewski [4], Jacek Zwiernik [5] and Joanna Maria Harazny [4,6]

1 Department of Emergency Medicine, School of Medicine, University of Warmia and Mazury, 10-719 Olsztyn, Poland

2 Students' Research Group, Department of Human Physiology and Pathophysiology, School of Medicine, University of Warmia and Mazury, 10-719 Olsztyn, Poland; aleksandra.bieniecka@student.uwm.edu.pl (A.B.); 158580@student.uwm.edu.pl (M.J.); patryk.michel@student.uwm.edu.pl (P.S.M.)

3 School of Public Health, University of Warmia and Mazury, 10-719 Olsztyn, Poland; 146986@student.uwm.edu.pl

4 Department of Human Physiology and Pathophysiology, School of Medicine, University of Warmia and Mazury, 10-719 Olsztyn, Poland; mariusz.majewski@uwm.edu.pl (M.K.M.); joanna.harazna@uwm.edu.pl (J.M.H.)

5 Department of Neurology and Neurosurgery, School of Medicine, University of Warmia and Mazury, 10-719 Olsztyn, Poland; jacek.zwiernik@uwm.edu.pl

6 Clinical Research Center, Department of Nephrology and Hypertension, University Erlangen-Nuremberg, 91054 Erlangen, Germany

* Correspondence: rakesh.jalali@uwm.edu.pl

Abstract: Background: Stroke is one of the most misdiagnosed conditions that causes serious medical disabilities. Its early and accurate diagnosis by the emergency team is crucial for the patient's survival. This study aimed to determine the percentage of brain strokes incorrectly diagnosed by paramedic teams and to analyze the factors influencing incorrect diagnoses. Methods: The data of 103 patients, mean age of 68.4 ± 14.96 years, admitted in 2019 to hospital emergency departments of the two hospitals in Olsztyn, Poland, were analyzed retrospectively. All patient data were obtained from their information cards. The parameters of the patients misdiagnosed and accurately diagnosed by paramedics were analyzed with Odds Ratio (OR) calculations using IBM SPSS version 23 software. Results: Stroke and transient ischemic attack were recognized in 77 cases (74.8%). In 26 patients (25.2%), the diagnosis made in the ambulance differed from that made in the hospital ward. The analysis of the Odds Ratio (OR) has shown that typical stroke risk factors, if present in a patient, facilitate the correct diagnosis. The greatest source of misdiagnosis of stroke by the paramedic team was the lack of hemiplegia (OR = 6.0). Conclusions: The absence of typical stroke risk factors and neurological stroke symptoms, such as smoking, hemiplegia, aphasia, hypercholesterolemia, arrhythmia, diabetes or a drooping corner of the mouth, constitutes a high risk of misdiagnosing stroke by the paramedic team.

Keywords: stroke; stroke risk factors; emergency medicine; neurological stroke symptoms; incorrect diagnosis

1. Introduction

Stroke remains the second leading cause of death and, when adjusted for disability-adjusted life years (DALYs), the third leading cause of death and disability combined worldwide [1,2]. Shortly before the SARS-CoV-2 pandemic in 2019, 81,182 patients were admitted to hospitals in Poland due to stroke. Data from 2010 to 2019 reveal that 86.2% of those hospitalized for stroke had an ischemic stroke (IS) and 13.8% had a hemorrhagic stroke (HS) [3].

Paramedics have to rely on the patient's medical history, risk factors and physical examination to diagnose a stroke. Despite having a variety of different stroke diagnosis tools, such as the Face, Arms, Speech, Time (FAST) test or Cincinnati Prehospital Stroke Scale, in a considerable number of cases the primary diagnosis does not match the actual condition of the patient [4]. According to many studies, stroke in a large number of patients is suspected based on stroke mimics [5–11].

It is up to the paramedic team to determine the exact time that has elapsed since the onset of symptoms. This is important because it affects the eligibility of patients for thrombolytic therapy, and a prompt administration of recombinant tissue plasminogen activator (rt-PA) increases its benefit. Early recognition is associated with markedly shorter time until arrival at the stroke unit and it is a key to a successful treatment [4,12].

The aim of this study was to determine the percentage of incorrectly diagnosed strokes by paramedics and to analyze the risk factors contributing to a misdiagnosis.

2. Materials and Methods

2.1. Design and Study Population

The study was a retrospective cohort analysis. The retrospective study "The lack of stroke risk factors was the risk of incorrect diagnosis of stroke patients by the paramedics in 2019 in Olsztyn", based on decision no. 2/2024 of the Ethics Committee of the University of Warmia and Mazury in Olsztyn, which operates in accordance with the principles of Good Clinical Practice and applicable law, did not require the consent of the Bioethics Committee for this type of research. The data of patients admitted to emergency departments (EDs) in two hospitals in Olsztyn, Poland, in 2019, in whom paramedics suspected a stroke, were analyzed. This was the last year in Olsztyn before the SARS-CoV-2 pandemic, which excluded the impact of this virus on the study results. The study population included 103 patients: 49 from the Ministry of Internal Affairs and Administration Hospital (the MSWiA Hospital) in Olsztyn and 54 from the Regional Specialist Hospital (the WSS Hospital) in Olsztyn, aged 23 to 97, with a mean age of 68.4 $\pm$ 14.96 years. There were 49 women (47.6%) and 54 men (52.4%). The managing directors of both hospitals provided written consent to use patient files to conduct the analyses. The data were encoded by generating individual patient ID codes before analysis.

2.2. Imaging in Stroke Patients

Both hospitals participating in the study had a CT scanner as well as an MRI scanner. The decision to perform a specific examination was made by a neurologist. As is standard, a CT scan without contrast was performed, and in the case of a high NIHSS score, it was supplemented with an angioCT scan of the cerebral arteries, and in the case of possible mechanical thrombectomy, a post-processing assessment of cerebral perfusion was performed using the Brainomix system. MRI was performed in patients with wake-up stroke symptoms and in doubtful cases suggesting, for example, posterior circulation stroke. If the CT or MRI scan performed on the day of admission did not show a stroke, then after 48–72 h, an MRI scan was performed if possible or CT if there were contraindications to MRI.

2.3. Data Collection

The data were retrieved from the medical archives of both hospitals. The criteria for including patients in the analyses were a diagnosis of "stroke" without a stroke specification made by paramedics and patients with a final diagnosis (ischemic or hemorrhagic) or transient ischemic attack (TIA) made in the hospital ward. No patients were excluded from either group. All patient data were obtained from patients' information cards, medical rescue cards, hospital ED cards and hospital discharge cards. The collected data included: gender; place of residence (urban or rural area); age; clinical signs (consciousness, visual disturbances, anisocoria, hemiplegia, aphasia, a drooping corner of the mouth or orientation) and the side of their occurrence, if applicable; initial prehospital and hospital discharge diagnoses (ICD-10); diagnosis consistency (correct or incorrect); presence of comorbidities; time since the last stroke; vital parameters measured before admission to the hospital ward (SBP—systolic blood pressure, DBP—diastolic blood pressure, MAP—mean arterial pressure, PP—pulse pressure, HR—heart rate, SaO2—oxygen saturation, RR—respiratory rate, BGL—blood glucose level); smoking; hospitalization ward; and death (yes or no). No sensitive data were included in the tables.

2.4. Data Analysis

Statistical analyses were performed with the use of the IBM SPSS Statistics version 23 software (IBM, New York, NY, USA). The Kolmogorov–Smirnov test was used to test the normality of variable distributions. To compare the means of the analyzed parameters with the normal distribution (age, PP) between the groups of patients, the *t*-Student test was used. For unpaired measurements with a non-normal distribution of results (other parameters), the differences in median values were compared with the non-parametric U-Mann–Whitney test. Correlation analyses were performed using Pearson's correlation coefficient and Spearman's correlation coefficient in the case of non-normal distribution. The Odds Ratio (OR) was calculated for the analyzed risk parameters of an incorrect diagnosis by paramedics. The description of the OR calculation can be found in the Supplementary Materials.

To determine significant differences (p_{chiQ}) in the categorical binary variables (yes/no), a Chi-Square test was used.

The result of the analyses was considered statistically significant at $p < 0.05$.

3. Results

3.1. Gender Distribution

The study population consisted of 103 patients: 54 males (52.4%) and 49 females (47.6%). The differences between male and female patients were not significant. The only clinical parameter that varied significantly ($p = 0.04$) between genders was RR. The mean RR was 15.17/min ± 2.50/min in females, while in males it was 16.65/min ± 2.75/min. Clinical characteristics of the study population collected by paramedics are presented in Table 1.

Table 1. Clinical characteristics of the study population collected by paramedics.

Parameter	N	Min	Max	Mean	SD	Median	IQR (25, 75)
Age [years]	103	23	97	68.40	14.96	70.00	(58, 78)
SBP [mmHg]	103	100	260	156.04	28.49	155.00	(137, 174)
DBP [mmHg]	103	54	150	87.72	17.25	88.00	(80, 95)
MAP [mmHg]	103	43	167	110.49	18.88	107.33	(98.33, 120.67)
PP [mmHg]	103	20	160	68.32	22.48	70.00	(50, 80)
HR [1/min]	103	55	150	83.60	17.71	80.00	(70, 94)
SaO_2 [%]	84	90	99	94.17	13.,87	97.00	(95, 98)
RR [1/min]	72	10	24	15.93	2.72	16.00	(14, 18)
BGL [mg/dL]	73	37	380	140.66	52.80	126.00	(111, 156.5)

SBP—systolic blood pressure, DBP—diastolic blood pressure, MAP—mean arterial pressure, PP—pulse pressure, HR—heart rate, SaO_2—oxygen saturation, RR—respiratory rate, BGL—blood glucose level, SD—standard deviation, IQR—inter quartile range (25th percentile, 75th percentile).

3.2. Comparison of Parameters Depending on the Place of Further Treatment

SBP was the only clinical parameter significantly ($p = 0.034$) different between patients treated in the MSWiA Hospital and the WSS Hospital in Olsztyn. Patients with higher SBP tended to be transported to and treated in the MSWiA Hospital. The mean SBP for patients hospitalized there was 161.2 mmHg ± 30.5 mmHg, while for patients treated in the WSS Hospital in Olsztyn it was 151.4 mmHg ± 26.0 mmHg. Gender and place of residence were not decisive factors in the distribution of patients to these hospitals. Age was the only parameter that differed between urban and rural residents. Patients with suspected stroke who lived in rural areas were tendentiously ($p = 0.068$) on average 5 years older than those who lived in cities (70.96 years ± 15.23 and 65.57 years ± 14.29, respectively).

3.3. Analysis of Prehospital Recognition of Stroke

Comparing the initial ICD-10 diagnosis made by the paramedics to the final ICD-10 diagnosis included in hospital discharge documents, the accuracy of the initial diagnosis was analyzed in two different variants:

(1) The number of entirely dissimilar diagnoses was assessed, i.e., it was analyzed whether the initial diagnosis and the final one referred to the same disease. The diagnosis of unspecified stroke (ICD-10 I64) was considered to match when the final diagnosis was also a specified type of stroke (ischemic or hemorrhagic) or transient ischemic attack (TIA) (Table 2).

Table 2. Compatibility between the initial (paramedics) and final (hospital) diagnoses.

Correct Diagnosis	n (N = 103)	[%]
yes	85	82.5
no	18	17.5

According to the data collected, 18 patients initially received an entirely different diagnosis than the one provided at hospital discharge. That group constituted 17.5% of cases. In the remaining 85 cases (82.5%), the initial diagnosis was accurate (Table 2).

The chosen hospital to which the patient was admitted did not affect the accuracy of the diagnoses made by paramedics, which differed from the one made in the hospital setting in all of those cases. The number of patients whose diagnoses differed is placed in brackets in each ICD-10 code category.

The diagnoses with the number of cases (N) made in the hospital setting that varied from the initial diagnosis of stroke by paramedics (ICD-10 I64) were as follows:

- G45.4 Transient global amnesia (N = 3);
- G45 Transient cerebral ischemic attacks and related syndromes (N = 4);
- G40.1 Localization-related (focal/partial) symptomatic epilepsy and epileptic syndromes with simple partial seizures (N = 1);
- R47.8 Other and unspecified speech disturbances (N = 1);
- G40.9 Epilepsy, unspecified (N = 2);
- Z30.9 Contraceptive management, unspecified (N = 1);
- G44.8 Other specified headache syndromes (N = 1);
- Z03.3 Observation for suspected nervous system disorder (N = 1);
- R47.8 Other and unspecified speech disturbances (N = 2);
- I63.5 Cerebral infarction due to unspecified occlusion or stenosis of cerebral arteries (N = 1);
- In one case, when the paramedics diagnosed a patient with fracture of the skull and facial bones (ICD-10 S02), the final hospital diagnosis was G45.9 Transient cerebral ischemic attack, unspecified (N = 1).

(2) It was assessed how many initial diagnoses of stroke without a precise distinction between the stroke type and TIA were confirmed in the hospital ward [1]. Among 103 analyzed patients, stroke was confirmed in the hospital setting in 62 cases (60.2%) and TIA in 15 (14.6%). A total of 26 cases (25.1%) were not diagnosed as cerebrovascular episodes at all (Table 3).

Table 3. Compatibility between the initial and final diagnoses of stroke or TIA.

Diagnosis	n (N = 103)	[%]
Stroke	62	60.2
TIA	15	14.6
CVA mimics	26	25.2

CVA mimics—other diseases that mimic symptoms of a cerebrovascular accident. The clinical parameters did not vary significantly between patients with accurate and inaccurate diagnoses of stroke or TIA.

The analysis of the group diagnosed with TIA revealed a statistically significant difference in assigning patients to the hospitals for further treatment ($p_{chiQ} = 0.005$), since 13 out of 15 patients with TIA (86.6%) were treated in the WSS Hospital in Olsztyn and only 2 out of 15 (13.33%) were admitted to the MSWiA Hospital. Among patients diagnosed with stroke and other diagnoses, there were no statistically significant differences in terms of choosing the hospital for further treatment (diagnosis of stroke: $p = 0.43$; unrecognized stroke: $p = 0.20$).

3.4. Factors Affecting the Diagnosis

The most important analysis performed in the study focused on factors that help recognize stroke in prehospital conditions and those that hinder the correct diagnosis. Diagnostic accuracy was not influenced by factors such as the age and gender of the patients, their place of residence and the hospital that the patient was transported to.

The study group, i.e., patients who were not diagnosed with stroke by paramedics, consisted of 26 people. The control group, in which the diagnosis of stroke/TIA was made correctly in prehospital care, included 77 patients. The total number of studied cases was 103 for each analyzed risk factor, apart from a drooping mouth corner and aphasia, where the documentation was incomplete in one case. For those factors, the studied population was 102 patients (Table 4, Figure 1).

Table 4. Factors influencing the diagnosis process by paramedic members.

	S_{yes}	C_{yes}	S_{no}	C_{no}	OR
No hemiplegia	13	11	13	66	6.00
No drooping mouth corner	21	37	5	39	4.43
Aphasia	17	23	9	53	4.35
Non-smoker	11	37	1	12	3.57
No arrhythmia	21	43	5	34	3.32
No hypercholesterolemia	23	54	3	23	3.27
No arterial hypertension	11	20	15	57	2.09
No diabetes mellitus	21	52	5	25	2.02
Conscious	24	66	2	10	1.82
No anisocoria	25	72	1	5	1.74
No previous stroke	21	55	5	22	1.68
Disturbed orientation	15	39	11	38	1.33
Visual disturbances	5	13	21	64	1.17
No visual disturbances	21	64	5	13	0.85
Preserved orientation	11	38	15	39	0.75
Previous stroke	5	22	21	55	0.60
Anisocoria	1	5	25	72	0.58
Unconscious	2	10	24	66	0.55
Diabetes mellitus	5	25	21	52	0.50
Arterial hypertension	15	57	11	20	0.48
Hypercholesterolemia	3	23	23	54	0.31
Arrhythmia	5	34	21	43	0.30

Table 4. *Cont.*

	S_{yes}	C_{yes}	S_{no}	C_{no}	OR
Smoker	1	12	11	37	0.28
No aphasia	9	53	17	23	0.23
Drooping mouth corner	5	39	21	37	0.23
Hemiplegia	13	66	13	11	0.17

S_{yes}—study group of patients with stroke symptoms or risk factors but incorrectly diagnosed by paramedics. S_{no}—study group of patients with no stroke symptoms or risk factors and incorrectly diagnosed by paramedics. C_{yes}—control group of patients with stroke symptoms or risk factors and correctly diagnosed by paramedics. C_{no}—control group of patients with no stroke symptoms or risk factors and correctly diagnosed by paramedics. OR—Odds Ratio.

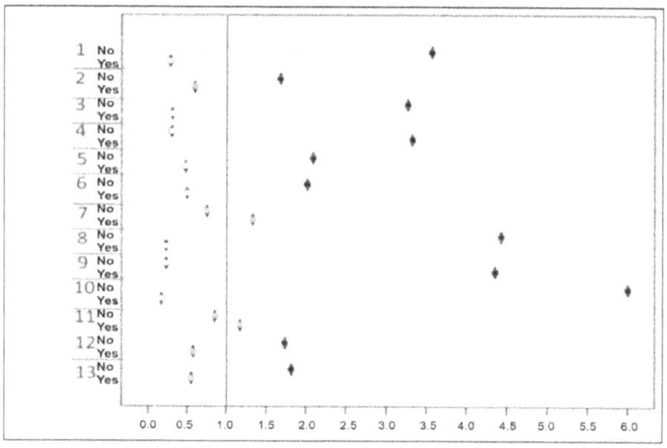

Figure 1. OR of making an incorrect diagnosis by paramedics. 1 smoking; 2 previous stroke; 3 hypercholesterolemia; 4 arrhythmia; 5 arterial hypertension; 6 diabetes mellitus; 7 preserved orientation; 8 drooping mouth corner; 9 aphasia; 10 hemiplegia; 11 visual disturbances; 12 anisocoria; 13 conscious. Circle in diamonds: white—OR $\leq$ 0.5; gray—0.5 < OR < 1.5; black OR $\geq$ 1.5.

Based on the analysis of the relative risk of an incorrect diagnosis of stroke or TIA by paramedics, the following observations were recorded:

- The consciousness of a patient was related to an increased risk of an incorrect diagnosis.
- The presence of anisocoria made it two-fold easier to recognize the stroke; however, its absence was related to an increased risk of an incorrect diagnosis.
- Vision deficiencies or their absence did not affect the diagnostic process.
- Hemiplegia occurred in nearly every case in which stroke was correctly recognized and turned out to be the most important factor in arriving at a correct diagnosis of stroke. Absence of hemiplegia was related to the highest risk of a misdiagnosis out of all the considered parameters.
- In the presence of aphasia, paramedics tended to make an incorrect diagnosis of stroke. On the other hand, aphasia was the most important factor that led to an inaccurate diagnosis as in the absence of aphasia the risk of an inaccurate diagnosis was low.
- A drooping corner of the mouth was a clinical sign associated with a high chance of paramedics and hospital staff members making the same diagnosis; the absence of a drooping corner of the mouth significantly increased the risk of an incorrect diagnosis in prehospital care.
- A disturbed orientation of the patient contributed to a misdiagnosis, but a preserved orientation did not influence the diagnostic process.
- If the patient was diabetic and their glucose level was high, a correct diagnosis was made more often.
- Among patients with hypertension, stroke was diagnosed correctly, while in patients with no hypertension, the risk of a misdiagnosis was high.

- Arrhythmia is an excellent indicator of an accurate diagnosis. Its presence facilitated making a correct diagnosis. In most cases, the detected arrhythmia was atrial fibrillation, which is an important risk factor for an ischemic stroke. Absence of arrythmia raised the risk of misdiagnosis.
- Hypercholesterolemia increased the possibility of a correct diagnosis, while the normal level of blood cholesterol in patients was related to a high risk of a mistake in the prehospital recognition of stroke.
- A previous cerebrovascular incident had no influence on the diagnostic process; however, if it was the first cerebrovascular incident in the patient's history, the risk of an inaccurate diagnosis was high.
- If a patient was a cigarette smoker, the chances of a correct diagnosis were high, while being a non-smoker lowered the probability of a recognition of stroke in prehospital care.

4. Discussion

Time plays a crucial role in stroke recognition. An inaccurate diagnosis prolongs the time that elapses from the onset of symptoms to hospital admission, and this can disqualify a patient from receiving lifesaving rt-PA that can be administered only within the first 4–5 h and maximally up to 6 h [4,12–14].

Our study established that, in 2019, the percentage of correct initial diagnoses made by paramedics in Olsztyn was high and amounted to 82.5%, and in the case of stroke or TIA it was 74.8%. A similar study performed in Poland by Karliński et al. revealed that the work of paramedics in prehospital conditions showed a high diagnostic sensitivity and positive predictive value (PPV), but lower than that of ambulance physicians and higher than that of non-ambulance physicians. A diagnosis made by paramedics was characterized by a sensitivity of 85% and a PPV of 72% [15]. Similar results were obtained in previous studies [16–22], but it is important to consider the differences in organizational structures of prehospital care among various countries.

The data presented above indicate that the absence of hemiplegia and the presence of aphasia are associated with the highest probability of a misdiagnosis. For example, aphasia was diagnosed to be associated with disorders of consciousness or dementia. This is also reflected in the calculated CI values. Diagnostic accuracy was not influenced by factors such as age, gender, place of residence and the hospital that the patient was transported to. The presence of common risk factors for stroke—such as hypertension, diabetes, arrhythmia, smoking and high cholesterol levels—facilitated an accurate diagnosis. Some of the conditions that paramedics considered a stroke included epilepsy, dementia, aphasia related to mental disorders and other vascular abnormalities affecting large arteries.

The analyses presented in the study raise the questions that need to be addressed for correct diagnosis of stroke, including: how should paramedics correctly recognize a stroke in patients who do not present with typical stroke symptoms? This is an important question because these patients may have a greater chance of surviving a stroke or even making a full recovery if the correct diagnosis is made promptly. In our opinion, prehospital assessment scales, such as FAST, the Los Angeles Motor Scale or the Cincinnati Prehospital Stroke Scale, designed to quickly identify patients eligible for thrombolytic therapy, rely mainly on symptoms resulting from circulatory disorders in the middle cerebral artery (MCA) or internal carotid artery (ICA) vascularization. These scales neglect the symptoms of posterior circulation stroke and do not help in detecting symptoms of lacunar stroke. On the other hand, paramedics who deal with patients with many different conditions daily may have difficulty mastering more complex assessment scales, such as the National Institutes of Health Stroke Scale (NIHSS) [23,24].

Additionally, a high workload causes burnouts and a tendency for paramedics to think schematically, making it easier for them to suspect stroke in patients with typical stroke symptoms. In our opinion, in addition to searching for more sensitive clinical assessment scales, the continuous education of paramedics is important [25,26]. In our centers, this is achieved by performing a neurological examination of the patient, carried out by a neurologist already present in the ED at the time of patient's arrival, in the presence of paramedics and providing information to paramedics about the final diagnosis. While conducting this study, mandatory training for paramedics was organized in Poland by the Ministry of Health under the name of Good Practices in Managing a Patient with Suspected Stroke, which unified the standard of practice for paramedics https://www.gov.pl/web/zdrowie/dobre-praktyki-postepowania-z-pacjentem-z-podejrzeniem-udaru-mozgu (accessed on 31 December 2019).

Limitations

The limitation of this work is that it is focused on analysis of the risk of incorrect diagnosis when diagnosing patients with suspected stroke by paramedics. In our study, the subgroup of patients with an incorrect diagnosis by paramedics was particularly small for a detailed comparative analysis of neurological symptoms and stroke risk factors in patients. In the future, the scope of these analyses could be deepened in a larger research group. The impact of the SARS-Cov-2 pandemic could also be taken into account in subsequent studies, including multicenter studies. The Supplementary Materials include tables with the results of analyses of neurological symptoms and stroke risk factors in the entire study group of patients and in subgroups with correct and incorrect diagnosis by paramedics. A significant limitation of these studies is the lack of information about stroke patients who were not diagnosed with stroke by paramedics and were not transported to hospital for further evaluation. This limitation should be addressed in future studies.

5. Conclusions

The absence of typical risk factors and symptoms for stroke in a patient, such as smoking, hemiplegia, aphasia, hypercholesterolemia, arrhythmia, diabetes or a drooping corner of the mouth, constituted a high risk of stroke misrecognition by paramedics in 2019 in Olsztyn. Development of more sensitive scales for stroke assessment is required for eliminating stroke misdiagnosis.

Supplementary Materials: The following supporting information can be downloaded at: https://www.mdpi.com/article/10.3390/jpm14090964/s1, Table S1: Significance of chi square differences (pchiQ) in YES/NO responses in the study group of patients. Upper and lower limits of the 95% confidence interval (CI 95%) were calculated using the Monte Carlo method; Table S2: Significance of chi square differences (pchiQ) in YES/NO responses in the subgroups of patients with correct und incorrect diagnosis. Upper and lower limits of the 95% confidence interval (CI 95%) were calculated using the Monte Carlo method.

Author Contributions: Conceptualization, R.J., M.P. and J.M.H.; data curation, M.P.; formal analysis, M.P. and J.M.H.; investigation, R.J., M.P. and J.M.H.; methodology, R.J. and J.M.H.; project administration, R.J.; resources, R.J., M.K.M. and J.M.H.; supervision, R.J. and J.Z.; validation, R.J. and M.K.M.; visualization, R.J.; writing—original draft, A.B., M.J. and P.S.M.; writing—review and editing, R.J. and J.Z. All authors have read and agreed to the published version of the manuscript.

Funding: This research received no external funding.

Institutional Review Board Statement: Decision No. 2/2024 of Ethics Committee of the University of Warmia and Mazury in Olsztyn. Consent No. DSDM.0721.59.19 from the Regional Specialist Hospital (the WSS Hospital) in Olsztyn. Consent No. 01/2020 from the Ministry of Internal Affairs and Administration Hospital (the MSWiA Hospital) in Olsztyn.

Informed Consent Statement: Not applicable. The correctness of the diagnosis was examined retrospectively. Hospital staff and paramedics were fully anonymous. Hospital directors gave written consent for these studies.

Data Availability Statement: All the analyzed data have been included in the manuscript.

Conflicts of Interest: The authors declare no conflicts of interest.

References

1. Błażejewska-Hyżorek, B.; Czernuszenko, A.; Członkowska, A.; Ferens, A.; Gasecki, D.; Kaczorowski, R.; Karaszewski, B.; Karliński, M.; Kazmierski, R.; Kłysz, B.; et al. Wytyczne postępowania w udarze mózgu. *Polski Prz. Neurol.* **2019**, *15*, 1–156. [CrossRef]
2. GBD 2019 Stroke Collaborators. Global, regional, and national burden of stroke and its risk factors, 1990–2019: A systematic analysis for the Global Burden of Disease Study 2019. *Lancet Neurol.* **2021**, *20*, 795–820. [CrossRef] [PubMed]
3. Jermakow, N.; Maluchnik, M.; Sienkiewicz-Jarosz, H.; Karaszewski, B.; Wierzchowska-Cioch, E.; Ryglewicz, D. Trends of stroke hospitalisation and fatality rates in young vs. elderly people in Poland during 2010–2019 decade. *Neurol. Neurochir. Polska* **2022**, *56*, 417–427. [CrossRef] [PubMed]
4. Magnusson, C.; Herlitz, J.; Sunnerhagen, K.S.; Hansson, P.O.; Andersson, J.O.; Jood, K. Prehospital recognition of stroke is associated with a lower risk of death. *Acta Neurol. Scand.* **2022**, *146*, 126–136. [CrossRef]
5. Newman-Toker, D.E.; Moy, E.; Valente, E.; Coffey, R.; Hines, A.L. Missed diagnosis of stroke in the emergency department: A cross-sectional analysis of a large population-based sample. *Diagnosis* **2014**, *1*, 155–166. [CrossRef]
6. Arch, A.E.; Weisman, D.C.; Coca, S.; Nystrom, K.V.; Wira, C.R., III; Schindler, J.L. Missed Ischemic Stroke Diagnosis in the Emergency Department by Emergency Medicine and Neurology Services. *Stroke* **2016**, *47*, 668–673, Erratum in *Stroke* **2016**, *47*, e59. [CrossRef]
7. Kozera-Strzelińska, D.; Karliński, M.; Rak, G.; Wojdacz, M.; Sienkiewicz-Jarosz, H.; Kurkowska-Jastrzębska, I. Stroke and TIA mimics in patients referred to a neurological emergency department by non-ambulance physicians, ambulance physicians and paramedics. *Neurol. Neurochir. Polska* **2019**, *53*, 83–89. [CrossRef]
8. Moulin, S.; Leys, D. Stroke mimics and chameleons. *Curr. Opin. Neurol.* **2019**, *32*, 54–59. [CrossRef]
9. Bakradze, E.; Liberman, A.L. Diagnostic Error in Stroke—Reasons and Proposed Solutions. *Curr. Atheroscler. Rep.* **2018**, *20*, 11. [CrossRef]
10. McClelland, G.; Rodgers, H.; Flynn, D.; Price, C.I. The frequency, characteristics and aetiology of stroke mimic presentations: A narrative review. *Eur. J. Emerg. Med.* **2019**, *26*, 2–8. [CrossRef]
11. Gibson, L.M.; Whiteley, W. The differential diagnosis of suspected stroke: A systematic review. *J. R. Coll. Physicians Edinb.* **2013**, *43*, 114–118. [CrossRef] [PubMed]
12. Hacke, W.; Donnan, G.; Fieschi, C.; Kaste, M.; von Kummer, R.; Broderick, J.P.; Brott, T.; Frankel, M.; Grotta, J.C.; Haley, E.C., Jr.; et al. Association of outcome with early stroke treatment: Pooled analysis of ATLANTIS, ECASS, and NINDS rt-PA stroke trials. *Lancet* **2004**, *363*, 768–774. [PubMed]
13. Saver, J.L.; Fonarow, G.C.; Smith, E.E.; Reeves, M.J.; Grau-Sepulveda, M.V.; Pan, W.; Olson, D.M.; Hernandez, A.F.; Peterson, E.D.; Schwamm, L.H. Time to treatment with intravenous tissue plasminogen activator and outcome from acute ischemic stroke. *JAMA* **2013**, *309*, 2480–2488. [CrossRef] [PubMed]
14. Fothergill, R.T.; Williams, J.; Edwards, M.J.; Russell, I.T.; Gompertz, P. Does use of the recognition of stroke in the emergency room stroke assessment tool enhance stroke recognition by ambulance clinicians? *Stroke* **2013**, *44*, 3007–3012. [CrossRef] [PubMed]
15. Karliński, M.; Kozera-Strzelińska, D.; Sienkiewicz-Jarosz, H.; Kurkowska-Jastrzębska, I.; Członkowska, A. Reliability of prehospital diagnosis of acute cerebrovascular accident. *Neurol. Neurochir. Polska* **2022**, *56*, 89–95. [CrossRef]
16. Andersson, E.; Bohlin, L.; Herlitz, J.; Sundler, A.J.; Fekete, Z.; Andersson Hagiwara, M. Prehospital Identification of Patients with a Final Hospital Diagnosis of Stroke. *Prehosp. Disaster Med.* **2018**, *33*, 63–70. [CrossRef]
17. Brandler, E.S.; Sharma, M.; McCullough, F.; Ben-Eli, D.; Kaufman, B.; Khandelwal, P.; Helzner, E.; Sinert, R.H.; Levine, S.R. Prehospital Stroke Identification: Factors Associated with Diagnostic Accuracy. *J. Stroke Cerebrovasc. Dis.* **2015**, *24*, 2161–2166. [CrossRef]
18. Wiszniewska, M.; Kobayashi, A.; Czlonkowska, A. Postępowanie w udarze mózgu Skrót Wytycznych Grupy Ekspertów Sekcji Chorób Naczyniowych Polskiego Towarzystwa Neurologicznego z 2012 roku. *Polski Prz. Neurol.* **2012**, *8*, 161–175.
19. Oostema, J.A.; Konen, J.; Chassee, T.; Nasiri, M.; Reeves, M.J. Clinical predictors of accurate prehospital stroke recognition. *Stroke* **2015**, *46*, 1513–1517. [CrossRef]
20. Pohl, M.; Hesszenberger, D.; Kapus, K.; Meszaros, J.; Feher, A.; Varadi, I.; Pusch, G.; Fejes, E.; Tibold, A.; Feher, G. Ischemic stroke mimics: A comprehensive review. *J. Clin. Neurosci.* **2021**, *93*, 174–182. [CrossRef]
21. Buck, B.H.; Akhtar, N.; Alrohimi, A.; Khan, K.; Shuaib, A. Stroke mimics: Incidence, aetiology, clinical features and treatment. *Ann. Med.* **2021**, *53*, 420–436. [CrossRef] [PubMed]
22. Mould-Millman, N.K.; Meese, H.; Alattas, I.; Ido, M.; Yi, I.; Oyewumi, T.; Colman, M.; Frankel, M.; Yancey, A., II. Accuracy of Prehospital Identification of Stroke in a Large Stroke Belt Municipality. *Prehosp. Emerg. Care* **2018**, *22*, 734–742. [CrossRef] [PubMed]
23. Alijanpour, S.; Mostafazdeh-Bora, M.; Ahmadi Ahangar, A. Different Stroke Scales; Which Scale or Scales Should Be Used? *Casp. J. Intern. Med.* **2021**, *12*, 1–21.
24. Kolankoh, F.A.; Mozaffari, N.; Dashti-Kalantar, R.; Mahammadi, M.M. The Relationship Between Acute Stroke Management and the Knowledge of Evidence-based Care and Attitudes Toward Stroke Care Among Emergency Nurses and Emergency Medical Services Personnel in Ardabil City in 2021. *Turk. J. Neurol.* **2023**, *29*, 52–59. [CrossRef]

25. Blek, N.; Szarpak, L. Profile of practices and knowledge on stroke among Polish emergency medical service staff. *Disaster Emerg. Med. J.* **2021**, *6*, 55–62. [CrossRef]
26. Chmielewski, J.; Wojciechowska, M.; Chirico, F.; Criescenzo, P.; Rizzo, A.; Starz, R.; Yıldırım, M.; Olcay, Z.F.; Szarpak, Ł.; Strzelecka, A.; et al. Job burnout in a sample of Polish paramedics–role of work experience, age and health behaviours. *Ann. Agric. Environ. Med.* **2024**. Available online: https://www.aaem.pl/pdf-191526-112920?filename=Job%20burnout%20in%20a%20sample.pdf (accessed on 2 August 2024).

Journal of *Personalized Medicine*

MDPI

Review

Mechanical Thrombectomy via Transbrachial Approach in the Emergency Management of Acute Ischemic Stroke Patients with Aortic Pathologies: Our Experience and Literature Review

Aida Iancu [1,2], Raluca Tudor [2,3,*], Dana Simona Chita [4], Catalin Juratu [1,2], Anca Tudor [5], Florina Buleu [2,6], Daian Popa [6,7] and Silviu Brad [1]

1 Department of Radiology, "Victor Babes" University of Medicine and Pharmacy, E. Murgu Square no. 2, 300041 Timisoara, Romania; aida.parvu@umft.ro (A.I.); catalin.juratu@umft.ro (C.J.); bradsilviu@yahoo.com (S.B.)
2 County Emergency Clinical Hospital "Pius Brinzeu", 300732 Timisoara, Romania; buleu.florina@gmail.com
3 Department of Neurology, "Victor Babes" University of Medicine and Pharmacy, E. Murgu Square no. 2, 300041 Timisoara, Romania
4 Department of Neurology, Faculty of General Medicine, "Vasile Goldis" Western University of Arad, 310025 Arad, Romania; chita.dana-simona@uvvg.ro
5 Department of Functional Sciences, "Victor Babes" University of Medicine and Pharmacy, E. Murgu Square no. 2, 300041 Timisoara, Romania; atudor@umft.ro
6 Department of Cardiology, "Victor Babes" University of Medicine and Pharmacy, E. Murgu Square no. 2, 300041 Timisoara, Romania; daian-ionel.popa@umft.ro
7 Department of Surgery, Emergency Discipline, "Victor Babes" University of Medicine and Pharmacy, 300041 Timisoara, Romania
* Correspondence: tudor.raluca@umft.ro; Tel.: +40-745-843-808

Abstract: Study design: Mechanical thrombectomy (MT) via the transbrachial approach (TBA) is a very rare option used in cases of patients with aortic pathologies and acute ischemic stroke (AIS) due to the insufficient evidence in the literature, the difficulty from a technical point of view and the result of this technique influenced by the complications that frequently accompany it. Background: Only a few cases of patients with aortic pathologies and acute ischemic stroke where MT via TBA were reported in the literature, and its application in the emergency management of AIS has still not been dealt with in detail. Objectives: Out of a need to clarify and clearly emphasize the effectiveness of this approach in emergency MT via TBA in patients with AIS and aortic pathologies, this literature review and case report has the following objectives: the first one is the presentation of an emergency MT via transbrachial approach performed in a 44-year-old patient with AIS and diagnosed aortic coarctation during transfemural approach (TFA), with successful reperfusion in our department and the second one is to review the cases reports of patients with different aortic pathologies and AIS reperfusion therapy performed by MT via TBA from the literature. Methods: A total of nine cases (one personal case and eight published cases) were revised in terms of aortic pathologies type, reperfusion therapy type, and the complication of both mechanical thrombectomy and local transbrachial approach. Results: Mechanical thrombectomy through the transbrachial approach was the first choice in more than half of these cases (55.55%, n = 5 cases) in the treatment of acute ischemic stroke in the presence of previously diagnosed aortic pathologies. In one-third of all cases (33.33%, n = 3, our case and 2 case reports from the literature), the transbrachial approach was chosen after attempting to advance the guiding catheter through the transfemoral approach and intraprocedural diagnosis of aortic pathology. In only one case, after an ultrasound evaluation of the radial artery that showed a monophasic flow, MT was performed via TBA. Local transbrachial complication was reported in one case, and in two other cases, it was not stated if there were such complications. Hemorrhagic transformation of AIS was reported in two cases that underwent MT-only cerebral reperfusion via TBA, one with acute aortic dissection type A and our case of previously undiagnosed aortic coarctation. In the cases in whom short and long-term follow-up was reported, the outcome of treatment, which was not exclusively endovascular (77.77% cases with only MT and 33.33% with association of first thrombolysis and after MT), was good (six from nine patients). In two case reports, the outcomes were not stated, and one patient died after a long hospitalization in the intensive care unit from respiratory complications (our patient). Conclusions: Being a clinical emergency, acute ischemic stroke requires urgent medical intervention. In patients with aortic pathologies, where acute ischemic stroke emergency care is a challenge, mechanical thrombectomy via the transbrachial approach is a safe alternative method for cerebral reperfusion.

Keywords: acute ischemic stroke emergency management; aortic pathologies; mechanical thrombectomy; case report; literature review

1. Introduction

Mechanical thrombectomy (MT) has proven its importance in improving outcomes after acute ischemic stroke (AIS) over the past decade, a fact increasingly emphasized by large, multi-center, randomized, controlled clinical trials [1–4]. According to these, the conventional transfemoral approach is the basic approach for MT due to optimal intraoperative catheterization and immediate access to large-diameter devices (which provides more confidence when inserting high-profile catheters/sheaths) or due to the higher frequency complications of other vascular approaches or because of the absence of formal training in medical schools [1–5].

However, TFA has some reported limitations. In patients with type III aortic arch, extensive atherosclerotic disease involving the arch and descending aorta, ilio-femoral athero-occlusive disease, atypical branching patterns, coarctation or dissections of the aorta that limit blood flow, cannulation of the aortic arch vessels using TFA may be a challenge [6]. Apart from these limitations, access-site complications such as groin hemorrhages and hematomas, pseudoaneurysms, retroperitoneal hematomas, peripheral artery occlusions, femoral nerve injuries, and access-site infections. All these complications have been reported (5.13% in non-randomized control trials, while in randomized control trials the rate is 2.78%) in a systematic review that included 16 randomized clinical trials (RCTs) and 17 non-randomized cohort studies [7].

When faced with challenging situations in acute ischemic stroke emergency management where MT via TFA may pose difficulties, it becomes essential to utilize alternative puncture techniques like transradial, transbrachial, or direct carotid puncture to successfully achieve vascular and thrombic access, despite the limited documentation surrounding their efficacy [8].

In other to provide clarity and emphasize the effectiveness of utilizing the transbrachial approach in emergency mechanical thrombectomy for patients with acute ischemic stroke and aortic pathologies, this literature review and case report aims to achieve the following objectives: firstly, to present a case from our own experience involving a 44-year-old hypertensive patient with AIS and previously undiagnosed aortic coarctation, in which we successfully performed emergency MT via the transbrachial approach; and secondly, to review case reports from the literature on patients with various aortic pathologies and acute ischemic stroke who underwent mechanical thrombectomy via TBA.

2. Case Report and Literature Review

2.1. Case Presentation

A 44-year-old man with a history of essential hypertension was brought into the emergency department (ED) by an ambulance with a doctor with left hemiparesis, inability to talk, and anarthria with an onset of approximately 150 min. The patient's stroke-related neurological deficit assessment with the National Institute of Health Stroke Scale (NIHSS) was 15.

The non-contrast computed tomography (CT) scan and the CT angiography (CTA) of the head and neck (Figure 1) multiphase performed at the ED admission detected a dense right middle cerebral artery (MCA) sign with a right M1 occlusion visibility from the emergence of the carotid artery over a length of approximately 1 cm and reinjection into M2. The dense MCA sign has a crucial role in diagnosing acute stroke. It often becomes visible on CT imaging before other signs of infarct, indicating an occlusion of a large artery within the brain and the resulting infarct [9].

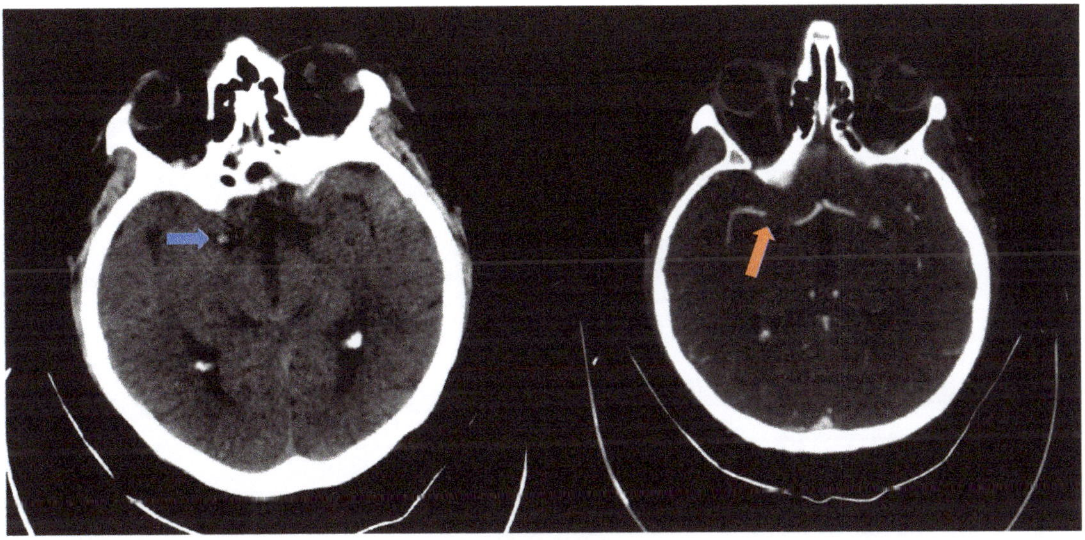

Figure 1. The left image displays the initial CT scan of the head, revealing no significant indications of ischemic or hemorrhagic events. The PC-ASPECTS score was 10. A hyperdense right middle cerebral artery is visible, indicated by a blue arrow. The right image shows a multiphase head angiography-CT, confirming the presence of a thrombus at the level of the MCA as segment M1, as indicated by a red arrow.

No clinically significant stenotic lesions were identified in the common carotid artery or internal or external carotid arteries bilaterally. The right vertebral artery was hypoplastic, with the right vertebral artery dominant and the bilateral basilar artery permeable. No acute cerebral hemorrhagic lesions were constituted, with an Alberta Stroke Program Early CT Score (PC-ASPECTS) of 10. All laboratory analyses were normal.

Under general anesthesia, emergency MT was conducted at almost 6 h following the onset of stroke symptoms. A transfemoral approach was obtained in order to perform mechanical thrombectomy. During the advancement with the guide catheter, aortic coarctation was discovered, which remained undiagnosed until that moment, and the initial standard femoral artery approach was abandoned.

The procedure involved secondly a transbrachial approach using an 8F sheath. Selective cannulation of the right common carotid artery was performed, followed by inserting a 0.035-inch guidewire. With a single retrieval attempt using a 4×20 mm stent, the thrombus was successfully extracted. Puncture resulted in complete revascularization of the occluded arterial territory (see Figure 2). Throughout the procedure, no clinical or technical complications were encountered immediately.

With unassisted breathing, full awareness, and orientation, the patient was relocated to the neurology department. A day following the mechanical thrombectomy procedure, the patient experienced a significant improvement in neurological function. A subsequent CT scan revealed no cerebral ischemia in the revascularized area, scoring a perfect ASPECT 10 (Figure 3).

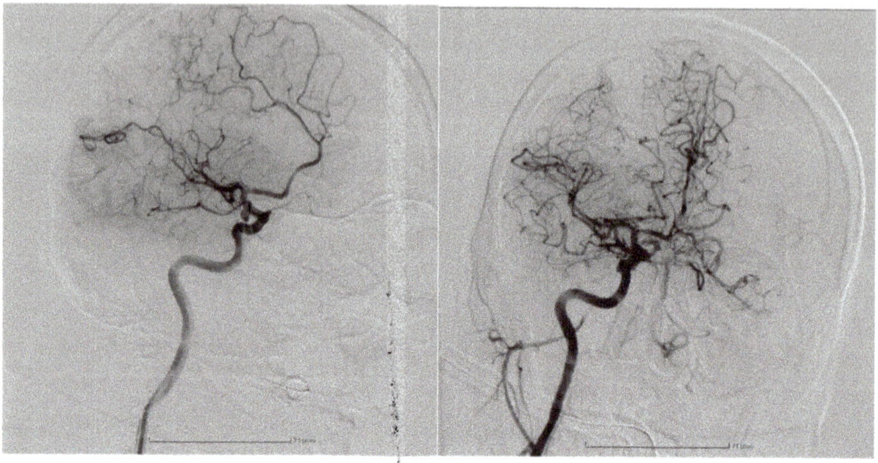

Figure 2. The lateral view of the digital subtraction angiography shows the occlusion of the right anterior cerebral artery (MCA) before the endovascular thrombectomy (left image). After the procedure (right image), a complete revascularization of the previously occluded arterial territory was successfully achieved.

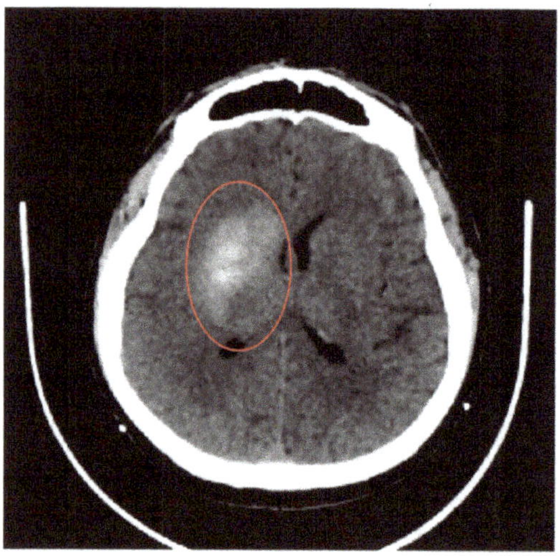

Figure 3. Head CT scan performed at 24 h after mechanical thrombectomy showed residual contrast substance in the nucleus basalis after revascularization—without established cerebral ischemia (red circle). The PC-ASPECTS was 10.

At the head CT examination 7 days post-procedural (Figure 4), compared to the previous examinations, it was observed the disappearance of the contrast substance residues from the nucleus basalis, as well as an extended ischemic hypodensity in the superficial right MCA (fronto-temporal) and in the lateral lenticulostriate arteries; ischemic hypodensity also occurred at the level of the right caudate nucleus.

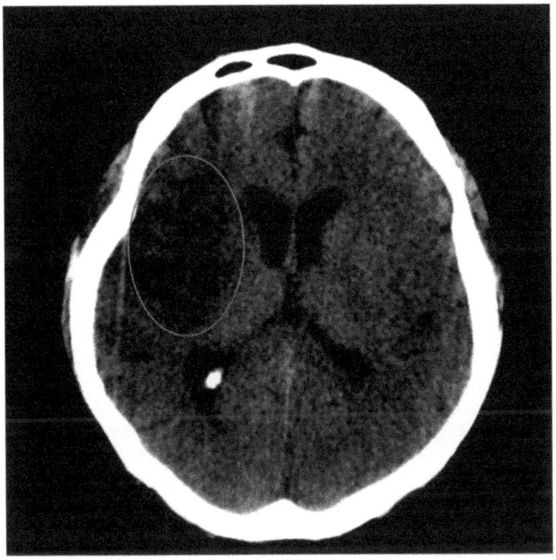

Figure 4. Head CT scan perform at 7 days after MT showed ischemia in the vascularized territory (lentiform nucleus and in the fronto-temporal-insular right lobe) (red circle).

On the morning of the 8th admission day, he was found to have a sudden onset of conscious disturbance and left hemiparesis with an NIHSS score of 22. EKG showed atrial fibrillation with rapid response. Embolic occlusion due to atrial fibrillation was highly suspected, and the patient received anticoagulant therapy with good neurological evolution. The patient developed respiratory complications due to a severe pulmonary infection. On the 31st day of hospitalization, the patient had a cardiac arrest that was successfully resuscitated, followed by patient transfer to the intensive care unit. During hospitalization in the intensive care unit, the patient had a fluctuating evolution, and despite the treatment (medication, kinetotherapy, hydroelectrolyte rebalance solutions), the patient's condition was deteriorating and required vasopressor support and mechanical ventilation. Six days after admission into the intensive care unit, the patient had cardiac arrest through asystole and did not respond to resuscitation maneuvers.

2.2. Literature Review

In general, the aortic arch has three major branches from proximal to distal: the brachiocephalic trunk, the left common carotid artery, and the left subclavian artery. These branches supply blood to the head, neck, and upper chest. The most common branching pattern, known as the standard arch, consists of the right brachiocephalic, left common carotid, and left subclavian arteries from right to left. According to a systematic review and meta-analysis of 51 articles (n = 23,882), the prevalence of standard arches is 80.9% [10]. Inanc et al. [11] identified three variations in the standard arch. The most common type, Type I, was found in 60.7% of patients, Type II (the bovine aortic arch) was seen in 34.3% of patients, and Type III was seen only in 4.8% of patients. Among the most common congenital malformations that occur in approximately 1% of all live births, aortic coarctation represents a proportion of 6–8% of these, according to the study performed by Hoffman and Kaplan [12].

Individuals with variations in the aortic arch and aortic coarctation may be more susceptible to atherosclerosis, leading to an increased risk of stroke due to the potential formation of blood clots. The alteration of hemodynamics could potentially occur due to the abnormal origin of arteries from the aortic arch or narrowing of the aorta, as hypothesized by Satti et al. [13].

Aortic pathologies present challenges during endovascular acute stroke treatment procedures, as highlighted in a study by Ribo et al. in 2013. The presence of these pathologies leads to prolonged procedure time and makes tasks such as carotid artery cannulation and stenting particularly difficult [14].

In fact, in patients with aortic pathologies and AIS, it is unclear how often alternative access is used in clinical practice and whether outcomes differ between patients who underwent MT through alternative (radial, carotidian, or brachial) versus transfemoral access [15].

Further, we conducted a literature review. Inclusion criteria were as follows: papers reporting cases with mechanical thrombectomy via transbrachial approach in patients with acute ischemic stroke and aortic pathologies, written in the English language and with full-text availability. We performed a comprehensive literature search of four electronic databases (PubMed, Scopus, Web of Science, Google Scholar) from inception until the first of November, 2023, using this search query ("Transbrachial" OR "TBA") AND ("case report" or "case reports") AND ("Mechanical thrombectomy" OR "MT" OR "Endovascular thrombectomy" OR "acute stroke") AND ("aortic pathologies" OR "aortic"). All duplicates were removed, and all references in the included case reports were screened manually for any eligible studies. Additionally, we cross-referenced the bibliographies of retrieved articles and review papers to ensure that we captured all case reports that met our research terms. Moreover, we performed a manual search for conference abstracts and/or posters or case reports in other databases to include in our review.

Ultimately, eight articles met the criteria for inclusion in this review, and one was excluded due to the unavailability of our data regarding the criteria followed (lack of concrete data about the included patients). Notably, all seven articles were case reports discussing TBA in patients with AIS and aortic pathologies, as summarized in Table 1.

Table 1. Summary of case reports of patients with acute ischemic stroke and aortic pathologies who underwent mechanical thrombectomy via transbrachial approach.

Number of Case Reports	Authors/Year	Sex/Age	Artery Occlusion Location	Reperfusion Therapy	Aortic Pathologies	MT Complications	Transbrachial Approach Local Complications	Outcomes
1.	Okawa et al., 2016 [16]	Not stated	Left terminal internal carotid artery	MT	Bovine aortic arch variant	No	No	Not stated
2.	Yamaguchi et al., 2017 [17]	Male, 94 years	Right middle cerebral artery	MT	Aortic arch type III	Hemorrhagic infarction of basal ganglia	Not stated	Alive, partially recovered
3.	Balci et al., 2019 [18]	Male, 57 years	Left middle cerebral artery m1 segment	MT	Thrombus protruding into the aortic arch	No	No	Alive, partially recovered
		Male, 60 years	Right middle cerebral artery m1 segment	MT	Thrombus protruding into the aortic arch	No	Moderate focal spasm at the entry site	Alive, partially recovered
4.	Kehara et al., 2020 [19]	Male/55 years	Right middle cerebral artery	MT	Acute aortic dissection type A	Right-sided hemorrhagic stroke	Not stated	Alive, recovered
5.	Proença et al., 2020 [20]	Male, 47 years	Mid-basilar artery	Intravenous thrombolysis + MT	History of type A aortic dissection (with previous endovascular stent graft surgery), intervention in the ascending and hemiarch aortic segment, ascending aortic aneurysm	No	No	Alive, recovered
6.	Bhatia et al., 2022 [21]	Female/51 years	Left middle cerebral artery	MT	Aortic bifurcation occlusion	Not stated	Not stated	Not stated
7.	Shimizu et al., 2023 [22]	Female/58 years	The left middle cerebral artery	Intravenous thrombolysis + MT	Aortic arch type III and Marfan syndrome	occlusion of the right internal carotid artery	No	Alive, partially recovered

3. Discussion

To the best of our knowledge, a literature review of aortic pathologies type, reperfusion therapy type, and the complication of both mechanical thrombectomy and local transbrachial approach in patients with acute ischemic stroke has not been previously published in the literature. Only a few cases of patients with aortic pathologies and acute ischemic stroke where MT via TBA was performed are reported [16–22], and this technique application in emergency management of AIS reperfusion has still not been dealt with in detail. So, we conducted a literature review, and after we analyzed these similar cases and from our case experience, we believe that TBA can be a feasible alternative route in AIS patients with aortic pathologies where the transfemoral approach cannot be used.

In interventional neuroradiology, the transfemoral artery approach remained the preferred arterial access site for most of the doctors who performed MT [6]. Only in cases where TFA has limitations [6], like coarctation of the aorta, a congenital malformation that typically presents in childhood, the other approach sites are used. Clinically, these patients present hypertension that appears in youth with a difference in blood pressure between the upper and lower extremities [23].

We present our case, where, unusually, the patient's aortic pathologies remained undiagnosed until his fortieth decade. Moreover, although he was hypertensive, with values most often difficult to control, only at the time of performing the MT via transfemoral approach the aortic coarctation was diagnosed. During the procedure, the interventional neuroradiologist decided to use the transbrachial approach for MT in order not to delay reperfusion management and for the patient not to leave the MT time window (<6 h). In this particular case, anticipating the possibility of inserting a larger caliber catheter (8F) for aspiration, the transbrachial approach was chosen instead of the radial. Also, based on his experience, the interventional neuroradiologist decided on this approach.

It is uncommon to incidentally discover aortic coarctation in adult patients, especially in association with AIS, particularly in adult and elderly patients who have not undergone correction for coarctation. The survival rate for patients with aortic coarctation is generally low [24], and there is ongoing debate regarding the best management strategies for such cases, particularly when other conditions like AIS complicate it.

When combined with secondary arterial hypertension, aortic coarctation increase the likelihood of developing premature coronary artery disease, aortic aneurysms, and cerebrovascular diseases, which not only affect prognosis but also have a significant impact on morbidity and disability [25]. The current guidelines strongly recommend the early detection and proactive management of aortic coarctation [23]. Despite advancements in surgical and interventional treatments for aortic coarctation, there have been reported cases of neurological complications, particularly paraplegia. These complications can arise from direct injury to spinal segmental arteries or inadequate oxygen supply to the spinal cord during the surgery correction process, leading to palsy or paralytic syndromes [26].

Two years ago, Trenk et al. [25] analyzed the results of a nationwide report based on 11,907 patients with coarctation of the aorta hospitalized between 1997 and 2015 in England. Late neurological complications (e.g., cerebral infarction and subarachnoid hemorrhage) occurred in 225 patients out of almost 150,000 patients followed annually during the study period (rate of 0.15%/patient-year). Subarachnoid hemorrhage occurred in 59.4% (n = 37 patients, 22 men) and at a median age of 28.7 years (IQR 20.2–44.5 years). Of these, prior to inclusion, only one patient had a diagnosis of cerebral arterial aneurysm. Ischemic stroke occurred in 188 patients. The median age at which they developed acute AIS was 56.1 years (IQR 43.6–68.1 years). Thirteen patients (6.9%) died during hospital admission, and the one-year mortality after stroke was 20%. Univariate conditional logistic regression analysis compared with patients matched for age, sex, and ethnicity showed that hypertension (odds ratio 4.00, $p = 0.0014$), dyslipidemia (odds ratio 4.50, $p = 0.007$), active smoking (odds ratio 11.00, $p = 0.02$), and diabetes mellitus (odds ratio 9.00, $p = 0.037$) were significantly related to the risk of AIS development. In multivariate analysis, only hypertension and smoking remained significantly related to the risk of ischemic stroke.

In the literature, there are few studies or case series studies that analyzed the transbrachial approach in emergency management of AIS [3,27,28]. When the brachial approach was compared with transradial or femoral approaches, it was noted to be more likely to have minor complications, with an overall access-site complication rate for noncoronary procedures of 10%. The authors concluded that both transradial and transbrachial approaches can be good alternative access routes when TFA is not appropriate in various neurointerventional procedures [28].

Local complications associated with transbrachial approach were reported until now, more frequent in percutaneous coronary intervention. In a study conducted by Kiemeneij et al. [29], the risk of complications (median nerve palsy and pseudoaneurysm due to subcutaneous hematoma in the puncture site) associated with brachial artery access was 2.3%, a higher risk than that of the transfemoral approach. Webber et al. [30] observed that inserting a larger than 8-Fr sheath might increase the frequency of pseudoaneurysms. With our patient, no local complication due to TBA was observed.

Small studies on transbrachial mechanical thrombectomy in acute ischemic stroke [3,31,32] concluded also that there were no technical difficulties or complications with this technique. Only a study conducted by Lu et al. on the safety and efficacy of the transbrachial approach for endovascular thrombectomy that included only 19 patients who had undergone MT for acute large vessel occlusion stroke concluded that the total procedure duration tended to be longer when the TBA was used after failure of the TFA (n = 6, 32%, median: 60.5 min) than when the TBA was used as the first side approach (n = 13, 68%, median: 22 min). Moreover, local complications were observed only in 2 cases: in one, a brachial artery pseudoaneurysm, and in the other, a brachial artery occlusion [3].

Regarding other access sites, mechanical thrombectomy via transradial and/or transbrachial approach in patients with AIS has recently been reported for both anterior and posterior circulation in the literature [27,33,34]. A systematic review and meta-analysis conducted by Kobeissi et al. that examine the feasibility of and outcomes following a transradial artery approach for posterior circulation large vessel occlusion strokes, observed a successful recanalization in almost all cases (98.69% rate, 93.50 to 100 cases) and a pooled meantime of puncture to recanalization of 29.19 min (24.05 to 35.42), concluding that transradial artery access for mechanical thrombectomy for this type of stroke displays early promise and feasibility [33]. After retrospectively analyzing five cases where the transbrachial approach was used for performing MT in acute stroke, Tsuji et al. observed that successful reperfusion was achieved in four out of five cases, and no access-site complications associated with this approach were reported in any case; however, death due to symptomatic intracranial hemorrhage was recorded [27]. When the transradial approach was compared with the transfemoral one, analyzing a homogeneous population in terms of the approach, which included a total of 2161 patients undergoing mechanical thrombectomy (446 patients that performed MT by transradial approach and 1715 patients by transfemoral approach), no significant differences across the two groups were found in terms of successful recanalization ($p = 0.36$), complete recanalization ($p = 0.73$), access-to-reperfusion time (mean difference, −3.92 min; $p = 0.17$), or symptomatic intracranial hemorrhage ($p = 0.62$). However, regarding access site complications, a significantly lower frequency in the transradial approach group was observed compared with the TFA group ($p = 0.001$) [35]. A low complication rate associated with transradial access, with only 1.4% ± 0.7% of stroke cases, was also noted by Peterson et al. after analyzing a number of 309 patients in which MT was performed via transradial approach from the studies included in their meta-analysis. Furthermore, when comparing studies that used the transradial approach with contemporary randomized clinical trials that used standard transfemoral access, no significant differences were found in puncture-to-reperfusion time, mortality, and/or site complications access of the transradial approach [36].

Two other alternative methods are available for patients who have experienced failed access for intracranial interventions: transcervical [37] (direct carotid puncture) and the recently introduced transvenous/transseptal access [38] (used to access the supra-aortic arteries from the venous side in cases where traditional transarterial access pathways, such as transfemoral, transradial/brachial routes, or direct carotid puncture, are expected to be unsuccessful). However, it is essential to note that direct carotid puncture carries the risk of serious complications such as neck hematoma, which could potentially compromise the airway. On the other hand, the two last methods, in emergency situations like AIS reperfusion, can be challenging. Transvenous/transseptal access presents logistical challenges and would not be suitable for patients with aortic pathologies, especially in aortic coarctation, as it would still require catheter manipulation in the aorta. The direct carotid approach in patients with AIS and coarctation of the aorta has been reported as a successful procedure in the literature so far, only by Roche et al. [39], who performed direct right common carotid puncture following the administration of the intravenous tissue plasminogen activator, in a 73-year-old woman with a large aortic arch saccular aneurysm measuring approximately 8 cm. But, also this approach technique, has disadvantages for patients with acute ischemic stroke. The primary issue commonly encountered with the cervical direct access technique is post-removal bleeding from the puncture site. To prevent the formation of cervical hematomas and the potential for obstruction of the upper airway, it is advisable to administer protamine after the procedure, apply manual compression, and, in some instances, utilize hemostatic closure devices.

After performing MT via TBA in our patient case and reviewing the literature (see Table 1) [16–22], both TBA advantages and disadvantages for patients with acute ischemic stroke can be outlined. One drawback of this approach, in comparison to the transradial approach, is that the brachial artery is functionally an "end artery", meaning that its blockage can lead to ischemia in the upper extremity. Fortunately, a surgical treatment is available for this condition, which can be performed immediately after intracranial thrombectomy. Additionally, based on our experience, achieving hemostasis is more challenging with the brachial approach than the radial approach. However, it is essential to note that the brachial artery is larger than the radial artery and has a lower risk of occlusion, mainly when the procedure is conducted under anticoagulation. Another advantage of the brachial approach is that it allows the operator to use shorter sheaths due to the closer proximity to the origins of the supra-aortic significant trunks [3].

Mechanical thrombectomy through the transbrachial approach was the first choice in more than half of these literature cases [18–20,22] (55.55%, n = 5 cases) in the treatment of acute ischemic stroke due to the presence of previously diagnosed aortic pathologies. In one-third of these cases (33.33%, our case and 2 case reports in the literature) [16,17], the transbrachial approach was chosen after attempting to advance the guiding catheter through the transfemoral approach and intraprocedural diagnosis of aortic pathology. In only one case [21], a patient with acute aortic dissection, after an ultrasound evaluation of the radial artery that showed a monophasic flow that could have caused difficulties and complications during the procedure, MT was performed via TBA. Local transbrachial complication was reported in one case [18], and in two other cases, it was not stated if there were such complications [19,21]. Hemorrhagic transformation of AIS was reported in two cases that underwent MT-only cerebral reperfusion via TBA, one with acute aortic dissection type A [19] and our case of previously undiagnosed aortic coarctation. In the cases in whom short and long-term follow-up was reported, the outcome of treatment, which was not exclusively endovascular (77.77% cases with only MT and 33.33% with association of first thrombolysis and after MT), was good (six from nine patients). In two case reports, the outcomes were not stated, and one patient died after a long hospitalization in the intensive care unit from respiratory complications (our patient).

In our case, the transbrachial approach allowed us to successfully rapidly reperfuse the patient's brain, thus reducing access-to-reperfusion time. So, we advise that the emergency imaging of patients with acute stroke should include the assessment of the aortic arch and that it be analyzed in detail, especially in very young patients or elderly who may have aortic pathology. Our case and also the other 2 cases [16,17] in the literature in which the switch to alternative access was imposed by previously undiagnostic aortic pathology have emphasized the fact that neurointerventionalists must be familiar with alternative access routes because an urgent need for such access may occur during acute AIS treatment.

Limitations

However, some issues may affect the generalizability of our findings. Compared to other large studies that included all patients with AIS and MT via transbrachial approach [3], our analysis only included case reports of patients with AIS and MT via TBA and aortic pathologies. Because there are several alternative approaches for patients with AIS, we believe that a larger study that includes a comparison between all these approaches already used in clinical practice in patients with AIS would help to choose the better approach for these types of patients, as well as studying the causes and risk factors that would affect the outcomes. For example, we cannot exclude the possibility that another approach type for MT is superior to TBA in patients with aortic pathology and AIS.

4. Conclusions

The MT through the transbrachial approach is a treatment option that should be considered as the first choice, especially in aortic coarctation patients, where the transfemoral approach is difficult due to anatomical issues. Interventional neuroradiologists should familiarize themselves with the transbrachial approach, especially as the use of MT is increasing during the acute phase treatment of stroke. Moreover, during MT, it is crucial to optimize all strategies that have the potential to prevent delays and ensure prompt initiation of stroke treatment.

In addition, in young hypertensive patients, unresponsive to antihypertensive treatment and admitted to the emergency department with acute stroke symptoms, we believe that the identification of an aortic pathology is essential. However, whether these patients should be routinely screened for aortic pathologies remains a matter of debate.

Author Contributions: Conceptualization: A.I., C.J. and F.B.; Data curation: A.T. and D.P.; Visualization: R.T. and D.S.C.; Writing—original draft: A.I. and F.B.; Writing—review and editing: D.S.C., R.T. and S.B. All authors have read and agreed to the published version of the manuscript.

Funding: This research received no external funding.

Institutional Review Board Statement: The study was conducted in accordance with the Declaration of Helsinki, and approved by the Ethics Committee of the County Emergency Hospital "Pius Brînzeu" Timisoara, Romania (approval certificate 385/2023).

Informed Consent Statement: The patient provided written informed consent in accordance with the Declaration of Helsinki.

Data Availability Statement: The data presented in this study are available on request from the corresponding author.

Conflicts of Interest: The authors declare no conflicts of interest.

References

1. Almallouhi, E.; Al Kasab, S.; Sattur, M.G.; Lena, J.; Jabbour, P.M.; Sweid, A.; Chalouhi, N.; Gooch, M.R.; Starke, R.M.; Peterson, E.C.; et al. Incorporation of transradial approach in neuroendovascular procedures: Defining benchmarks for rates of complications and conversion to femoral access. *J. Neurointerv. Surg.* **2020**, *12*, 1122–1126. [CrossRef]
2. Joshi, K.C.; Beer-Furlan, A.; Crowley, R.W.; Chen, M.; Munich, S.A. Transradial approach for neurointerventions: A systematic review of the literature. *J. NeuroInterv. Surg.* **2020**, *12*, 886–892. [CrossRef]
3. Lu, C.-J.; Lin, Y.-H.; Chu, H.-J.; Tang, S.-C.; Lee, C.-W. Safety and efficacy of the transbrachial approach for endovascular thrombectomy in patients with acute large vessel occlusion stroke. *J. Formos. Med. Assoc.* **2021**, *120 Pt 3*, 705–712. [CrossRef] [PubMed]
4. Bendszus, M.; Fiehler, J.; Subtil, F.; Bonekamp, S.; Aamodt, A.H.; Fuentes, B.; Gizewski, E.R.; Hill, M.D.; Krajina, A.; Pierot, L.; et al. Endovascular thrombectomy for acute ischaemic stroke with established large infarct: Multicentre, open-label, randomised trial. *Lancet* **2023**, *402*, 1753–1763. [CrossRef] [PubMed]
5. Ahuja, C.K.; Agarwal, V.; Vyas, S.; Gupta, V. Access Route for Endovascular Neurointervention—Transfemoral to Transradial: Is it Worth the Effort and are we Ready for the Change? *J. Clin. Interv. Radiol. ISVIR* **2021**, *06*, 184–189. [CrossRef]

6. Ghaith, A.K.; El Naamani, K.; Mualem, W.; Ghanem, M.; Rajjoub, R.; Sweid, A.; Yolcu, Y.U.; Onyedimma, C.; Tjoumakaris, S.I.; Bydon, M.; et al. Transradial versus Transfemoral Approaches in Diagnostic and Therapeutic Neuroendovascular Interventions: A Meta-Analysis of Current Literature. *World Neurosurg.* **2022**, *164*, e694–e705. [CrossRef] [PubMed]
7. Oneissi, M.; Sweid, A.; Tjoumakaris, S.; Hasan, D.; Gooch, M.R.; Rosenwasser, R.H.; Jabbour, P. Access-Site Complications in Transfemoral Neuroendovascular Procedures: A Systematic Review of Incidence Rates and Management Strategies. *Oper. Neurosurg.* **2020**, *19*, 353–363. [CrossRef] [PubMed]
8. Mokin, M.; Snyder, K.V.; Levy, E.I.; Hopkins, L.N.; Siddiqui, A.H. Direct carotid artery puncture access for endovascular treatment of acute ischemic stroke: Technical aspects, advantages, and limitations. *J. Neurointerv. Surg.* **2015**, *7*, 108–113. [CrossRef] [PubMed]
9. Leys, D.; Pruvo, J.P.; Godefroy, O.; Rondepierre, P.; Leclerc, X. Prevalence and significance of hyperdense middle cerebral artery in acute stroke. *Stroke* **1992**, *23*, 317–324. [CrossRef]
10. Popieluszko, P.; Henry, B.M.; Sanna, B.; Hsieh, W.C.; Saganiak, K.; Pękala, P.A.; Walocha, J.A.; Tomaszewski, K.A. A systematic review and meta-analysis of variations in branching patterns of the adult aortic arch. *J. Vasc. Surg.* **2018**, *68*, 298–306.e10. [CrossRef]
11. İnanç, Y.; İnanç, Y.; Ay, H. The effect of demographic features on aortic arch anatomy and its role in the etiology of cerebrovascular disease. *Neuropsychiatr. Dis. Treat.* **2018**, *14*, 29–35. [CrossRef]
12. Hoffman, J.I.; Kaplan, S. The incidence of congenital heart disease. *J. Am. Coll. Cardiol.* **2002**, *39*, 1890–1900. [CrossRef]
13. Satti, S.R.; Cerniglia, C.A.; Koenigsberg, R.A. Cervical vertebral artery variations: An anatomic study. *AJNR Am. J. Neuroradiol.* **2007**, *28*, 976–980.
14. Ribo, M.; Flores, A.; Rubiera, M.; Pagola, J.; Mendonca, N.; Rodriguez-Luna, D.; Piñeiro, S.; Meler, P.; Alvarez-Sabin, J.; Molina, C.A. Difficult catheter access to the occluded vessel during endovascular treatment of acute ischemic stroke is associated with worse clinical outcome. *J. Neurointerv. Surg.* **2013**, *5* (Suppl. S1), i70–i73. [CrossRef]
15. Reznik, M.E.; Espinosa-Morales, A.D.; Jumaa, M.A.; Zaidi, S.; Ducruet, A.F.; Jadhav, A.P. Endovascular thrombectomy in the setting of aortic dissection. *J. Neurointerv. Surg.* **2017**, *9*, 17–20. [CrossRef]
16. Okawa, M.; Tateshima, S.; Liebeskind, D.; Ali, L.K.; Thompson, M.L.; Saver, J.; Duckwiler, G.R. Successful recanalization for acute ischemic stroke via the transbrachial approach. *J. Neurointerv. Surg.* **2016**, *8*, 122–125. [CrossRef]
17. Yamaguchi, S.; Horie, N.; Morofuji, Y.; Satoh, K.; Suyama, K. Rapid Recanalization Using TrevoProVue through a 4.2 Fr Catheter without a Guiding Catheter via Transbrachial Approach: A Case Report. *NMC Case Rep. J.* **2017**, *4*, 97–99. [CrossRef]
18. Balci, S.; Arsava, E.M.; Topcuoglu, M.A.; Arat, A. Floating Aortic Thrombus: A Rare Cause of Acute Ischemic Stroke Necessitating Modification of Access Route for Thrombectomy. *J. Stroke Cerebrovasc. Dis.* **2019**, *28*, 104291. [CrossRef]
19. Kehara, H.; Urashita, S.; Gomibuchi, T.; Komatsu, K.; Takahashi, K.; Tsukioka, K.; Terasaki, T.; Kono, T.; Wada, N.; Kakizawa, Y.; et al. Mechanical Thrombectomy for Postoperative Stroke in a Patient with Acute Aortic Dissection Type A. *NMC Case Rep. J.* **2020**, *7*, 71–74. [CrossRef]
20. Proença, F.B.; Madureira, F.R.J.B.; Campos, C.; Teotónio, P.; Neto, L. Transbrachial Basilar Artery Thrombectomy in a Patient with Aortic Dissection. *ACTA Radiológica Portuguesa* **2020**, *32*, 25–28.
21. Bhatia, V.; Choudhary, N.; Prabhakar, A.; Kumar, A.; Khurana, D. Transbrachial access for mechanical thrombectomy in a case of acute ischemic stroke with aortic bifurcation occlusion. *J. Stroke Med.* **2022**, *5*, 91–95. [CrossRef]
22. Shimizu, T.; Sakamoto, M.; Kamitani, H.; Kurosaki, M. Transbrachial Mechanical Thrombectomy for Acute Ischemic Stroke in Marfan's Syndrome: A Case Report. *J. Neuroendovasc. Ther.* **2023**, *17*, 68–72. [CrossRef] [PubMed]
23. Baumgartner, H.; De Backer, J.; Babu-Narayan, S.V.; Budts, W.; Chessa, M.; Diller, G.-P.; Lung, B.; Kluin, J.; Lang, I.M.; Meijboom, F.; et al. 2020 ESC Guidelines for the management of adult congenital heart disease: The Task Force for the management of adult congenital heart disease of the European Society of Cardiology (ESC). Endorsed by: Association for European Paediatric and Congenital Cardiology (AEPC), International Society for Adult Congenital Heart Disease (ISACHD). *Eur. Heart J.* **2020**, *42*, 563–645.
24. Kim, Y.Y.; Andrade, L.; Cook, S.C. Aortic Coarctation. *Cardiol. Clin.* **2020**, *38*, 337–351. [CrossRef] [PubMed]
25. Trenk, L.; Lammers, A.E.; Radke, R.; Baumgartner, H.; Wort, S.J.; Gatzoulis, M.A.; Diller, G.P.; Kempny, A. Neurological complications in aortic coarctation: Results of a Nationwide analysis based on 11,907 patients. *Int. J. Cardiol.* **2021**, *322*, 114–120. [CrossRef] [PubMed]
26. Costello, T.G.; Fisher, A. Neurological complications following aortic surgery. Case reports and review of the literature. *Anaesthesia* **1983**, *38*, 230–236. [PubMed]
27. Tsuji, Y.; Miki, T.; Kakita, H.; Sato, K.; Yoshida, T.; Shimizu, F. Mechanical Thrombectomy for Large Vessel Occlusion via the Transbrachial Approach: Case Series. *Neurointervention* **2020**, *15*, 89–95. [CrossRef] [PubMed]
28. Lee, D.G.; Lee, D.H.; Shim, J.H.; Suh, D.C. Feasibility of the Transradial or the Transbrachial Approach in Various Neurointerventional Procedures. *Neurointervention* **2015**, *10*, 74–81. [CrossRef]
29. Kiemeneij, F.; Laarman, G.J.; Odekerken, D.; Slagboom, T.; van der Wieken, R. A randomized comparison of percutaneous transluminal coronary angioplasty by the radial, brachial and femoral approaches: The access study. *J. Am. Coll. Cardiol.* **1997**, *29*, 1269–1275. [CrossRef]
30. Webber, G.W.; Jang, J.; Gustavson, S.; Olin, J.W. Contemporary management of postcatheterization pseudoaneurysms. *Circulation* **2007**, *115*, 2666–2674. [CrossRef]

31. Shibata, T.; Oomura, M.; Nishikawa, Y.; Mase, M. Direct Brachial Approach for Acute Basilar Artery Occlusion: Technical Note and Preliminary Clinical Experience. *Neurointervention* **2020**, *15*, 31–36. [CrossRef]
32. Park, S.; Kwak, J.H.; Baek, H.J.; Park, J.W.; Kim, J.S.; Suh, D.C. The Use of Protection Device in Landmark-wire Technique of Symptomatic Subclavian Artery Occlusion with Combined Approach via Trans-femoral vs. Trans-brachial Arteries: Technical note. *Neurointervention* **2011**, *6*, 89–94. [CrossRef]
33. Kobeissi, H.; Ghozy, S.; Liu, M.; Adusumilli, G.; Bilgin, C.; Kadirvel, R.; Kallmes, D.F.; Brinjikji, W. Mechanical Thrombectomy via Transradial Approach for Posterior Circulation Stroke: A Systematic Review and Meta-Analysis. *Cureus* **2022**, *14*, e26589. [CrossRef]
34. Verhey, L.H.; Orozco, A.R.; Oliver, M.; Lyons, L.; Sewell, A.P.; Tsai, J.P.; Mazaris, P.; Khan, M.; Singer, J.A. Transradial versus transfemoral access for mechanical thrombectomy in acute ischemic stroke: A retrospective cohort study. *J. Stroke Cerebrovasc. Dis.* **2023**, *32*, 107282. [CrossRef]
35. Elfil, M.; Ghaith, H.S.; Doheim, M.F.; Aboutaleb, P.E.; Romeo, D.; Salem, M.M.; Aladawi, M.; Jankowitz, B.T.; Burkhardt, J.K.; Nguyen, T.N.; et al. Transradial Versus Transfemoral Access for Mechanical Thrombectomy: A Systematic Review and Meta-Analysis. *Stroke Vasc. Interv. Neurol.* **2023**, *3*, e000758. [CrossRef]
36. Peterson, C.; Waldau, B. Transradial access for thrombectomy in acute stroke: A systematic review and meta-analysis. *Clin. Neurol. Neurosurg.* **2020**, *198*, 106235. [CrossRef]
37. Blanc, R.; Piotin, M.; Mounayer, C.; Spelle, L.; Moret, J. Direct cervical arterial access for intracranial endovascular treatment. *Neuroradiology* **2006**, *48*, 925–929. [CrossRef] [PubMed]
38. Orlov, K.; Arat, A.; Osiev, A.; Berestov, V.; Aytemir, K.; Topcuoglu, M.A.; Arsava, E.M. Transvenous Treatment of Carotid Aneurysms Through Transseptal Access. *World Neurosurg.* **2019**, *124*, 459–463.e2. [CrossRef] [PubMed]
39. Roche, A.D.; Murphy, B.; Adams, N.; Sheahan, R.; Brennan, P.; Looby, S. Direct Common Carotid Artery Puncture for Endovascular Treatment of Acute Large Vessel Ischemic Stroke in a Patient with Aortic Coarctation. *J. Stroke Cerebrovasc. Dis.* **2017**, *26*, e211–e213. [CrossRef] [PubMed]

Journal of
Personalized
Medicine

MDPI

Article

Code Stroke Alert: Focus on Emergency Department Time Targets and Impact on Door-to-Needle Time across Day and Night Shifts

Florina Buleu [1], Daian Popa [2,3,*], Carmen Williams [4], Anca Tudor [5], Dumitru Sutoi [2,3], Cosmin Trebuian [2,3], Covasala Constantin Ioan [6], Aida Iancu [7], Gabriel Cozma [4,8], Ana-Maria Marin [9], Ana-Maria Pah [1], Ion Petre [3,5] and Ovidiu Alexandru Mederle [2,4]

1 Department of Cardiology, "Victor Babes" University of Medicine and Pharmacy, E. Murgu Square No. 2, 300041 Timisoara, Romania; florina.buleu@umft.ro (F.B.); anamaria.pah@umft.ro (A.-M.P.)
2 Department of Surgery, Emergency Discipline, "Victor Babes" University of Medicine and Pharmacy, 300041 Timisoara, Romania; dumitru.sutoi@umft.ro (D.S.); trebuian.cosmin@umft.ro (C.T.); mederle.ovidiu@umft.ro (O.A.M.)
3 Doctoral School, Faculty of General Medicine, "Victor Babes" University of Medicine and Pharmacy Timisoara, 300041 Timisoara, Romania; petre.ion@umft.ro
4 Emergency Municipal Clinical Hospital, 300254 Timisoara, Romania; drcarmen.williams@yahoo.com (C.W.); gabriel.cozma@umft.ro (G.C.)
5 Department of Functional Sciences, "Victor Babes" University of Medicine and Pharmacy, E. Murgu Square No. 2, 300041 Timisoara, Romania; atudor@umft.ro
6 Emergency Clinical Hospital, 310003 Arad, Romania; covasala.constantin@gmail.com
7 Department of Radiology, "Victor Babes" University of Medicine and Pharmacy, E. Murgu Square No. 2, 300041 Timisoara, Romania; aida.parvu@umft.ro
8 Department of Surgical Semiology, Faculty of Medicine, "Victor Babes" University of Medicine and Pharmacy Timisoara, 300041 Timişoara, Romania
9 Department of Parasitology and Parasitic Diseases, University of Life Sciences "King Mihai I" from Timisoara, Calea Aradului 119, 300645 Timisoara, Romania; anamaria.marin@usvt.ro
* Correspondence: daian-ionel.popa@umft.ro; Tel.: +40-746-912-660

Abstract: Background and objectives: To minimize stroke-related deaths and maximize the likelihood of cerebral reperfusion, medical professionals developed the "code stroke" emergency protocol, which allows for the prompt evaluation of patients with acute ischemic stroke symptoms in pre-hospital care and the emergency department (ED). This research will outline our experience in implementing the stroke code protocol for acute ischemic stroke patients and its impact on door-to-needle time (DTN) in the ED. Methods: Our study included patients with a "code stroke alert" upon arrival at the emergency department. The final sample of this study consisted of 258 patients eligible for intravenous (IV) thrombolysis with an onset-to-door time < 4.5 h. ED admissions were categorized into two distinct groups: "day shift" (from 8 a.m. to 8 p.m.) (n = 178) and "night shift" (from 8 p.m. to 8 a.m.) (n = 80) groups. Results: An analysis of ED time targets showed an increased median during the day shift for onset-to-ED door time of 310 min (IQR, 190–340 min), for door-to-physician (emergency medicine doctor) time of 5 min (IQR, 3–9 min), for door-to-physician (emergency medicine doctor) time of 5 min (IQR, 3–9 min), and for door-to-physician (neurologist) time of 7 min (IQR, 5–10 min), also during the day shift. During the night shift, an increased median was found for door-to-CT time of 21 min (IQR, 16.75–23 min), for door-to-CT results of 40 min (IQR, 38–43 min), and for door-to-needle time of 57.5 min (IQR, 46.25–60 min). Astonishingly, only 17.83% (n = 46) of these patients received intravenous thrombolysis, and the proportion of patients with thrombolysis was significantly higher during the night shift ($p = 0.044$). A logistic regression analysis considering the door-to-needle time (minutes) as the dependent variable demonstrated that onset-to-ED time ($p < 0.001$) and door-to-physician (emergency medicine physicians) time ($p = 0.021$) are predictors for performing thrombolysis in our study. Conclusions: This study identified higher door-to-CT and door-to-emergency medicine physician times associated with an increased DTN, highlighting further opportunities to improve acute stroke care in the emergency department. Further, door-to-CT and door-to-CT results showed statistically significant increases during the night shift.

Keywords: emergency department; ED time targets; door-to-needle time; acute ischemic stroke; rt-PA

1. Introduction

The incidence of acute ischemic stroke (AIS) is similar to the incidence of acute coronary syndromes. Thus, acute ischemic syndromes are responsible for the majority of cardiovascular-related deaths and, therefore, overall mortality in most countries [1, 2]. AIS represents the second leading cause and a significant reason for disability and related costs [3]. According to stroke statistical reports from 2015, Romania emerged as the European country with the highest incidences of new strokes and stroke-related fatalities [4].

To increase and optimize the chances of cerebral reperfusion to reduce stroke-related fatalities, the "code stroke" was created, which is an emergency protocol for the immediate assessment of patients with suspected cerebrovascular events [5,6]. This protocol aims to increase the administration of currently available reperfusion therapies for ischemic stroke. However, only a small percentage of stroke patients received intravenous thrombolysis in the first 4.5 h after symptom onset. The primary reason for the low rate of administration is either the delayed arrival of patients at the emergency department [7,8] or the absence of a dedicated stroke team/unit in most hospitals [9].

Although this information is available, there needs to be more awareness and implementation of it among medical personnel when it comes to meeting time targets for ED admissions of AIS patients in hospitals without specialized stroke teams or units. Therefore, it is crucial to explore ways to increase the rate of rt-PA administration, especially considering that in Romania, the Romanian Neurology Society board introduced the National Program of Priority Actions in the Interventional Treatment of Patients with Acute Cerebral Vascular Accident (PA-CVA) document in 2018 [5], report that the thrombolysis rate is less than 10% (around 5.4%), with a notable increase in the last five years from 0.8% [9].

For this reason, this study aims to analyze ED time targets and their impact on the DTN time in the county's largest hospital, which has a specialist team ready to respond to a "code stroke alert".

2. Methods

2.1. Study Population and Inclusion and Exclusion Criteria

We conducted an observational study on patients referred to the Emergency County Clinical Hospital in Arad, Romania, between 1 January 2020 and 31 December 2023 with a "Code Stroke Alert". This hospital has an annual influx of over 70,000 patients, is the largest hospital in the county, and coordinates residency programs in neurology and emergency medicine.

Our acute stroke protocol begins with emergency medical services (EMS) personnel identifying a patient with a "code stroke alert" transported by ambulance or the identification of this patient by the triage assistant/emergency physician upon their admission to the ED. Our prehospital acute stroke screening protocol focuses on dispatchers, and paramedics must be able to diagnose stroke using simple tools such as the FAST (Face, Arms, Speech, and Time) indicators, baseline functional status, and current anticoagulants [5]. Immediately after the patient's admission to the ED, a "code stroke alert" is announced, and the on-duty neurologist examines the patient together with the emergency medicine physician. During this study, our institution had 24/7 coverage by a team consisting of a neurologist, an emergency medicine physician, a radiologist, and an emergency medicine nurse. Moreover, this team could mobilize before the patient's arrival when the pre-hospital notification was received. The patient is transported to a designated "stroke bed" on arrival. The thrombolytic dose is calculated based on the patient's weight and prepared if the patient qualifies for thrombosis. The patient's blood is obtained for laboratory analysis upon admission to the ED, and an intravenous administration of thrombolytics is performed in the ED if the patient meets the criteria for thrombolysis.

We analyzed consecutive patients who had complete medical records (both electronic and paper) and who were labeled with a "code stroke alert" in the emergency department. Of the initial sample of 345 patients, only 258 patients met the criteria for inclusion and exclusion in our study (not eligibility criteria for IV thrombolysis). According to the local protocol, intravenous thrombolysis with rt-PA was initiated within 4.5 h from the onset of the first symptoms of stroke. Patients below 18 years old, those with an initial diagnosis of intracerebral hemorrhage or brain tumor, and those who arrived at the emergency department more than 4.5 h from the onset of stroke symptoms were excluded from our analysis.

Upon admission, the medical staff recorded the precise moment at which stroke symptoms first appeared, as well as the mode and time of the patient's arrival at the ED. The patients themselves or their family members provided information on when the initial stroke-related symptoms were, which was noted as the "onset time". For individuals who experienced symptoms while sleeping, symptom onset was determined as the last period when they were stroke-symptom-free. Ten patients with neurological deficits upon awakening from sleep were considered to have had wake-up strokes. Since it was impossible to assess the exact time of deficit onset, according to our national protocol, these patients were not eligible for IV thrombolysis [5]. The arrival time at the ED was defined as when the patient's registration was completed at the ED triage office. The onset-to-needle time was calculated as the interval between symptom onset and when IV thrombolysis was performed. All time measurements were expressed in minutes.

Our national protocol [5] recommends the following time targets for stroke management:

- Onset-to-needle time $\leq$ 4.5 h;
- Door-to-physician time $\leq$ 10 min (an initial evaluation by both emergency medicine physician and neurologist that includes the time last known to be well, eligibility for IV thrombolysis, and the evaluation of stroke severity);
- Door-to-CT time $\leq$ 25 min;
- Door-to-CT results $\leq$ 45 min;
- Door-to-needle time $\leq$ 60 min.

To accurately establish the patients' arrival time in the emergency department, we utilized the initial registration time at the ED triage office. This allowed us to categorize ED admissions into two distinct groups: a "day shift" (from 8 a.m. to 8 p.m.) and "night shift" (from 8 p.m. to 8 a.m.). We categorized the mode of arrival—whether it was through EMS or if the patient walked or drove in. We chose these two factors (arrival mode and type of shift) because they are within our realm of influence and have the potential to be modified.

Moreover, by dividing the final sample into two subgroups consisting of 178 patients during the day shift and 80 patients during the night shift, we aimed to analyze the impact of various factors and the management time for acute stroke in the ED on the rate of intravenous rt-PA administration.

As shown in the study flowchart represented in Figure 1, a total of 345 patients with "code stroke alert" and a symptom onset time of less than 4.5 h were screened in the ED for eligibility for intravenous reperfusion therapy.

Only patients who satisfied the inclusion and exclusion criteria (n = 258) were selected in the final sample of this study. Of these patients, 26 received IV thrombolysis during the day shift; only 20 received IV thrombolysis during the night shift.

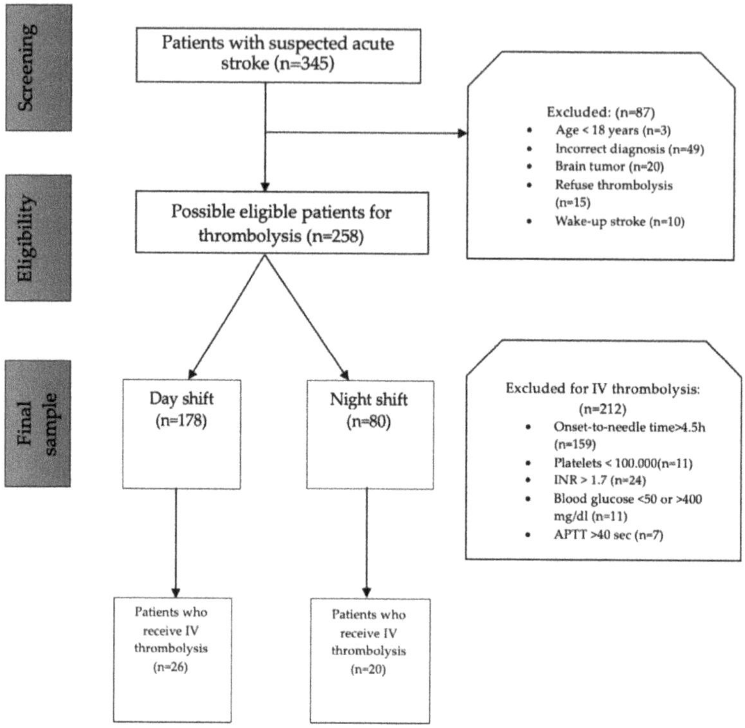

Figure 1. Study flowchart.

2.2. Evaluation of Stroke

Immediately following admission to the emergency department, all patients undergo a comprehensive medical evaluation which includes a cerebral computed tomography (CT) scan with or without contrast, as well as a complete blood count, international normalized ratio (INR), and prothrombin time, partial prothrombin time, blood glucose, and electrolyte tests. It is important to note that patients without medical data were not included in this evaluation. In conjunction with the emergency medicine physician and neurologist, the radiologist collaboratively assessed the stroke's subtype, severity, and location based on the brain imaging and clinical examination results according to the stroke definition established by The World Health Organization in 1970, which is still used today [10].

The neurologist on duty assessed neurological deficits and stroke severity in the first clinical evaluations of patients in the ED and categorized them using the National Institutes of Health Stroke Scale (NIHSS) at the following intervals: at admission, 1 h, 2 h, and 24 h [11].

2.3. Ethics

This study was conducted following the Declaration of Helsinki, and the protocol was approved by the Ethics Committee of the Arad County Emergency Clinical Hospital (no. 11687/27 March 2024). The collected data were identified before a statistical analysis was performed. All patients signed the informed consent.

2.4. Statistical Analysis

Mean and standard deviation or median and interquartile range (IQR) values were used to present continuous variables, while frequencies and percentages were used for categorical variables. The distribution of continuous variables was assessed using the Shapiro–Wilk test. Unpaired t-tests or Mann–Whitney U and Chi-square tests were employed to compare the characteristics of patients who received thrombolysis and those who did not. Several multivariate logistic regression models were used to determine the independent factors associated with the administration of thrombolysis. For the sample size calculation, we conducted a power analysis test using the GPower3.1 application for the t-test family—the Wilcoxon–Mann–Whitney test (two groups) with two tails, a normal parent distribution and 95% power, taking 0.05 as the level of significance and 0.5 as the effect size.

The results were presented as odds ratios with 95% confidence intervals. A *p*-value of less than 0.05 was considered statistically significant. Data analysis was conducted using JASP v0.18.3 (a free and open-source program for statistical analysis supported by the University of Amsterdam).

3. Results

3.1. Baseline Characteristics of Patients Who Arrived at the Emergency Department

The final sample included 258 patients eligible for IV thrombolysis who were admitted to the ED with a stroke alert. The following results were obtained after dividing them into two subgroups according to their arrival time: those admitted during the day shift (n = 178) and the night shift (n = 80).

Table 1 shows the patients' demographic and clinical characteristics according to the shift type. There were statistically significant differences, with changed values observed only in terms of lower patient height values in the day shift group ($p = 0.004$), lower hemoglobin values in the day shift group ($p < 0.001$), values of increased INR in the night shift group ($p = 0.039$), and a higher prothrombin time in the night shift group ($p < 0.001$). (Table 1, Figures 2 and 3A,B).

Figure 2 shows the baseline parameters analyzed in Table 1 which decreased statistically significantly during the day shift.

Figure 3 shows the baseline parameters analyzed in Table 1 that increased statistically significantly during the night shift.

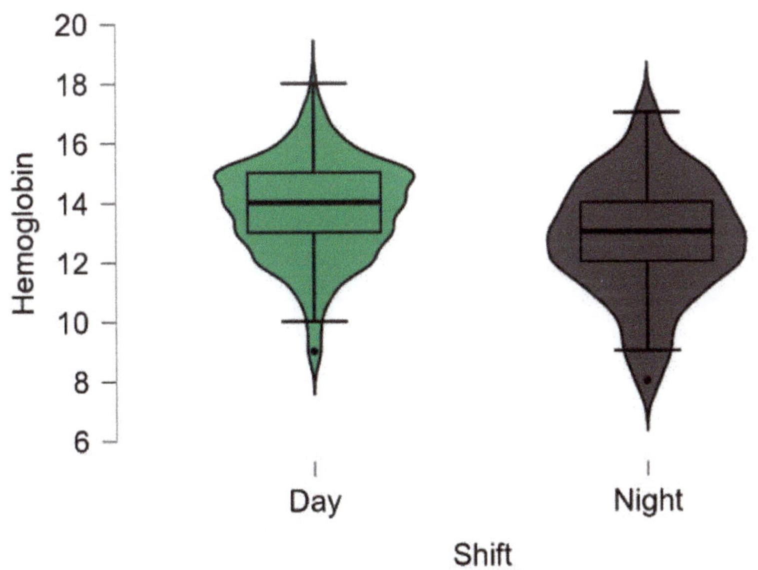

Figure 2. Violin plots of the values of the hemoglobin (mg/dL) between the two types of ED shift ($p < 0.001$). The boxplots inside the violin represent the median and interquartile ranges.

Table 1. Characteristics of analyzed group according to day shift (n = 178) and night shift (n = 80).

Variable	Shift	Valid	Mean ± SD	Median (IQR)	*p*
Physical characteristics					
Age, years	Day	178	67.29 ± 11.8	68 (61–75)	0.054
	Night	80	69.83 ± 12.68	71 (64–79)	
Height, cm	Day	178	171.52 ± 8.3	170 (165–178)	0.004 *
	Night	80	168.35 ± 7.35	168 (164.5–173.25)	
Weight, kg	Day	178	77.49 ± 12.45	79 (70–85)	0.157
	Night	80	75.15 ± 11.85	75 (68.75–81)	
SBP, mmHg	Day	178	156.56 ± 21.01	160 (140–170)	0.072
	Night	80	150.88 ± 19.44	150 (135–166.25)	
DBP, mmHg	Day	178	82.19 ± 13.13	80 (75–90)	0.166
	Night	80	79.69 ± 12.46	80 (70–90)	
GCS	Day	178	13.16 ± 3.36	15 (12–15)	0.269
	Night	80	12.61 ± 3.9	15 (12–15)	
NIHSS at presentation	Day	178	14.21 ± 5.34	14 (10–18)	0.331
	Night	80	14.8 ± 5.78	15 (10.75–19)	
Blood test sample results					
Platelets count, $\times 10^9$ µL	Day	178	224.19 ± 70.84	220 (175–254.75)	0.519
	Night	80	217.15 ± 64.61	218 (170.75–252)	
Hemoglobin, mg/dL	Day	178	13.74 ± 1.65	14 (13–15)	<0.001 *
	Night	80	12.75 ± 1.99	13 (12–14)	
Blood Glucose, mg/dL	Day	178	138.72 ± 48.25	125.5 (104–163.75)	0.925
	Night	80	138.43 ± 43.78	123 (105–175.25)	
Total Cholesterol, mg/dL	Day	178	188.93 ± 44.66	187.5 (162.5–220)	0.705
	Night	80	191.33 ± 51.35	189.5 (148.75–230.25)	
INR	Day	178	1.53 ± 1.41	1.14 (1.03–1.39)	0.039 *
	Night	80	1.79 ± 1.87	1.25 (1.1–1.44)	
Partial thromboplastin time, s	Day	178	29.62 ± 15.72	26.05 (23.5–30.2)	0.895
	Night	80	28.07 ± 9.23	26.3 (23.98–29.2)	
Prothrombin time, s	Day	178	16.11 ± 15.98	12.9 (12–14.38)	<0.001 *
	Night	80	19.38 ± 21.42	14.15 (12.8–15.55)	

* significant difference. SBP, systolic blood pressure; DBP, diastolic blood pressure; GCS, Coma Glasgow Score; INR, international normalized ratio. Values are expressed as means ± standard deviation (SD), by median (interquartile range), or by number (%).

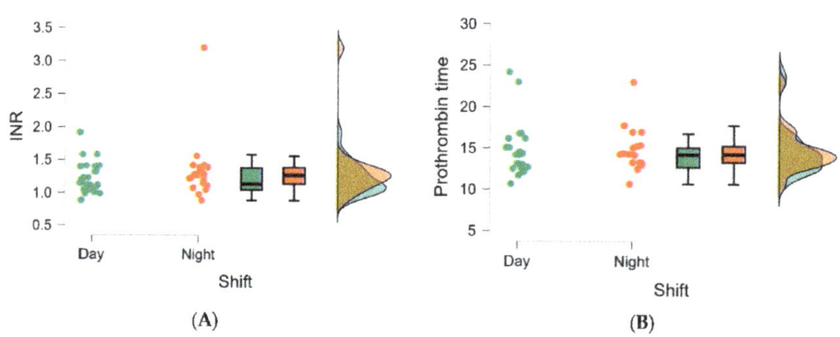

Figure 3. (**A**) Raincloud plots of INR values between the two types of ED shift ($p = 0.039$). (**B**) Raincloud plots of the values of prothrombin time (seconds) between the two types of ED shift ($p < 0.001$).

The onset-to-ED door time, the door-to-physician time for both emergency medicine and neurology physicians, the door-to-blood test time, the door-to-CT time, the door-to-CT results, and the door-to-needle time were calculated for the two groups (the "day shift", and "night shift" groups). The door-to-needle time was similar in all groups ($p = 0.533$). The door-to-CT and door-to-CT results were 19 and 39 min for the day shift, respectively, and 21 and 40 min for the night shift. The Shapiro–Wilk test confirmed normal distribution in all groups, and the unpaired t-test revealed statistically significant differences between the two groups (p= 0.037 and p = 0.02, respectively). The arrival mode in ED, with EMS or arrival via walk-in, was similar between the two ED shifts. (Table 2).

Table 2. Time targets and arrival mode in the emergency department according to day shift (n = 178) and night shift (n = 80).

Variable	Shift	Valid	Mean ± SD	Median (IQR)	p
		ED Time Targets (minutes)			
Onset-to-ED door time	Day	178	274.27 ± 101.33	310 (190–340)	0.082
	Night	80	248.25 ± 115.16	300 (127.5–330)	
Door-to-physician time (ED doctor)	Day	178	6.58 ± 5.12	5 (3–9)	0.232
	Night	80	5.453 ± 3.33	5 (3–8)	
Door-to-physician time(neurologist)	Day	178	8.15 ± 5.18	7 (5–10)	0.468
	Night	80	7.21 ± 3.02	7 (5–9)	
Door-to-blood samples	Day	178	8.06 ± 2.44	10 (5–10)	0.411
	Night	80	7.81 ± 2.62	10 (5–10)	
Door-to-CT	Day	178	19.12 ± 8.07	19 (13–22)	0.037 *
	Night	80	19.85 ± 4.84	21 (16.75–23)	
Door-to-CT results	Day	178	38.52 ± 7.76	39 (34.25–42)	0.02 *
	Night	80	39.84 ± 4.67	40 (38–43)	
Door-to-needle time	Day	26	55.19 ± 10.15	57.5 (46.25–60)	0.533
	Night	20	54 ± 6.41	55 (50–60)	
		Arrival Mode			
Emergency medical services (EMS)	Day	178	(91) 51.12%		0.894
	Night	80	(41) 51.25%		
Arrival via walk-in	Day	178	(87) 48.87%		0.878
	Night	80	(39) 48.75%		

* significant difference.

The door-to-CT and door-to-CT results times were increased statistically significantly during the night shift. (Figure 4A,B).

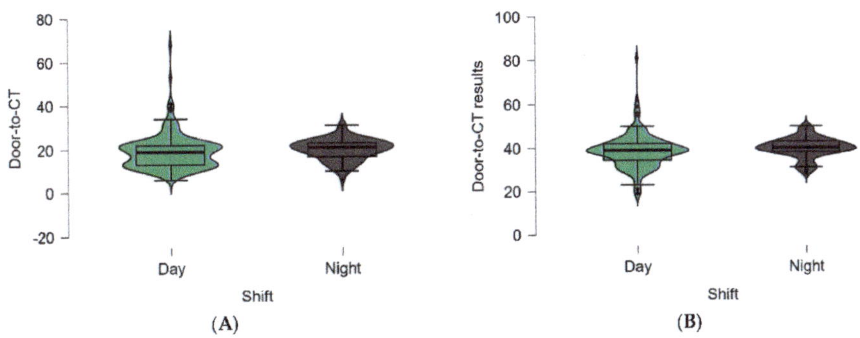

Figure 4. (**A**). Violin plot of the values of the door-to-CT time (minutes) between the two groups of patients (p = 0.037). (**B**) Violin plot of the values of the door-to-CT results time (minutes) between the two groups of patients (p = 0.02). The box plots inside the violins represent the median and interquartile ranges.

3.2. *Analysis of Administration of Intravenous rt-PA during Day Shift or Night Shift*

Three hundred forty-five patients with code stroke alert activations were recorded between 2020 and 2023, with a total of forty-six patients receiving IV thrombolysis. We also noted that in our study, the proportion of patients receiving thrombolysis was significantly higher during the night shift ($p = 0.044$) (Table 3).

Table 3. Analysis of IV thrombolysis administration between emergency department across day and night shifts.

Shift		Thrombolysis No	Thrombolysis Yes	Total
Day	Count	152	26	178
	% within row	85.393%	14.607%	100.000%
Night	Count	60	20	80
	% within row	75.000%	25.000%	100.000%
Total	Count	212	46	258
	% within row	82.171%	17.829%	100.000%
$p = 0.044$				

3.3. The Analysis of ED Times Targets

A logistic regression analysis considering the door-to-needle time (minutes) as the dependent variable demonstrated that the onset-to-ED time ($p < 0.001$) and door-to-physician (emergency medicine physicians) time ($p = 0.021$) are predictors for performing thrombolysis; the shorter the times for these two variables are, the more significantly increased the chance of thrombolysis is. (Table 4).

Table 4. Logistic regression (using the enter method) considers door-to-needle time as a dependent variable.

Variables in the Equation	B	S.E.	Wald	df	Sig.	Exp(B)	95% C.I.for EXP(B) Lower	95% C.I.for EXP(B) Upper
Onset-to-ED door (minutes)	−0.031	0.005	30.942	1	<0.001 *	0.97	0.959	0.98
Door-to-physician (ED doctor) (minutes)	−0.422	0.183	5.328	1	0.021 *	0.655	0.458	0.938
Door-to-neurologist (minutes)	0.289	0.193	2.258	1	0.133	1.336	0.916	1.948
Door-to-blood-samples (minutes)	−0.015	0.118	0.015	1	0.902	0.986	0.781	1.243
Door-to-CT (minutes)	−0.102	0.067	2.306	1	0.129	0.903	0.793	1.03
Door-to-CT results (minutes)	−0.081	0.058	1.901	1	0.168	0.923	0.823	1.035
Constant	9.235	2.225	17.235	1	<0.001	10,250.746		

* significant association; Cox and Snell R-Square = 0.44.

Moreover, the dependence of the door-to-needle time (minutes) on the door-to-CT results (minutes) is significant, direct, and weak ($p = 0.010$, r = 0.377). (Figure 5).

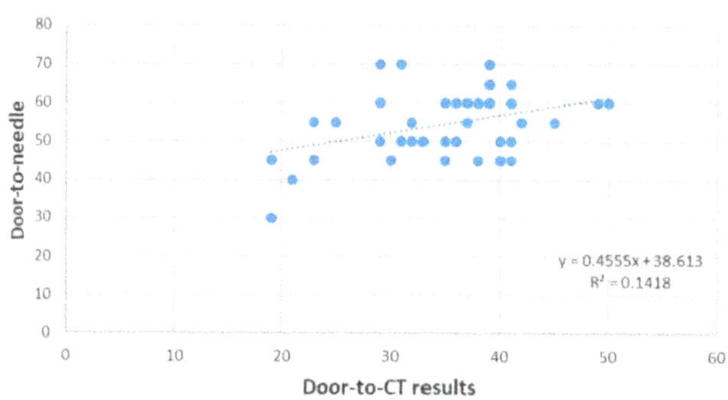

Figure 5. Linear regression plot.

4. Discussion

Evidence from previous studies indicates a direct relationship between the importance of stroke management times and the thrombolysis rate. We can state that patients with ischemic stroke in the ED are a priority, and compliance with these ED target times is directly correlated with their outcome and the thrombolysis rate [12–14]. Our study observed statistically significant differences in the ED time targets for code stroke alert management times between patients admitted during two ED shifts, a day shift (n = 178) and a night shift (n = 80). Our results show that admission to the emergency department during the night shift resulted in longer management times for door-to-CT and door-to-CT results. However, there was no delay in treatment delivery, with the proportion of patients receiving thrombolysis significantly higher during the night shift ($p = 0.044$).

Despite the stroke protocol remaining consistent throughout the day, our data revealed a notable increase in door-to-CT and door-to-CT results during night shift hours. There are several potential explanations for this finding. Firstly, the fatigue experienced by the medical staff, including the 24 h on-call neurologist, can lead to longer reaction times when responding to code stroke alerts. Additionally, the reduced number of senior radiology residents available during night shifts means that all medical personnel have a more significant workload, which can contribute to delays in the overall process. Due to legislation in our country, it is only possible to preregister patients after they arrive in our jurisdiction. This legislation prohibits the transmission of patient-identifiable information by EMS while en route. Another aspect is that our study also covers the COVID-19 period. In recent years, the DTN time has improved significantly in Romania; however, the COVID-19 pandemic has affected this time measure. In 2017, the average of this time was 67 min, which decreased to 43 min in 2020. Yet, in 2023, it increased again to 60 min. The declaration of a state of emergency in Romania on 16 March 2020 did not initially affect the DTN time recorded in our national register for that month. As a result, the challenges faced by the healthcare system, including EMS and ED staff, over 30 months of disrupted processes and exhausted medical staff led to longer door-to-needle times. Our national stroke data analysis reflects this [9]. The improved time during the COVID-19 pandemic may be because physicians treated AIS as the same emergency as before or because during that period, the number of patients presenting for all diseases in the ED decreased after government restrictions, impacting first the door-to-physician (ED doctors) time. During that time, access and assessments of AIS patients with COVID-19 in the ED followed the same protocol; the only factor that could interfere with prolonged ED time targets was the requirement for physicians to wear mandatory personal protective equipment when monitoring and treating these patients.

Additionally, the health system protocol in our country requires confirmation from the patient or a witness before registration [5]. Unfortunately, this poses a challenge for stroke patients who may not be able to identify themselves due to aphasia or impaired consciousness. As a result, there is often a delay of 10 to 15 min as physicians search for a witness to identify the patient. CT imaging cannot be ordered as the patient must still be registered in the electronic entry system. We have been informed that many other hospitals experience similar delays in which imaging can only be ordered once the patient is electronically registered (personal communications).

Ganti et al. conducted a study with a similar design to ours, also aiming to identify what factors in the emergency department impact the door-to-needle time in acute stroke patients eligible for intravenous thrombolysis and classifying their cohort as either "day shift" (6 a.m.–6 p.m.) or "night shift" (6 p.m.–6 a.m.) patients. Nearly half of the cohort, 49%, arrived during the daytime; 24% presented during the night shift, and the remaining 27% presented on the weekend. The majority, 85%, were brought to the hospital by EMS, while 15% of patients walked in. When examining the median DTN time, it was found that during the day shift, it took approximately 37 min (with an interquartile range of 26–51 and a range of 10–117). On the other hand, during the night shift, the median DTN time increased to 59 min (with an interquartile range of 39–89 and a range of 34–195).

Interestingly, when a dedicated stroke team was present, the median DTN time significantly decreased to 36 min compared to 51 min when no one was available. The median door-to-CT time was also 24 min (with an interquartile range of 18–31 min). Univariate analyses revealed that arriving during the night shift ($p < 0.0001$), arriving as a walk-in ($p = 0.0080$), and experiencing a longer time to CT scan ($p < 0.0001$) were all associated with a longer DTN time. Conversely, the presence of a dedicated stroke team was associated with a significantly shorter DTN time ($p < 0.0001$) [15].

Within this examination of consecutive patients experiencing acute ischemic stroke and admitted within 4.5 h of symptom onset, a total of 258 individuals were eligible for thrombolysis. Astonishingly, only 17.83% (n = 46) of these patients received intravenous thrombolysis. This highlights the global underutilization of rt-PA administration, as recent international studies estimate that only 10–20% of eligible patients receive this treatment [16]. It is worth noting that Romania, according to the PA-CVA document, reports a mean national rt-PA administration rate lower than 10% (approximately 8.7%), making our study's thrombolysis rate comparatively higher [17,18]. Similarly, China reports an alarmingly low national thrombolysis rate of only 2.4%, with intravenous rt-PA usage at a mere 1.6% [19].

Among the factors associated with the lack of performing thrombolysis in our study, no statistically significant correlation was found between the two shifts regarding the mode of arrival at the ED, whether it was via EMS ($p = 0.894$) or walk-in ($p = 878$), or risk factors such as the presence of high blood glucose ($p = 0.925$) or low platelets ($p = 0.519$).

This lack of correlation is consistent with the literature, which reports different distributions of arrival modes and risk factors between the groups. For example, previous studies have shown a significant association between arriving during the night shift ($p < 0.0001$) and arriving without the emergency medical system ($p = 0.0080$) [20]. In a different study, about 18.1% of patients reported arriving at the ED by ambulance, while most arrived in private cars [21]. We consider the fact that there is no statistically significant difference in arrival mode types between our day and night shifts a strength of this study as it allows us to better analyze the impact of ED time targets on the administration of IV thrombolysis and which ED time is a predictor for an increased DTN time.

Therefore, our data show that for day shifts, medians increased, for an onset-to-ED door time of 310 min (IQR, 190–340 min), a door-to-physician (emergency medicine doctor) time of 5 min (IQR, 3–9 min), and a door-to-physician (neurologist) time of 7 min (IQR, 5–10 min). For the night shift, the medians increased for a door-to-CT time of 21 min (IQR, 16.75–23 min), a door-to-CT results time of 40 min (IQR, 38–43 min), and a DTN time of 57.5 min (IQR, 46.25–60 min). Our study's mean door-to-CT time of 21 min is under the recommended target of $\leq$25 min. A much-increased value of door-to-CT time (49.4 min) was registered in a study from Lebanon [21].

A comprehensive study was conducted over three years on patients diagnosed with acute stroke in the emergency departments of three Victorian hospitals, and it was found that out of all patients included, 71% (n = 2509) arrived by ambulance, while the remaining 29% (n = 1039) used private transport. Several factors were found to be significantly associated with ambulance arrival, including older age ($p < 0.001$), being born in Australia ($p < 0.001$), and speaking English at home ($p = 0.003$). The study also revealed that arriving by ambulance was independently linked to receiving prompt stroke care in the emergency department, coming within 2 h from symptom onset, being treated at an advanced stroke service center that offers thrombolysis, being triaged specifically for stroke, undergoing medical assessment within 25 min, and being referred for a CT scan within 45 min [22].

A study based on a project called HASTE (Hurry Acute Stroke Treatment and Evaluation) consisting of three study phases evaluated the effectiveness of four specific strategies in reducing the DTN time for intravenous alteplase in acute ischemic stroke patients. Employing a prospective pre- and post-intervention design, the study accounted for each strategy, secular trends, and patient characteristics. Notably, significant improvements in door-to-needle times were observed throughout the different phases of HASTE. Phase I involved a year-long data collection period and an analysis to assess the existing performance of the DTN. In Phase II, which spanned two years, a triage system was implemented to prioritize severe stroke cases within 4.5 h of onset. This approach aimed to concentrate the efforts of the stroke team on patients with the highest likelihood of requiring alteplase despite the high volume of milder or subacute stroke assessments encountered in their busy ED (with over 1500 stroke service admissions annually). During the HASTE phase III study, a new protocol was introduced to streamline the process for patients with a code stroke alert. Instead of being transferred to an ED bed, these patients were taken directly from the EMS stretcher to the CT scanner. Upon arrival at the emergency department, ED physicians swiftly evaluated the patient's medical stability and neurological signs before promptly transporting the patient to the scanner on the same stretcher. After implementing these strategies, they observed significant enhancements in the DTN time. The administration of alteplase in the diagnostic imaging area led to a remarkable 32% reduction in the DTN time. Similarly, transferring the patient to the diagnostic imaging area using Emergency Medical Services stretcher resulted in a substantial 30% decrease in the DTN time. Registering the patient as unknown before their complete identification by family members or an informant yielded a 12% reduction in the DTN time. Additionally, employing simultaneous notification through a group pager for incoming patients with high stroke severity contributed to a statistically significant decrease in the DTN time of 11% [23].

In our analysis, we conducted a logistic regression to examine the impact of different ED times on the DTN time. We found that the onset-to-ED ($p < 0.001$) and door-to-physician (emergency medicine physician) times were significant predictors for the administration of thrombolysis. Specifically, we observed that shorter times for these two variables were associated with a significantly higher likelihood of receiving thrombolysis, as shown in Table 4. Recent research has indicated a correlation between decreased healthcare professionals and longer door-to-physician and DTN times [24]. Encouragingly, our findings revealed that the distribution of the capacity limitations for stroke patients arriving at the emergency department mirrored what happened in emergency shifts overall. We believe the factors contributing to the low rate of intravenous thrombolysis in our study are the following: delays during the triage and initial assessment of stroke patients in the emergency department, as can be observed in the results of our study.

Furthermore, stroke symptoms can sometimes be subtle or mimic other conditions, and this can be worsened when the initial assessment is conducted by a resident rather than an ED specialist, leading to a delay in stroke identification and treatment, as we can note from our observations. It may be beneficial to conduct further investigations to gain a deeper understanding of how staffing models and the timing of patient arrival in the ED contribute to delays in stroke care, particularly during periods of increased ED crowding. Additionally, exploring the reasons behind neurologists' decisions to not perform IV thrombolysis in eligible patients admitted to the ED during the time window could provide valuable insights, considering our research primarily focuses on ED management and time targets.

The findings of this study have significant implications for medical practice, specifically in raising awareness about the importance of timely intervention for AIS patients through stroke code alerts. By analyzing ED time targets, this study has the potential to enhance acute stroke management in countries like Romania, where stroke incidence and mortality rates are alarmingly high. By identifying areas for improvement, we can optimize emergency department protocols and make a positive impact on stroke care not only nationally but also internationally. It is worth noting that this study examined the time window for AIS treatment and identified weaknesses that can be addressed to improve the thrombolysis procedure during emergency department management. So, we believe that the implementation of a process to bring the patient directly to the CT scanner from the emergency medical services stretcher or to start IV thrombolysis at the CT scanner are changes that can be implemented to shorten door-to-needle times and thereby increase reperfusion therapy rates as well as patient outcomes.

5. Study Limitations

It is essential to acknowledge the limitations of this study. While we conducted a retrospective analysis and obtained all timing information from patient medical records, there is still a possibility of unmeasured factors influencing our estimates. Despite our efforts to control for known variables associated with the DTN time, other potentially confounding variables may exist. We did not specifically investigate individual patient reasons for outliers, such as cases in which the stroke initially appeared mild but later worsened. However, a previous study conducted by our team, which focused on an emergency department located 3.5 km away from a thrombolysis hospital with a neurology department, did not find any significant statistical differences regarding ED time targets between patients who received thrombolysis and those who did not [12].

Further research will be required to address the predictors for the DTN time and understand the generalizability of our study's results. This study was conducted in a high-volume academic center, and we anticipate that future studies will need to be carried out in different centers with varying acute stroke protocols. It is crucial to investigate why specific interventions were not implemented by documenting the reasons behind their omission. Although we did not collect data on stroke mimics or risk factors related to performed IV thrombolysis or a lack of IV thrombolysis, previous research suggests that only reducing the DTN time does lower the risk of complications [25]. It is important to note that specific changes may vary depending on hospital policies and structures. However, the impact of meeting or shortening these time targets can be assessed in other hospitals to determine their effect on the DTN time. Unfortunately, we could not analyze whether the same level of attention was consistently given to patients with code stroke alerts during different shifts or if they burdened the stroke team and CT or ED resources excessively. Nevertheless, it is crucial to assess the capacity of stroke programs in other centers based on their available resources. However, it is essential to remember that we did not include in this study patients in whom mechanical thrombectomy could probably have been performed after exceeding the 4.5 h target for IV thrombolysis [5] or patients with wake-up stroke due to the impossibility of performing a neuroimaging assessment using advanced techniques such as CT perfusion (CTP), which is available in only one hospital in Romania, or magnetic resonance imaging (MRI), which is not available for acute stroke.

6. Conclusions

This study identified higher door-to-CT and door-to-emergency medicine physician times associated with an increased DTN time. Further, door-to-CT and door-to-CT results times showed statistically significant increases during the night shift. These findings need to be considered when conducting quality improvements of hospital acute stroke protocols as they represent factors that can be addressed operationally.

Author Contributions: Conceptualization: F.B., D.P., D.S., C.C.I. and A.I.; methodology: D.P., A.-M.P., D.S., C.W., O.A.M., A.T., C.T. and F.B.; software: A.T., F.B., D.S., A.-M.M., I.P. and C.C.I., validation: O.A.M., A.I., F.B., G.C., C.T., I.P. and C.W.; investigation: D.P., A.I., G.C. and O.A.M.; resources: D.P., A.-M.P., C.C.I. and F.B.; writing—original draft preparation: D.P., A.I., C.T., and F.B.; writing—review and editing: F.B., C.W., C.C.I., G.C., D.S., A.I. and O.A.M.; visualization: O.A.M., D.S., A.-M.P., A.-M.M., G.C., C.W. and A.T.; supervision: O.A.M., A.-M.P., A.-M.M., I.P. and A.I. All authors have read and agreed to the published version of the manuscript.

Funding: We would like to acknowledge the Victor Babes University of Medicine and Pharmacy Timisoara for covering the publication costs for this research paper.

Institutional Review Board Statement: This study was conducted following the Declaration of Helsinki, and the protocol was approved by the Ethics Committee of the Arad County Emergency Clinical Hospital (no. 11687/27 March 2024).

Informed Consent Statement: Informed consent was obtained from all subjects involved in the study.

Data Availability Statement: The datasets are not publicly available, but de-identified data may be provided upon request from Popa Daian.

Conflicts of Interest: The authors declare no conflicts of interest.

References

1. Wafa, H.A.; Wolfe, C.D.A.; Emmett, E.; Roth, G.A.; Johnson, C.O.; Wang, Y. Burden of Stroke in Europe: Thirty-Year Projections of Incidence, Prevalence, Deaths, and Disability-Adjusted Life Years. *Stroke* **2020**, *51*, 2418–2427. [CrossRef] [PubMed]
2. Di Cesare, M.; Perel, P.; Taylor, S.; Kabudula, C.; Bixby, H.; Gaziano, T.A.; McGhie, D.V.; Mwangi, J.; Pervan, B.; Narula, J.; et al. The Heart of the World. *Glob. Heart* **2024**, *19*, 11. [CrossRef] [PubMed]
3. Feigin, V.L.; Stark, B.A.; Johnson, C.O.; Roth, G.A.; Bisignano, C.; Abady, G.G.; Abbasifard, M.; Abbasi-Kangevari, M.; Abd-Allah, F.; Abedi, V.; et al. Global, regional, and national burden of stroke and its risk factors, 1990–2019: A systematic analysis for the Global Burden of Disease Study 2019. *Lancet Neurol.* **2021**, *20*, 795–820. [CrossRef] [PubMed]
4. Stroke Alliance for Europe. The Burden of Stroke in Europe—Challenges for Policy Makers. Available online: https://www.stroke.org.uk/sites/default/files/the_burden_of_stroke_in_europe_-_challenges_for_policy_makers.png (accessed on 14 January 2022).
5. Priority Action for Interventional Treatment of Patients with Acute Stroke. Standard Operating Procedure Regarding the Patient Track and Therapeutic Protocol in Romania. Available online: https://legislatie.just.ro/Public/DetaliiDocument/209994 (accessed on 12 October 2023).
6. Manners, J.; Khandker, N.; Barron, A.; Aziz, Y.; Desai, S.M.; Morrow, B.; Delfyett, W.T.; Martin-Gill, C.; Shutter, L.; Jovin, T.G. An interdisciplinary approach to inhospital stroke improves stroke detection and treatment time. *J. NeuroInterventional Surg.* **2019**, *11*, 1080–1084. [CrossRef] [PubMed]
7. Maestroni, A.; Mandelli, C.; Manganaro, D.; Zecca, B.; Rossi, P.; Monzani, V.; Torgano, G. Factors influencing delay in presentation for acute stroke in an emergency department in Milan, Italy. *Emerg. Med. J.* **2008**, *25*, 340–345. [CrossRef] [PubMed]
8. Terecoasă, E.O.; Radu, R.A.; Negrilă, A.; Enache, I.; Cășaru, B.; Tiu, C. Pre-Hospital Delay in Acute Ischemic Stroke Care: Current Findings and Future Perspectives in a Tertiary Stroke Center from Romania—A Cross-Sectional Study. *Medicina* **2022**, *58*, 1003. [CrossRef] [PubMed]
9. Tiu, C.; Terecoasă, E.O.; Tuță, S.; Bălașa, R.; Simu, M.; Sabău, M.; Stan, A.; Radu, R.A.; Tiu, V.; Cășaru, B.; et al. Quality of acute stroke care in Romania: Achievements and gaps between 2017 and 2022. *Eur Stroke J* **2023**, *8*, 44–51. [CrossRef] [PubMed]
10. Aho, K.; Harmsen, P.; Hatano, S.; Marquardsen, J.; Smirnov, V.E.; Strasser, T. Cerebrovascular disease in the community: Results of a WHO collaborative study. *Bull. World Health Organ.* **1980**, *58*, 113. [PubMed]
11. Goldstein, L.B.; Bertels, C.; Davis, J.N. Interrater reliability of the NIH stroke scale. *Arch. Neurol.* **1989**, *46*, 660–662. [CrossRef]
12. Popa, D.; Iancu, A.; Petrica, A.; Buleu, F.; Williams, C.G.; Sutoi, D.; Trebuian, C.; Tudor, A.; Mederle, O.A. Emergency Department Time Targets for Interhospital Transfer of Patients with Acute Ischemic Stroke. *J. Pers. Med.* **2024**, *14*, 13. [CrossRef]
13. Jones, S.; Moulton, C.; Swift, S.; Molyneux, P.; Black, S.; Mason, N.; Oakley, R.; Mann, C. Association between delays to patient admission from the emergency department and all-cause 30-day mortality. *Emerg. Med. J.* **2022**, *39*, 168–173. [CrossRef] [PubMed]
14. Jones, E.M.; Boehme, A.K.; Aysenne, A.; Chang, T.; Albright, K.C.; Burns, C.; Beasley, T.M.; Martin-Schild, S. Prolonged emergency department length of stay as a predictor of adverse outcomes in patients with intracranial hemorrhage. *J. Crit. Care Med.* **2015**, *2015*, 526319. [CrossRef] [PubMed]
15. Ganti, L.; Mirajkar, A.; Banerjee, P.; Stead, T.; Hanna, A.; Tsau, J.; Khan, M.; Garg, A. Impact of emergency department arrival time on door-to-needle time in patients with acute stroke. *Front. Neurol.* **2023**, *14*, 1126472. [CrossRef] [PubMed]
16. De Souza, A.C.; Sebastian, I.A.; Zaidi, W.A.W.; Nasreldein, A.; Bazadona, D.; Amaya, P.; Elkady, A.; Gebrewold, M.A.; Vorasayan, P.; Yeghiazaryan, N.; et al. Regional and national differences in stroke thrombolysis use and disparities in pricing, treatment availability, and coverage. *Int. J. Stroke* **2022**, *17*, 990–996. [CrossRef] [PubMed]
17. Uivarosan, D.; Bungau, S.; Tit, D.M.; Moisa, C.; Fratila, O.; Rus, M.; Bratu, O.G.; Diaconu, C.C.; Pantis, C. Financial burden of stroke reflected in a pilot center for the implementation of thrombolysis. *Medicina* **2020**, *56*, 54. [CrossRef] [PubMed]
18. Sabau, M.; Bungau, S.; Buhas, C.L.; Carp, G.; Daina, L.G.; Judea-Pusta, C.T.; Buhas, B.A.; Jurca, C.M.; Daina, C.M.; Tit, D.M. Legal medicine implications in fibrinolytic therapy of acute ischemic stroke. *BMC Med. Ethics* **2019**, *20*, 70. [CrossRef] [PubMed]
19. Dong, Q.; Dong, Y.; Liu, L.; Xu, A.; Zhang, Y.; Zheng, H.; Wang, Y. The Chinese Stroke Association scientific statement: Intravenous thrombolysis in acute ischaemic stroke. *Stroke Vasc. Neurol.* **2017**, *2*, 147–159. [CrossRef]
20. Dimitriou, P.; Tziomalos, K.; Christou, K.; Kostaki, S.; Angelopoulou, S.M.; Papagianni, M.; Ztriva, E.; Chatzopoulos, G.; Savopoulos, C.; Hatzitolios, A.I. Factors associated with delayed presentation at the emergency department in patients with acute ischemic stroke. *Brain Inj.* **2019**, *33*, 1257–1261. [CrossRef]
21. El Sayed, M.J.; El Zahran, T.; Tamim, H. Acute stroke care and thrombolytic therapy use in a tertiary care center in Lebanon. *Emerg. Med. Int.* **2014**, *2014*, 438737. [CrossRef]
22. Kinsella, D.; Mosley, I.; Braitberg, G. A Retrospective Study Investigating: Factors associated with mode of arrival and emergency department management for patients with acute stroke. *Australas. Emerg. Care* **2018**, *21*, 99–104. [CrossRef]

23. Kamal, N.; Holodinsky, J.K.; Stephenson, C.; Kashayp, D.; Demchuk, A.M.; Hill, M.D.; Vilneff, R.L.; Bugbee, E.; Zerna, C.; Newcommon, N.; et al. Improving Door-to-Needle Times for Acute Ischemic Stroke: Effect of Rapid Patient Registration, Moving Directly to Computed Tomography, and Giving Alteplase at the Computed Tomography Scanner. *Circ. Cardiovasc. Qual. Outcomes* **2017**, *10*, e003242. [CrossRef] [PubMed]
24. Jaffe, T.A.; Goldstein, J.N.; Yun, B.J.; Etherton, M.; Leslie-Mazwi, T.; Schwamm, L.H.; Zachrison, K.S. Impact of Emergency Department Crowding on Delays in Acute Stroke Care. *West. J. Emerg. Med.* **2020**, *21*, 892–899. [CrossRef] [PubMed]
25. Man, S.; Solomon, N.; Grory, B.M.; Alhanti, B.; Uchino, K.; Saver, J.L.; Smith, E.E.; Xian, Y.; Bhatt, D.L.; Schwamm, L.H.; et al. Shorter Door-to-Needle Times Are Associated With Better Outcomes After Intravenous Thrombolytic Therapy and Endovascular Thrombectomy for Acute Ischemic Stroke. *Circulation* **2023**, *148*, 20–34. [CrossRef] [PubMed]

Journal of
Personalized
Medicine

MDPI

Article

Better Performance of Modified Scoring Systems to Predict the Clinical Outcomes of *Vibrio* Bacteremia in the Emergency Department: An Observational Study

Chia-Ming Hsieh [1,2,3,4], Sung-Yuan Hu [1,2,3,4,5,*], Ming-Shun Hsieh [5,6,7], Shih-Che Huang [4,8,9], Chia-Hui Shen [1] and Yi-Chun Tsai [1]

1 Department of Emergency Medicine, Taichung Veterans General Hospital, Taichung 40705, Taiwan; chiaming.hsieh1204@gmail.com (C.-M.H.); aa1239076@gmail.com (C.-H.S.); rosa87324@gmail.com (Y.-C.T.)
2 Department of Post-Baccalaureate Medicine, College of Medicine, National Chung Hsing University, Taichung 402202, Taiwan
3 Institute of Medicine, School of Medicine, Chung Shan Medical University, Taichung 40201, Taiwan
4 School of Medicine, Chung Shan Medical University, Taichung 40201, Taiwan; cucu0214@gmail.com
5 School of Medicine, National Yang Ming Chiao Tung University, Taipei 11217, Taiwan; edmingshun@gmail.com
6 Department of Emergency Medicine, Taipei Veterans General Hospital, Taoyuan Branch, Taoyuan 330, Taiwan
7 Department of Emergency Medicine, Taipei Veterans General Hospital, Taipei 11217, Taiwan
8 Department of Emergency Medicine, Chung Shan Medical University Hospital, Taichung 40201, Taiwan
9 Lung Cancer Research Center, Chung Shan Medical University Hospital, Taichung 40201, Taiwan
* Correspondence: song9168@pie.com.tw; Tel.: +886-4-23592525 (ext. 3601); Fax: +886-4-23594065

Abstract: Background: *Vibrio* is a genus of Gram-negative bacteria found in various aquatic environments, including saltwater and freshwater. *Vibrio* bacteremia can lead to sepsis, a potentially life-threatening condition in which the immune system enters overdrive in response to the disease, causing widespread inflammation and damage to tissues and organs. *V. vulnificus* had the highest case fatality rate (39%) of all reported foodborne infections in the United States and a high mortality rate in Asia, including Taiwan. Numerous scoring systems have been created to estimate the mortality risk in the emergency department (ED). However, there are no specific scoring systems to predict the mortality risk of *Vibrio* bacteremia. Therefore, this study modified the existing scoring systems to better predict the mortality risk of *Vibrio* bacteremia. Methods: Cases of *Vibrio* bacteremia were diagnosed based on the results from at least one blood culture in the ED. Patient data were extracted from the electronic clinical database, covering January 2012 to December 2021. The primary outcome was in-hospital mortality.This study used univariate and multivariate analyses to evaluate the mortality risk. Results: This study enrolled 36 patients diagnosed with *Vibrio* bacteremia, including 23 males (63.9%) and 13 females (36.1%), with a mean age of 65.1 $\pm$ 15.7 years. The in-hospital mortality rate amounted to 25% (9/36), with 31.5% in *V. vulnificus* (6/19) and 17.6% in *V.* non-*vulnificus* (3/17). The non-survivors demonstrated higher MEDS (10.3 $\pm$ 2.4) than the survivors (6.2 $\pm$ 4.1) (p = 0.002). Concerning the qSOFA, the survivors scored 0.3 $\pm$ 0.5, and the non-survivors displayed a score of 0.6 $\pm$ 0.7 (p = 0.387). The AUC of the ROC for the MEDS and qSOFA was 0.833 and 0.599, respectively. This study modified the scoring systems with other predictive factors, including BUN and pH. The AUC of the ROC for the modified MEDS and qSOFA reached up to 0.852 and 0.802, respectively. Conclusion: The MEDS could serve as reliable indicators for forecasting the mortality rate of patients grappling with *Vibrio* bacteremia. This study modified the MEDS and qSOFA to strengthen the predictive performance of mortality risk for *Vibrio* bacteremia. We advocate the prompt initiation of targeted therapeutic interventions and judicious antibiotic treatments to curb fatality rates.

Keywords: *Vibrio*; bacteremia; mortality risk; scoring systems; seasonal distribution

1. Introduction

Vibrio is a genus of Gram-negative bacteria found in various aquatic environments, including saltwater and freshwater [1–4]. V. vulnificus can cause severe wound infections and sepsis in people with compromised immune systems [5,6]. People can become infected with *V. vulnificus* through two main routes: consuming contaminated seafood (particularly raw or undercooked shellfish) or directly exposing open wounds to seawater containing the bacterium. In population-based studies in the United States in the 1980s, the incidence of *V. vulnificus* infections was approximately 0.5/100,000 people per year [7–9].

Other pathogenic Vibrio species include *V. cholerae*, the causative agent of cholera, a severe diarrheal disease that can be fatal if left untreated [10,11]. *V. cholerae* non-O1 and non-O139 strains have been increasingly recognized as a cause of gastroenteritis and extraintestinal infections, although they are less commonly associated with the widespread outbreaks typical of the O1 and O139 serogroups. The transmission of non-O1 and non-O139 *V. cholerae* is typically associated with consuming contaminated water or undercooked seafood, especially in coastal areas [12].

Vibrio bacteremia is a condition in which Vibrio bacteria, usually *V. vulnificus* or *V. cholerae*, enter the bloodstream and cause an infection. In a previous study, *V. vulnificus* had the highest case fatality rate of 39% in all reported foodborne infections in the United States [13]. In Asia, studies from South Korea, Japan, and China have also shown a very high mortality rate from *Vibrio* infections [14–16]. Even in the limited data from Taiwan, the high fatality rate of *Vibrio* infections is consistently demonstrated [17,18].

Vibrio bacteria, particularly *V. vulnificus*, thrive in warm seawater temperatures, with optimal growth occurring between 20 °C and 30 °C (68 °F and 86 °F). As a result, *Vibrio* infections, including *Vibrio* bacteremia, tend to increase during the warmer months, particularly in areas with warm coastal waters [14,15,19,20]. One study, for example, found that the case fatality rate of *V. vulnificus* bacteremia was significantly higher during the summer months in the United States [21].

Otherwise, numerous scoring systems have been created to estimate the mortality risk in emergency departments (EDs) [22,23]. Their efficiency has been documented across various scenarios, including cases of infectious disease, length of stay (LOS), and hospital admission. In a literature review, there were no studies that used specific scoring systems to predict the mortality risk of *Vibrio* bacteremia. This study focused on modifying the existing scoring systems by adding the laboratory variables according to the results of the univariate analysis. The modified scoring systems demonstrated more powerful performance and could help clinicians to provide appropriate antibiotics and intervention as early as possible to lower the mortality of *Vibrio* bacteremia.

2. Materials and Methods

2.1. Study Design and Inclusion Criteria

The institutional review board at Taichung Veterans General Hospital (TCVGH) granted approval for our research (No. CE22240B), following the ethical guidelines of the Declaration of Helsinki. Nevertheless, the informed consent of the patients was waived because of the retrospective design. This observational research was carried out at a tertiary care center in Taiwan, which accommodates approximately 65,000 ED visits each year. We carried out this hospital-based study on patients with *Vibrio* bacteremia. Cases of confirmed *Vibrio* bacteremia were identified through the findings of at least one blood culture in the ED. Patient information was gathered from the electronic clinical database of TCVGH, spanning from January 2012 to December 2021. Data included demographics, laboratory investigations, and clinical outcomes. The primary outcome was in-hospital mortality. This study used univariate and multivariate analyses to evaluate the mortality risk.

2.2. Microbiological Diagnosis

In this study, the microbiological laboratory used VITEK® MS PRIME (bioMérieux, Lyon, France) to identify the microorganisms and VITEK® II for routine antimicrobial susceptibility testing (AST) to provide efficient workflow and faster AST results.

2.3. Scoring Systems

This study used the following clinical scoring systems to predict the clinical outcome and the risk of mortality (Table S1): Mortality in Emergency Department Sepsis (MEDS) Score, Worthing Physiological Scoring (WPS), Rapid Emergency Medicine Score (REMS), and quick Sepsis-related Organ Failure Assessment (qSOFA). According to the results of the univariate analysis, this study modified the systems mentioned above with blood urea nitrogen (BUN) and the potential of hydrogen (pH) to predict the mortality risk of *Vibrio* bacteremia again.

2.4. Statistic Analysis

In this study, continuous variables were presented as the mean ± standard deviation (SD), and categorical variables as number and percentages. To evaluate differences in categorical variables, chi-squared tests were used, whereas Mann–Whitney–Wilcoxon U tests were employed for continuous variables to compare the mortality risk between survivors and non-survivors. The study conducted univariate and multivariate analyses using the Cox regression model to identify potential mortality predictors, presenting the results as hazard ratios and confidence intervals. The predictive power of different scoring systems was compared using the area under the curve (AUC) of the receiver operating characteristic (ROC) curve. Cut-off points were utilized to categorize mortality risks based on sensitivity, specificity, negative predictive value (NPV), and positive predictive value (PPV). The population distribution and mortality risk according to cumulative points was calculated and plotted. Statistical significance was assigned to p-values < 0.05. Data analyses were carried out using the Statistical Package for the Social Science (IBM SPSS version 22.0; International Business Machines Corp., New York, NY, USA) and R (Version 4.1.3, R Foundation for Statistical Computing, Vienna, Austria).

3. Results

3.1. Demographics and Clinical Characteristics

This study summarized the demographics, comorbidities, and clinical findings of the 36 patients with *Vibrio* bacteremia in Table 1, including 23 males (63.9%) and 13 females (36.1%), with a mean age of 65.1 ± 15.7 years and an average LOS of 16.6 ± 12.7 days. The comorbidities for *Vibrio* bacteremia included liver cirrhosis, which showed the highest proportion (27.8%), followed by congestive heart failure (22.2%) and alcoholism (16.7%). None of the comorbidities showed significant differences in terms of mortality. The 30-day in-hospital mortality rate amounted to 25% (9/36), with 31.5% in *V. vulnificus* (6/19) and 17.6% in *V.* non-*vulnificus* (3/17).

Table 1. Characteristics, manifestations, clinical course, and management of patients with *Vibrio* bacteremia.

General Data	All (n = 36)	Survival (n = 27)	Mortality (n = 9)	p-Value
		Sex		0.235
Male	23 (63.9%)	19 (70.4%)	4 (44.4%)	
Female	13 (36.1%)	8 (29.6%)	5 (55.6%)	
Age	65.1 ± 15.7	62.3 ± 15.5	73.7 ± 13.6	0.081
		Pathogens		0.451
Vibrio vulnificus	19 (52.8%)	13 (48.2%)	6 (66.7%)	
Vibrio non-*vulnificus*	17 (47.2%)	14 (51.9%)	3 (33.3%)	

Table 1. *Cont.*

General Data	All (n = 36)	Survival (n = 27)	Mortality (n = 9)	p-Value
		Vital signs		
SBP	127.72 ± 28.13	128.81 ± 27.49	124.44 ± 31.46	0.865
DBP	70.58 ± 14.85	72.74 ± 15.12	64.11 ± 12.61	0.195
MAP	89.6 ± 17.8	91.4 ± 18.2	84.2 ± 16.3	0.433
HR	104.6 ± 25.4	107.6 ± 25.7	95.7 ± 23.5	0.138
RR	19.4 ± 2.40	19.2 ± 1.7	20.1 ± 3.8	0.761
BT	37.7 ± 1.2	37.9 ± 1.2	37.3 ± 1.2	0.195
		Symptoms		
Fever or chills	21 (58.3%)	15 (55.6%)	6 (66.7%)	0.705
Limb pain or swelling	10 (27.8%)	8 (29.6%)	2 (22.2%)	1.000
Abdominal pain or diarrhea	7 (19.4%)	6 (22.2%)	1 (11.1%)	0.652
		Comorbidities		
HCVD	5 (13.9%)	4 (14.8%)	1 (11.1%)	1.000
CAD	5 (13.9%)	4 (14.8%)	1 (11.1%)	1.000
CHF	8 (22.2%)	6 (22.2%)	2 (22.2%)	1.000
CVA	16 (44.4%)	12 (44.4%)	4 (44.4%)	1.000
DM	7 (19.4%)	5 (18.5%)	2 (22.2%)	1.000
Alcoholism	6 (16.7%)	4 (14.8%)	2 (22.2%)	0.627
Liver cirrhosis	10 (27.8%)	8 (29.6%)	2 (22.2%)	1.000
COPD	5 (13.9%)	3 (11.1%)	2 (22.2%)	0.581
Transplant	2 (5.6%)	0 (0%)	2 (22.2%)	0.057
Cancer	11 (30.6%)	8 (29.6%)	3 (33.3%)	1.000
		Clinical course		
Shock	7 (19.4%)	4 (14.8%)	3 (33.3%)	0.333
Intubation	15 (41.7%)	10 (37.0%)	5 (55.6%)	0.443
Urgent hemodialysis	4 (11.1%)	1 (3.7%)	3 (33.3%)	0.041 *
Hypotension	11 (30.6%)	5 (18.5%)	6 (66.7%)	0.012 *
Vasopressor	10 (27.8%)	5 (18.5%)	5 (55.6%)	0.079
		Management		
Antibiotics				0.024 *
Cephalosporins	19 (52.8%)	16 (59.3%)	3 (33.3%)	
Cephalosporins+Tetracyclines	7 (19.4%)	6 (22.2%)	1 (11.1%)	
Cephalosporins+Quinolone	5 (13.9%)	4 (14.8%)	1 (11.1%)	
Others	5 (13.9%)	1 (3.7%)	4 (44.4%)	
Surgery	11 (30.6%)	7 (25.9%)	4 (44.4%)	0.409
Drainage	6 (16.7%)	4 (14.8%)	2 (22.2%)	0.627
		Infection source		0.169
Primary	12 (33.3%)	7 (25.9%)	5 (55.6%)	
Wound or Marine	12 (33.3%)	9 (33.3%)	3 (33.3%)	
GI tract	12 (33.3%)	11 (40.7%)	1 (11.1%)	

Chi-squared test. Mann–Whitney U-test. * $p < 0.05$, statistically significant. Continuous data were expressed as mean ± SD. Categorical data were expressed as number and percentage. Abbreviations: BT, body temperature; CAD, coronary artery disease; CHF, congestive heart failure; COPD, chronic obstructive pulmonary disease; CVA, cerebrovascular accident; DBP, diastolic blood pressure; DM, diabetes mellitus; GI: gastrointestinal; HCVD, hypertensive cardiovascular disease; HR, heart rate; MAP, mean blood pressure; RR, respiratory rate; SBP, systolic blood pressure.

3.2. Laboratory Data

The laboratory data and scoring systems are shown in Table 2. White blood cell count (WBC) (12,280.7 ± 6517.3 vs. 6018.9 ± 2766.3, p = 0.009), absolute neutrophil count (ANC) (10,829.8 ± 6038.4 vs. 4720.0 ± 2002.0, p = 0.003), BUN (20.4 ± 14.1 vs. 40.0 ± 21.2, p = 0.005), potassium (K) (3.82 ± 0.73 vs. 4.64 ± 1.12, p = 0.038), maximum of creatine kinase (CK) (103.1 ± 92.2 vs. 1126.4 ± 1896.1, $p = 0.009$), and pH (7.40 ± 0.05 vs. 7.32 ± 0.09, $p = 0.016$) showed significant differences between the survivors and the non-survivors.

Table 2. Laboratory data of patients with *Vibrio* bacteremia.

Variables	All ($n = 36$)	Survival ($n = 27$)	Mortality ($n = 9$)	p-Value
		Complete blood cells		
WBC	10,715.3 ± 6392.5	12,280.7 ± 6517.3	6018.9 ± 2766.3	0.009 **
ANC	9302.3 ± 5933.1	10,829.8 ± 6038.4	4720.0 ± 2002.0	0.003 **
Hb	11.9 ± 2.2	12.0 ± 2.4	11.6 ± 1.7	0.559
PLT	162.9 ± 84.3	173.9 ± 89.0	131.4 ± 62.6	0.291
		Biochemistry		
BUN	25.6 ± 18.2	20.4 ± 14.1	40.0 ± 21.2	0.005 **
Cr	1.34 ± 0.76	1.20 ± 0.66	1.76 ± 0.92	0.111
Na	134.2 ± 4.9	133.9 ± 5.3	135.1 ± 3.8	0.621
K	4.03 ± 0.90	3.82 ± 0.73	4.64 ± 1.12	0.038 *
Total bilirubin	3.24 ± 4.94	3.15 ± 5.22	3.56 ± 4.23	0.820
GPT	60.4 ± 55.5	68.0 ± 57.9	36.0 ± 40.5	0.062
LDH	329.4 ± 143.0	334.9 ± 151.4	307.3 ± 127.5	1.000
CRP	4.59 ± 5.72	4.35 ± 5.76	5.33 ± 5.89	0.407
Lactate	33.6 ± 20.7	34.1 ± 21.4	32.5 ± 20.1	0.940
Glucose	142.2 ± 61.1	151.17 ± 66.27	115.38 ± 31.51	0.268
Maximum of CK	389.6 ± 1060.5	103.1 ± 92.2	1126.4 ± 1896.1	0.009 **
		Arterial blood gas		
pH	7.38 ± 0.07	7.40 ± 0.05	7.32 ± 0.09	0.016 *
PaO_2^-	53.05 ± 25.22	55.04 ± 24.31	46.21 ± 29.03	0.397
$PaCO_2^-$	22.79 ± 2.85	22.74 ± 2.91	22.93 ± 2.89	0.728
HCO_3^-	−2.10 ± 2.62	−1.83 ± 2.65	−3.01 ± 2.48	0.204

Chi-squared test. Mann–Whitney U-test. * $p < 0.05$, ** $p < 0.01$, statistically significant. Continuous data were expressed as mean ± SD. Abbreviations: ANC, absolute neutrophil count; BUN, blood urea nitrogen; CK, creatine kinase; CRP, C-reactive protein; Cr, creatinine; GPT, glutamic pyruvic transaminase; Hb, hemoglobin; K, potassium; LDH, lactate dehydrogenase; Na, sodium; PLT, platelet; WBC, white blood cell count.

3.3. Microbiology and Seasonal Distribution of Mortality Cases

Emergency physicians performed a bacterial culture on individual patients at least once. The microorganisms found in blood culture were distributed between *V. vulnificus* ($n = 19$) and *V.* non-*vulnificus* ($n = 17$), including *V. cholera*, non-O1, non-O139, ($n = 10$), *V. fluvialis* ($n = 5$), *V. cholerae* O1 ($n = 1$), and *V. alginolyticus* ($n = 1$) (Table 3). There was a trend association between the mortality cases of *Vibrio* bacteremia and seasonal distribution, with a trend of $p = 0.044$ (Figure 1).

Table 3. The microorganisms causing *Vibrio* bacteremia.

Microorganisms	Case Numbers (n)
Vibrio vulnificus	19
Vibrio non-*vulnificus*	17
Vibrio cholera non-O1, non-O139	10
Vibrio fluvialis	5
Vibrio cholerae O1	1
Vibrio alginolyticus	1

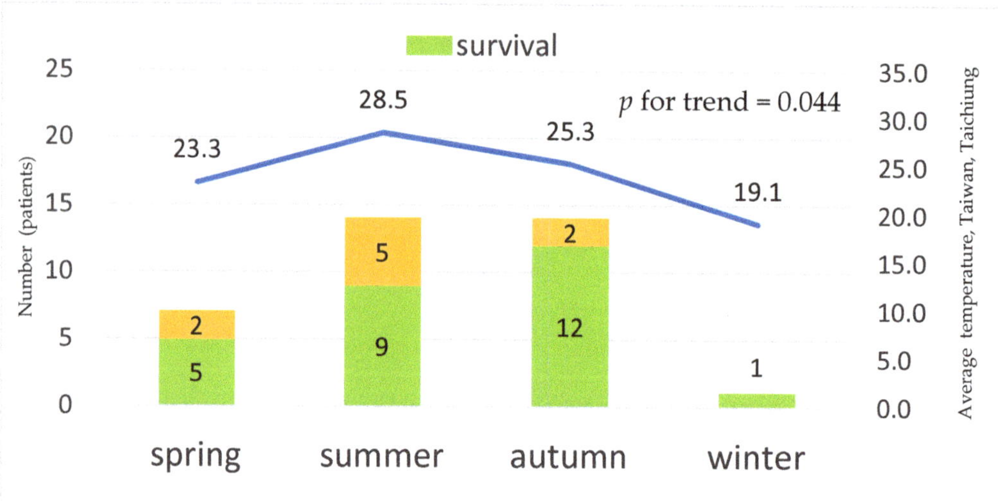

Figure 1. The trend association between the mortality cases of *Vibrio* bacteremia and seasonal distribution ($p = 0.044$).

3.4. Scoring Systems

The non-survivors had significantly higher scores in the original MEDS (10.3 ± 2.4) than the survivors (6.2 ± 4.1) ($p = 0.002$). The remaining scoring systems showed no different significance (Table 4).

Table 4. The scoring systems to predict the mortality risk of patients with *Vibrio* bacteremia.

Scores	All ($n = 36$)	Survival ($n = 27$)	Mortality ($n = 9$)	p-Value
MEDS	7.1 ± 4.2	6.2 ± 4.1	10.3 ± 2.4	0.002 **
WPS	2.4 ± 2.1	2.0 ± 1.6	3.4 ± 3.2	0.349
qSOFA	0 ± 0.6	0.3 ± 0.5	0.6 ± 0.7	0.387
REMS	6.0 ± 2.6	5.7 ± 2.2	6.9 ± 3.6	0.426

** $p < 0.01$, statistically significant. Continuous data were expressed as mean ± SD. Abbreviations: MEDS, Mortality in Emergency Department Sepsis; REMS, Rapid Emergency Medicine Score; qSOFA, quick Sepsis-related Organ Failure Assessment; WPS, Worthing Physiological Scoring system.

3.5. Univariateand Multivariate Analyses of Risk Factors

This study conducted univariate analyses for predisposing factors on clinical outcomes and the results are summarized in Table 5. Higher hazard ratios (HRs) were foundin the non-survivors, including hypotension, renal failure, urgent hemodialysis, organ transplant, and elevation of WBC, potassium, BUN, and creatinine. In univariate analysis, the MEDS and WPS showed significantly higher in the non-survivors (Table 6). Higher HR in the non-survivors regarding scores of the original MEDS ($p = 0.037$) in multivariate analysis was found (Table 6).

Table 5. Hazard ratios and 95% confidence interval of univariate analysis for patients with *Vibrio* bacteremia.

Variables	Hazard Ratios	95% Confidence Interval	*p*-Value
WBC	1.00	1.00–1.00	0.016 *
BUN	1.04	1.01–1.07	0.009 **
Cr	2.05	1.03–4.08	0.041 *
K	2.11	1.23–3.64	0.007 **
CK	1.00	1.00–1.00	0.011 *
pH	0.79	0.68–0.91	0.001 **
Transplant	11.41	2.19–59.39	0.004 **
Urgent hemodialysis	5.96	1.48–24.08	0.012 *
Hypotension	5.35	1.33–21.51	0.018 *
Renal failure	0.25	0.07–0.94	0.040 *

* $p < 0.05$, ** $p < 0.01$, statistically significant. Abbreviations: BUN, blood urea nitrogen; CK, creatine kinase; Cr, creatinine; K, potassium; WBC, white blood cell count.

Table 6. Hazard ratios and 95% confidence interval of univariate and multivariate analysesfor patients with *Vibrio* bacteremia.

	Univariate			Multivariate		
Variables	HR	95% CI	*p*-Value	HR	95% CI	*p*-Value
MEDS	1.23	1.05–1.44	0.011 *	1.28	1.02–1.62	0.037 *
WPS	1.38	1.03–1.84	0.030 *	1.08	0.45–2.61	0.863
qSOFA	1.88	0.74–4.72	0.182	2.21	0.13–38.98	0.588
REMS	1.22	0.96–1.56	0.100	1.48	0.91–2.40	0.111

* $p < 0.05$, statistically significant. Abbreviations: CI, conference interval; HR, hazard ratios; MEDS, Mortality in Emergency Department Sepsis; REMS, Rapid Emergency Medicine Score; qSOFA, quick Sepsis-related Organ Failure Assessment; WPS, Worthing Physiological Scoring system.

3.6. The Receiver Operating Characteristic Curve (ROC)

The ROC of the original MEDS, WPS, qSOFA, and REMS for accuracy in predicting the mortality riskswas analyzed, and the results are shown in Figure 2 and Table 7. The cut-off point of the MEDS was 10, and the AUC of the ROC measured up to 0.833, which had a sensitivity of 66.7% and a specificity of 92.6% ($p = 0.003$).

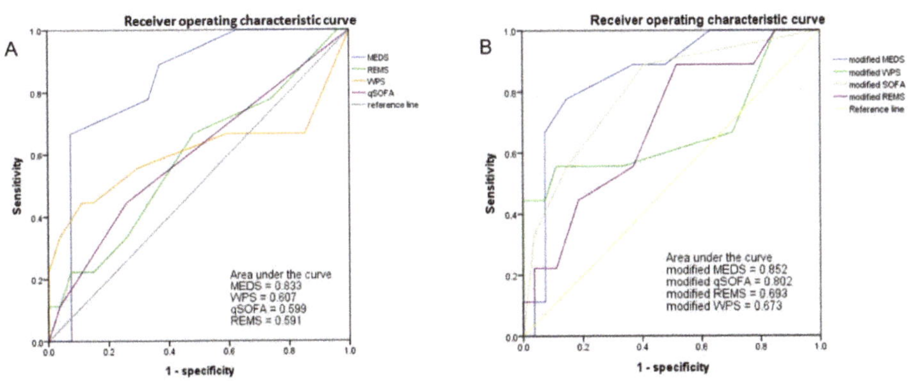

Figure 2. The AUC of ROC of the MEDS, WPS, qSOFA, and REMS in predicting the mortality risks of patients with *Vibrio* bacteremia (Panel **A**). The AUC of ROC of the modified MEDS, WPS, qSOFA, and REMS in predicting the mortality risks of patients with *Vibrio* bacteremia (Panel **B**). AUC = area under the curve; ROC = receiver operating characteristic curve.

Table 7. The AUC of the ROC, cut-off point (COP), sensitivity specificity, positive predictive value (PPV), negative predictive value (NPV), accuracy, and standard error (SE) of the original MEDS, WPS, qSOFA, and REMS to predict mortality risk.

Scores	AUC	COP	Sensitivity	Specificity	PPV	NPV	Accuracy	SE	p-Value
MEDS	0.833	10	66.7%	92.6%	75.0%	89.3%	86.1%	0.07	0.003 **
WPS	0.607	5	44.4%	88.9%	57.1%	82.8%	77.8%	0.14	0.342
qSOFA	0.599	1	44.4%	74.1%	36.4%	80.0%	66.7%	0.12	0.381
REMS	0.591	6	66.7%	51.9%	31.6%	82.4%	55.6%	0.11	0.422

** $p < 0.01$, statistically significant. Abbreviations: MEDS, Mortality in Emergency Department Sepsis; REMS, Rapid Emergency Medicine Score; qSOFA, quick Sepsis-related Organ Failure Assessment; WPS, Worthing Physiological Scoring system.

This study modified the original scoring systems with other predictive factors, including BUN (if BUN > 25, the modified score had one point added) and pH (if pH < 7.36, the modified score had one point added). We reveal the results in Figure 2 and Table 8. The cut-off point of the modified MEDS was 10, and the AUC of the ROC increased to 0.852 with a sensitivity of 77.8% and a specificity of 85.2% ($p = 0.002$). The cut-off point of the modified qSOFA was 1, and the AUC of the ROC reached up to 0.802, with a sensitivity of 88.9% and a specificity of 59.3% ($p = 0.007$).

Table 8. The AUC of ROC, cut-off point (COP), sensitivity specificity, positive predictive value (PPV), negative predictive value (NPV), accuracy, and standard error (SE) of the modified MEDS, WPS, qSOFA, and REMS to predict the mortality risk.

Modified Scores	AUC	COP	Sensitivity	Specificity	PPV	NPV	Accuracy	SE	p-Value
Modified MEDS	0.852	10	77.8%	85.2%	63.6%	92.0%	83.3%	0.07	0.002 **
Modified qSOFA	0.802	1	88.9%	59.3%	42.1%	94.1%	66.7%	0.09	0.007 **
Modified REMS	0.693	6	88.9%	48.1%	36.4%	92.9%	58.3%	0.10	0.086
Modified WPS	0.673	5	55.6%	88.9%	62.5%	85.7%	80.6%	0.13	0.125

** $p < 0.01$, statistically significant. If BUN > 25, the modified score had one point added; if pH < 7.36, the modified score had one point added. Abbreviations: MEDS, Mortality in Emergency Department Sepsis; REMS, Rapid Emergency Medicine Score; qSOFA, quick Sepsis-related Organ Failure Assessment; WPS, Worthing Physiological Scoring system.

3.7. Cumulative Survival Rates obtained by Kaplan–Meier and Discrimination Plot

This study analyzed the cumulative survival rates of patients with *Vibrio* bacteremia using Kaplan–Meier. The original MEDS and WPS demonstrated significant differences between the survivors and non-survivors ($p = 0.0012$ and $p < 0.0001$) if the cut-off points of the original MEDS and WPS were 10 and 5. Otherwise, the original qSOFA and REMS demonstrated no significant differences between the survivors and non-survivors ($p = 0.37$ and $p = 0.56$) if the cut-off points of the qSOFA and REMS were 1 and 6 (Figure 3). However, the modified MEDS, WPS, and qSOFA demonstrated significant differences between the survivors and non-survivors ($p < 0.0001$, $p = 0.00044$, and $p = 0.0034$) if the cut-off points of the modified MEDS, WPS, and qSOFA were 10, 5, and 1. Otherwise, the modified REMS demonstrated no significant differences between the survivors and non-survivors ($p = 0.28$) if the cut-off point of the REMS was 6 (Figure 4).The discrimination plots of patients with *Vibrio* bacteremia show that the mortality rates of the original MEDS, WPS, qSOFA, and REMS were 71.4%, 75.0%, 50.0%, and 30.0% if the cut-off points were more than 10, 5, 1, and 6, respectively (Figure 5). The mortality rates of the modified MEDS, WPS, qSOFA, and REMS were 75.0%, 66.7%, 55.6%, and 33.3% if the cut-off points were more than 10, 5, 1, and 6, respectively (Figure 6).

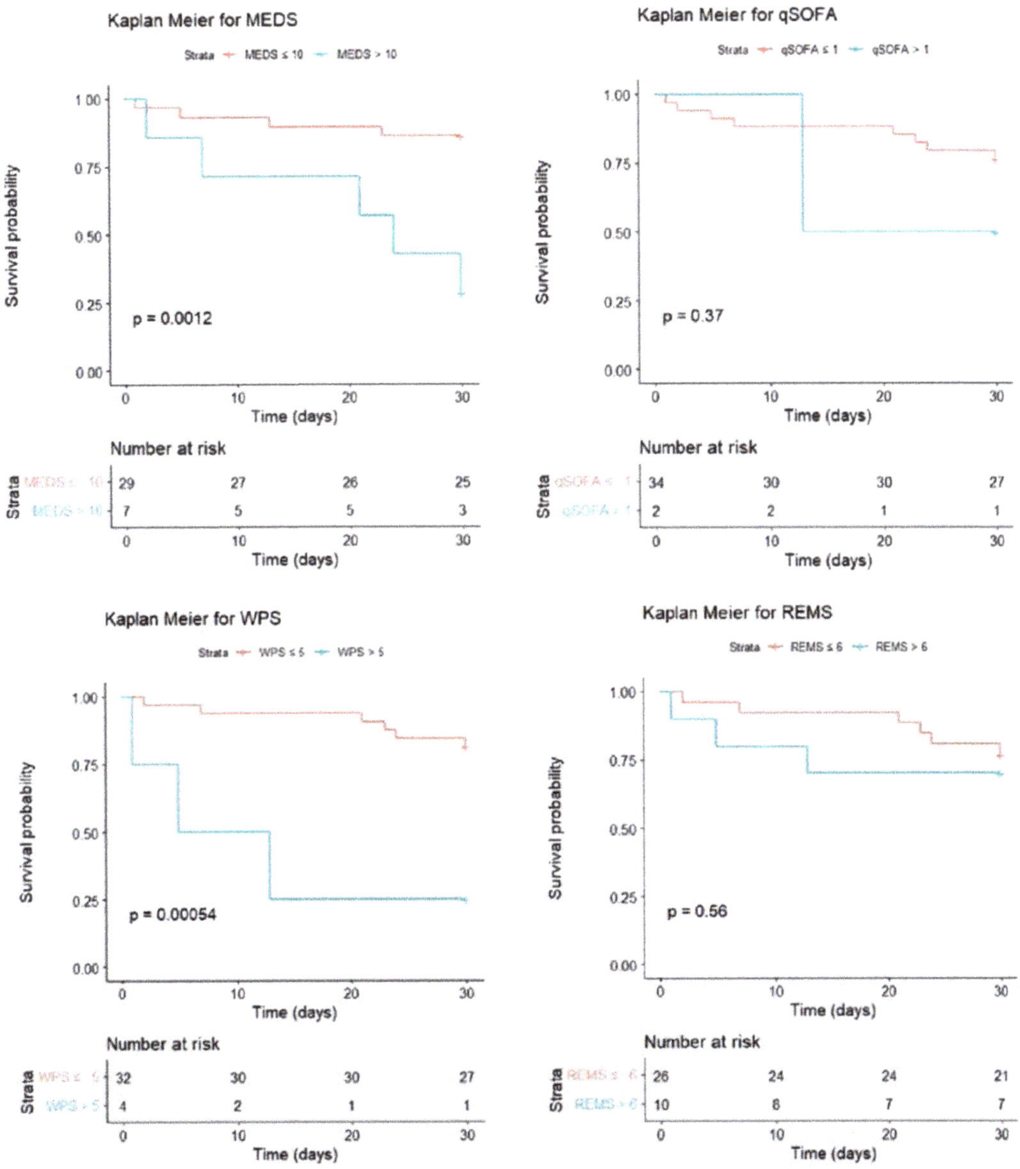

Figure 3. The cumulative 30-day survival rates of patients with *Vibrio* bacteremia were calculated by Kaplan–Meier. The cut-off points of the original MEDS, WPS, qSOFA, and REMS were 10, 5, 1, and 6. Abbreviations: MEDS, Mortality in Emergency Department Sepsis; REMS, Rapid Emergency Medicine Score; qSOFA, quick Sepsis-related Organ Failure Assessment; WPS, Worthing Physiological Scoring system.

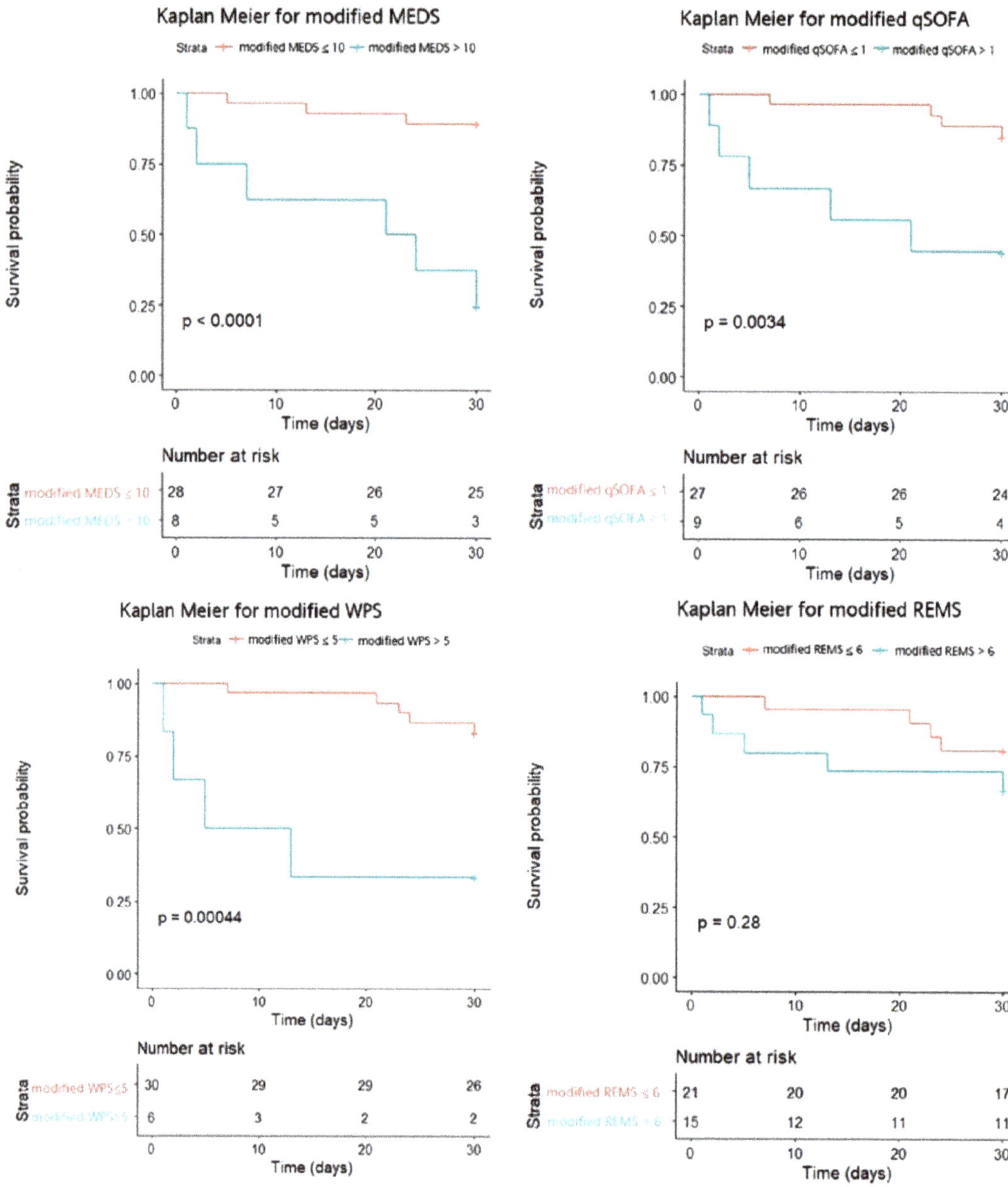

Figure 4. The cumulative 30-day survival rates of patients with *Vibrio* bacteremia were calculated by Kaplan–Meier. The cut-off points of the modified MEDS, WPS, qSOFA, and REMS were 10, 5, 1, and 6. Abbreviations: MEDS, Mortality in Emergency Department Sepsis; REMS, Rapid Emergency Medicine Score; qSOFA, quick Sepsis-related Organ Failure Assessment; WPS, Worthing Physiological Scoring system.

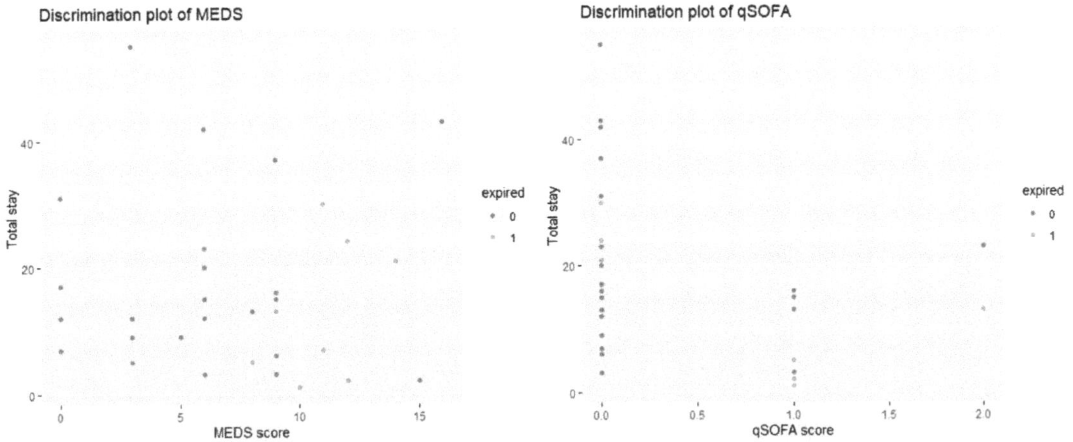

Cut-off point	MEDS ≤ 10	MEDS > 10
Mortality rate	13.8%	71.4%

Cut-off point	qSOFA ≤ 1	qSOFA > 1
Mortality rate	23.5%	50.0%

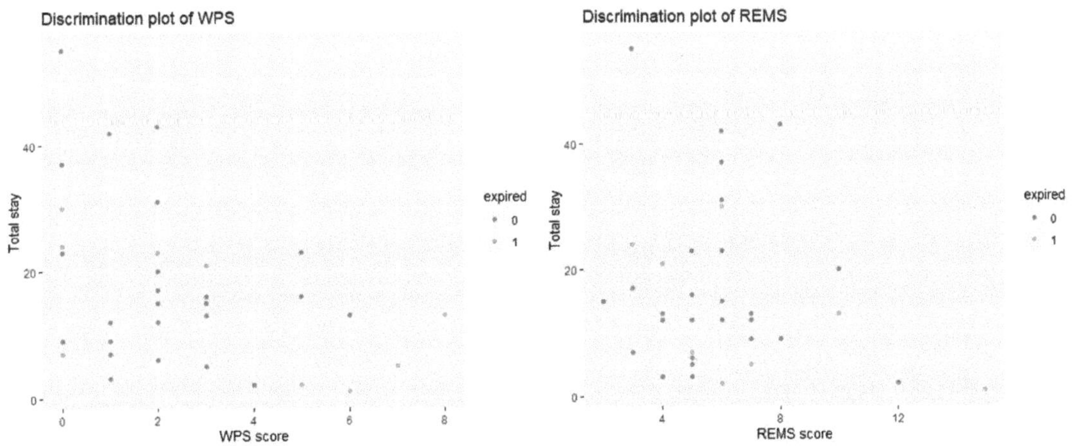

Cut-off point	WPS ≤ 5	WPS > 5
Mortality rate	18.8%	75.0%

Cut-off point	REMS ≤ 6	REMS > 6
Mortality rate	23.1%	30.0%

Figure 5. Discrimination plots showing the mortality rates of 71.4%, 75.0%, 50.0%, and 30.0% in the original scoring systems of the MEDS, WPS, qSOFA, and REMS if the cut-off points were more than 10, 5, 1, and 6, respectively. Abbreviations: MEDS, Mortality in Emergency Department Sepsis; REMS, Rapid Emergency Medicine Score; qSOFA, quick Sepsis-related Organ Failure Assessment; WPS, Worthing Physiological Scoring system.

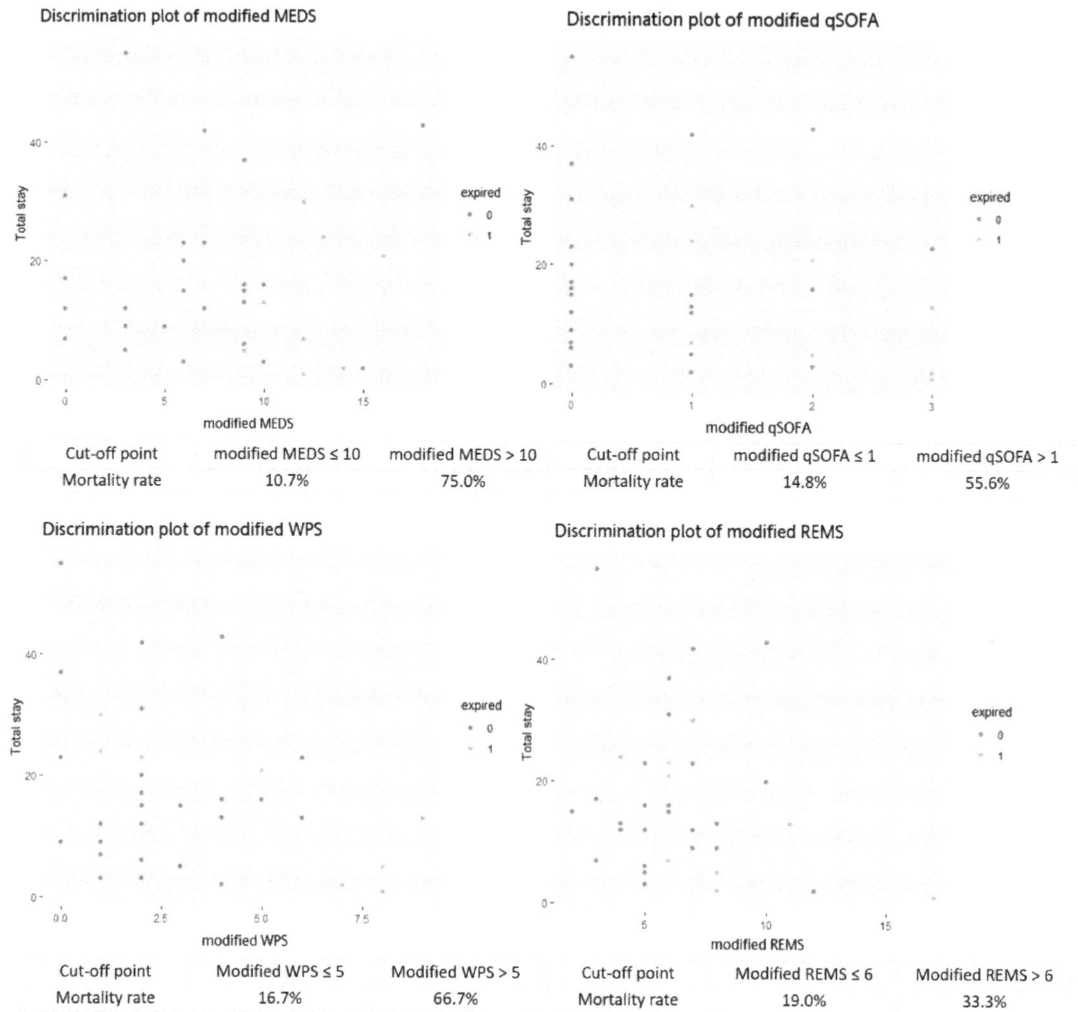

Figure 6. Discrimination plots showing the mortality rates of 75.0%, 66.7%, 55.6%, and 33.3% in the scoring systems of the modified MEDS, WPS, qSOFA, and REMS if the cut-off points were more than 10, 5, 1, and 6, respectively. Abbreviations: MEDS, Mortality in Emergency Department Sepsis; REMS, Rapid Emergency Medicine Score; qSOFA, quick Sepsis-related Organ Failure Assessment; WPS, Worthing Physiological Scoring system.

4. Discussion

Our study showed an overall mortality rate of 25%, with 31.5% due to *V. vulnificus* (n = 6/19). The reported mortality rate of *Vibrio* infection was about 19~39%, and 37% in another study in medical centers in Taiwan [6,13,16,24]. *V. vulnificus* was the most common cause of *Vibrio*-related illness and demonstrated high mortality; about 36% in a previous study in the United States [25].

In the previous studies, the ratio of male to female patients was 2:1 in Taiwan [26] and 3.6:1 (84.8%) in mainland China [27]. The results of these studies indicated that *Vibrio* infection is more likely to occur in males. Our study also demonstrated that cirrhosis was the most common comorbidity, accounting for 27.8%, and chronic liver disease represented

36.1%, similar to the previous research [8,25,28,29]. Liver diseases appeared more common in males [30], which might explain why the proportion of males with *Vibrio* bacteremia had a higher prevalence rate.

In the clinical course, hypotension was an unfavorable prognostic factor [31]. Hypotension indicated a more severe state of septic shock and was associated with an increased mortality rate [32,33]. Additionally, a significant increase in mortality was observed in cases when urgent hemodialysis was required. Previous studies already supported this finding [34,35]. Other interventions, such as intubation and vasopressor use, did not differ significantly.

The antibiotic treatment for *Vibrio* bacteremia typically involves a third-generation cephalosporin combined with tetracycline or fluoroquinolone [36–38]. *Vibrio* bacteremia often exhibited poor responsiveness to the treatment of penicillin. In our study, most cases received treatment with cephalosporins, including ceftriaxone or cefepime, upon arrival at the ED. However, there were six cases where an immediate assessment of the potential source of infection was not feasible due to clinical presentations or patient history inquiries. Consequently, these cases were treated with other broad-spectrum antibiotics—five with piperacillin and one with oxacillin. Notably, the mortality rate among this group of patients was significantly higher.

In microorganisms, *V. vulnificus* was the most common species causing *Vibrio* bacteremia [2,39]. This pathogen was prevalent in estuarine waters, aligning with the geographical environment of Taiwan—a seafood-rich island surrounded by the sea on all sides. The second most common species was *V.cholerae*, non-O1 and non-O139, predominant among *V.* non-*vulnificus*. *V. cholerae*, non-O1 and non-O139, was often associated with infectious diarrhea or contaminated water [40]. Taiwan, situated in the subtropics, possesses geographical features conducive to the growth of these bacterial strains.

A number of clinical scoring systems exist to quickly stratify patients and identify potentially severe conditions in both the ED and intensive care unit based on variable physiological parameters [22,41]. These simple and user-friendly clinical scoring systems enable physicians to quickly decide on the treatment plans for patients and start early goal-directed therapies, including the administration of suitable antibiotics.

The original MEDS score, developed by Shapiro et al. in 2003, incorporates various clinical parameters such as terminal disease, respiratory difficulty, septic shock, platelet count, band proportion, age, lower respiratory infection, nursing home residence, and altered mental status [42]. This scoring system has been shown to accurately estimate the risk of mortality in emergency department patients with suspected infectious conditions [43]. In Taiwan, the MEDS score is commonly utilized for predicting mortality among patients suffering from community-acquired bacteremia [44]. Higher original MEDS scores were found in the non-survivors in this single-center retrospective study. Moreover, the application of multivariate logistic regression revealed that the AUC of ROC for the original MEDS score was 0.833, alongside a sensitivity of 66.7% and a specificity of 92.6%. This highlights its capability to predict mortality in *Vibrio* bacteremia cases, using a cut-off point of 10.

This study modified the scoring systems by choosing the predictive factors, including BUN and pH, according to univariate and multivariate analyses. Previous studies have highlighted the predictive capability of BUN or the BUN-to-albumin ratio for the mortality rate in bacteremia [45–47]. A study in South Korea also suggested that pH levels can aid in estimating the mortality rate of *Vibrio* infections [48].

The original MEDS and qSOFA were designed for simplicity and ease of calculation, often excluding blood test data [49–51]. However, this simplicity came at the cost of some accuracy. In cases where blood test data were available, we enhanced these commonly used scoring systems with laboratory data (BUN and pH) to improve their predictive accuracy, specifically for *Vibrio* bacteremia. Although they lead to a few minutes' delay for the blood test results, the modified MEDS and qSOFA will significantly benefit from advancements in testing technologies—making such waits considerably shorter than before. This enhances our ability to predict a patient's condition's severity accurately. We believe that a few minutes' delay can bring advantages, such as more precise diagnoses, and can avoid unnecessary treatment expenses and the risks associated with delayed treatment, ultimately leading to significant long-term savings in healthcare costs.

5. Limitation

There were several limitations in this study. First, this was a single-center retrospective study with a relatively small sample size. This may have led to some analyses showing no significant difference and a selection bias or confounding variables not accounted for in the analysis. Second, *Vibrio* bacteremia is a rare clinical entity, so finding a control group without *Vibrio* bacteremia in this retrospective study was challenging. Third, compared to previous studies, we did not document or analyze data related to the source or site of infection in these *Vibrio* bacteremia patients. Fourth, our study modified those existing scoring systems, and while we did see improvements in sensitivity and specificity, it may still need to catch up to our ideal expectations.

6. Conclusions

The original MEDS could serve as reliable indicators for forecasting the mortality rate of patients grappling with *Vibrio* bacteremia. This study modified the MEDS and qSOFA by increasing the laboratory variables, including BUN and pH, to strengthen the predictive performance for the mortality risk of *Vibrio* bacteremia. It is advocated to promptly initiate targeted therapeutic interventions and judicious antibiotic treatments to curb fatality rates. Substantive, expansive investigations are requisite to engender deeper insights into the malady and ensure maximal patient well-being.

Supplementary Materials: The following supporting information can be downloaded at: https://www.mdpi.com/article/10.3390/jpm14040385/s1, Table S1: scoring systems. Refs [41–44,51] are cited in Supplementary Materials.

Author Contributions: Conceptualization, S.-Y.H. and S.-C.H.; methodology, M.-S.H. and S.-Y.H.; data curation, S.-Y.H., C.-H.S. and Y.-C.T.; writing—original draft preparation, C.-M.H. and S.-Y.H.; writing—review and editing, M.-S.H. and S.-Y.H.; project administration, S.-Y.H.; funding acquisition, S.-Y.H. All authors have read and agreed to the published version of the manuscript.

Funding: This work was supported by grants from the Taichung Veterans General Hospital (TCVGH), Taichung, Taiwan (TCVGH-1127203C, TCVGH-T1127801, TCVGH-1137203C, and TCVGH-T1137801), and the Taipei Veterans General Hospital, Taoyuan branch, Taoyuan, Taiwan (TYVH-10808, TYVH-10809, and TYVH-10902). The funders had no role in the study design, data collection, analysis, decision to publish, or preparation of the manuscript. No additional external funding was received for this study.

Institutional Review Board Statement: The institutional review board of Taichung Veterans General Hospital approved this study on 17 June 2022. (The study period ranged from 1 July 2021 to 30 June 2022.) (IRB file number: CE22240B).

Informed Consent Statement: Patient consent was waived because this study was retrospective, observational, and anonymous.

Data Availability Statement: Readers can access the data and material supporting the study's conclusion by contacting Sung-Yuan Hu at song9168@pie.com.tw.

Acknowledgments: We thank the Clinical Informatics Research and Development Center and Biostatistics Task Force of Taichung Veterans General Hospital. We thank Yu-Ju Chen, M.T., Center of Microbiological Laboratory, Department of Pathology and Laboratory Medicine, Taichung Veterans General Hospital, for providing the methodology of identification for *Vibrio* species.

Conflicts of Interest: The authors declare no conflicts of interest.

References

1. Morris, J.G., Jr.; Black, R.E. *Cholera* and other *vibrioses* in the United States. *N. Engl. J. Med.* **1985**, *312*, 343–350. [CrossRef] [PubMed]
2. Baker-Austin, C.; Oliver, J.D.; Alam, M.; Ali, A.; Waldor, M.K.; Qadri, F.; Martinez-Urtaza, J. *Vibrio* spp. infections. *Nat. Rev. Dis. Primers* **2018**, *4*, 8. [CrossRef] [PubMed]
3. Sampaio, A.; Silva, V.; Poeta, P.; Aonofriesei, F. *Vibrio* spp.: Life Strategies, Ecology, and Risks in a Changing Environment. *Diversity* **2022**, *14*, 97. [CrossRef]
4. Ina-Salwany, M.Y.; Al-Saari, N.; Mohamad, A.; Mursidi, F.A.; Mohd-Aris, A.; Amal, M.N.A.; Kasai, H.; Mino, S.; Sawabe, T.; Zamri-Saad, M. *Vibriosis* in Fish: A Review on Disease Development and Prevention. *J. Aquat. Anim. Health* **2019**, *31*, 3–22. [CrossRef] [PubMed]
5. Tacket, C.O.; Brenner, F.; Blake, P.A. Clinical features and an epidemiological study of *Vibrio vulnificus* infections. *J. Infect. Dis.* **1984**, *149*, 558–561. [CrossRef] [PubMed]
6. Coerdt, K.M.; Khachemoune, A. *Vibrio vulnificus*: Review of Mild to Life-threatening Skin Infections. *Cutis* **2021**, *107*, E12–E17. [CrossRef] [PubMed]
7. Klontz, K.C.; Lieb, S.; Schreiber, M.; Janowski, H.T.; Baldy, L.M.; Gunn, R.A. Syndromes of *Vibrio vulnificus* infections: Clinical and epidemiologic features in Florida cases, 1981–1987. *Ann. Intern. Med.* **1988**, *109*, 318–323. [CrossRef] [PubMed]
8. Johnston, J.M.; Becker, S.F.; McFarland, L.M. *Vibrio vulnificus*: Man and the sea. *JAMA* **1985**, *253*, 2850–2853. [CrossRef] [PubMed]
9. Hoge, C.W.; Watsky, D.; Peeler, R.N.; Libonati, J.P.; Israel, E.; Morris, J.G., Jr. Epidemiology and spectrum of *Vibrio* infections in a Chesapeake Bay community. *J. Infect. Dis.* **1989**, *160*, 985–993. [CrossRef]
10. Satitsri, S.; Pongkorpsakol, P.; Srimanote, P.; Chatsudthipong, V.; Muanprasat, C. Pathophysiological mechanisms of diarrhea caused by the *Vibrio cholerae* O1 El Tor variant: An in vivo study in mice. *Virulence* **2016**, *7*, 789–805. [CrossRef]
11. Montero, D.A.; Vidal, R.M.; Velasco, J.; George, S.; Lucero, Y.; Gómez, L.A.; Carreño, L.J.; García-Betancourt, R.; O'Ryan, M. *Vibrio cholerae*, classification, pathogenesis, immune response, and trends in vaccine development. *Front. Med.* **2023**, *10*, 1155751. [CrossRef] [PubMed]
12. Deshayes, S.; Daurel, C.; Cattoir, V.; Parienti, J.J.; Quilici, M.L.; de La Blanchardière, A. Non-O1, non-O139 *Vibrio cholera* bacteraemia: Case report and literature review. *Springerplus* **2015**, *4*, 575. [CrossRef]
13. Mead, P.S.; Slutsker, L.; Dietz, V.; McCaig, L.F.; Bresee, J.S.; Shapiro, C.; Griffin, P.M.; Tauxe, R.V. Food-related illness and death in the United States. *Emerg. Infect. Dis.* **1999**, *5*, 607–625. [CrossRef] [PubMed]
14. Kim, J.S.; Lee, E.G.; Chun, B.C. Epidemiologic Characteristics and Case Fatality Rate of *Vibrio vulnificus* Infection: Analysis of 761 Cases From 2003 to 2016 in Korea. *J. Korean Med. Sci.* **2022**, *37*, e79. [CrossRef]
15. Leng, F.; Lin, S.; Wu, W.; Zhang, J.; Song, J.; Zhong, M. Epidemiology, pathogenetic mechanism, clinical characteristics, and treatment of *Vibrio vulnificus* infection: A case report and literature review. *Eur. J. Clin. Microbiol. Infect. Dis.* **2019**, *38*, 1999–2004. [CrossRef] [PubMed]
16. Zhao, H.; Xu, L.; Dong, H.; Hu, J.; Gao, H.; Yang, M.; Zhang, X.; Chen, X.; Fan, J.; Ma, W. Correlations between Clinical Features and Mortality in Patients with *Vibrio vulnificus* Infection. *PLoS ONE* **2015**, *10*, e0136019. [CrossRef]
17. Tsao, C.H.; Chen, C.C.; Tsai, S.J.; Li, C.R.; Chao, W.N.; Chan, K.S.; Lin, D.B.; Sheu, K.L.; Chen, S.C.; Lee, M.C.; et al. Seasonality, clinical types and prognostic factors of *Vibrio vulnificus* infection. *J. Infect. Dev. Ctries.* **2013**, *7*, 533–540. [CrossRef]
18. Chen, S.C.; Chan, K.S.; Chao, W.N.; Wang, P.H.; Lin, D.B.; Ueng, K.C.; Kuo, S.H.; Chen, C.C.; Lee, M.C. Clinical outcomes and prognostic factors for patients with *Vibrio vulnificus* infections requiring intensive care: A 10-yr retrospective study. *Crit. Care Med.* **2010**, *38*, 1984–1990. [CrossRef]
19. DePaola, A.; Hopkins, L.H.; Peeler, J.T.; Wentz, B.; McPhearson, R.M. Incidence of *Vibrio parahaemolyticus* in US coastal waters and oysters. *Appl. Environ. Microbiol.* **1990**, *56*, 2299–2302. [CrossRef]
20. Archer, E.J.; Baker-Austin, C.; Osborn, T.J.; Jones, N.R.; Martínez-Urtaza, J.; Trinanes, J.; Oliver, J.D.; González, F.J.C.; Lake, I.R. Climate warming and increasing *Vibrio vulnificus* infections in North America. *Sci. Rep.* **2023**, *13*, 3893. [CrossRef]
21. Shapiro, R.L.; Altekruse, S.; Hutwagner, L.; Bishop, R.; Hammond, R.; Wilson, S.; Ray, B.; Thompson, S.; Tauxe, R.V.; Griffin, P.M. The role of Gulf Coast oysters harvested in warmer months in *Vibrio vulnificus* infections in the United States, 1988–1996. *J. Infect. Dis.* **1998**, *178*, 752–759. [CrossRef]
22. Wei, X.; Ma, H.; Liu, R.; Zhao, Y. Comparing the effectiveness of three scoring systems in predicting adult patient outcomes in the emergency department. *Medicine* **2019**, *98*, e14289. [CrossRef]
23. Chang, S.H.; Hsieh, C.H.; Weng, Y.M.; Hsieh, M.S.; Goh, Z.N.L.; Chen, H.Y.; Chang, T.; Ng, C.J.; Seak, J.C.; Seak, C.K.; et al. Performance assessment of the mortality in emergency department sepsis score, modified early warning score, rapid emergency medicine score, and rapid acute physiology score in predicting survival outcomes of adult renal abscess patients in the emergency department. *Biomed. Res. Int.* **2018**, *2018*, 6983568.
24. Chuang, Y.C.; Yuan, C.Y.; Liu, C.Y.; Lan, C.K.; Huang, A.H. *Vibrio vulnificus* infectionin Taiwan: Report of 28 cases and review of clinical manifestations and treatment. *Clin. Infect. Dis.* **1992**, *15*, 271–276. [CrossRef] [PubMed]
25. Dechet, A.M.; Yu, P.A.; Koram, N.; Painter, J. Nonfoodborne *Vibrio* infections: An important cause of morbidity and mortality in the United States, 1997–2006. *Clin. Infect. Dis.* **2008**, *46*, 970–976. [CrossRef]

26. Li, X.; Wu, Y.; Sun, X.; Ma, J.; Li, X.; Liu, C.; Xie, H. Non-O1/non-O139 *Vibrio cholera* bacteraemia in mainland China from 2005 to 2019: Clinical, epidemiological and genetic characteristics. *Epidemiol. Infect.* **2020**, *148*, e186. [CrossRef] [PubMed]
27. Zhang, X.; Lu, Y.; Qian, H.; Liu, G.; Mei, Y.; Jin, F.; Xia, W.; Ni, F. Non-O1, Non-O139 *Vibrio cholerae* (NOVC) bacteremia: Case report and literature review, 2015–2019. *Infect. Drug Resist.* **2020**, *13*, 1009–1016. [CrossRef]
28. Blake, P.A.; Merson, M.H.; Weaver, R.E.; Hollis, D.G.; Heublein, P.C. Disease caused by a marine *Vibrio*: Clinical characteristics and epidemiology. *N. Engl. J. Med.* **1979**, *300*, 1–5. [CrossRef]
29. Kitaura, S.; Okamoto, K.; Wakabayashi, Y.; Okada, Y.; Okazaki, A.; Ikeda, M.; Hakuta, R.; Nakai, Y.; Okugawa, S.; Koike, K.; et al. *Vibrio fluvialis* liver abscess and bacteremia in a sashimi lover: A case report and review of the literature. *Open Forum Infect. Dis.* **2020**, *7*, ofaa212. [CrossRef]
30. Williams, C.D.; Stengel, J.; Asike, M.I.; Torres, D.M.; Shaw, J.; Contreras, M.; Landt, C.L.; Harrison, S.A. Prevalence of nonalcoholic fatty liver disease and nonalcoholic steatohepatitis among a largely middle-aged population utilizing ultrasound and liver biopsy: A prospective study. *Gastroenterology* **2011**, *140*, 124–131. [CrossRef]
31. Liu, J.W.; Lee, I.K.; Tang, H.J.; Ko, W.C.; Lee, H.C.; Liu, Y.C.; Hsueh, P.R.; Chuang, Y.C. Prognostic factors and antibiotics in *Vibrio vulnificus* septicemia. *Arch. Intern. Med.* **2006**, *166*, 2117–2123. [CrossRef] [PubMed]
32. Rangel-Frausto, M.S.; Pittet, D.; Costigan, M.; Hwang, T.; Davis, C.S.; Wenzel, R.P. The natural history of the systemic inflammatory response syndrome (SIRS): A prospective study. *JAMA* **1995**, *273*, 117–123. [CrossRef] [PubMed]
33. Singer, M.; Deutschman, C.S.; Seymour, C.W.; Shankar-Hari, M.; Annane, D.; Bauer, M.; Bellomo, R.; Bernard, G.R.; Chiche, J.D.; Coopersmith, C.M.; et al. The third international consensus definitions for sepsis and septic shock (Sepsis-3). *JAMA* **2016**, *315*, 801–810. [CrossRef] [PubMed]
34. Lerstloompleephunt, N.; Tantawichien, T.; Sitprija, V. Renal failure in *Vibrio vulnificus* infection. *Ren. Fail.* **2000**, *22*, 337–343. [CrossRef] [PubMed]
35. Neveu, H.; Kleinknecht, D.; Brivet, F.; Loirat, P.; Landais, P. Prognostic factors in, acute renal failure due to sepsis. Results of a prospective multicentre study. *Nephrol. Dial. Transplant.* **1996**, *11*, 293–299. [CrossRef] [PubMed]
36. daSilva, L.V.; Ossai, S.; Chigbu, P.; Parveen, S. Antimicrobial and genetic profiles of *Vibrio vulnificus* and *Vibrio parahaemolyticus* isolated from the Maryland Coastal Bays, United States. *Front. Microbiol.* **2021**, *12*, 676249.
37. Chen, S.C.; Lee, Y.T.; Tsai, S.J.; Chan, K.S.; Chao, W.N.; Wang, P.H.; Lin, D.B.; Chen, C.C.; Lee, M.C. Antibiotic therapy for necrotizing fasciitis causedby *Vibrio vulnificus*: Retrospective analysis of an 8 year period. *J. Antimicrob. Chemother.* **2012**, *67*, 488–493. [CrossRef] [PubMed]
38. Kim, S.E.; Shin, S.U.; Oh, T.H.; Kim, U.J.; Darboe, K.S.; Kang, S.J.; Jang, H.C.; Jung, S.I.; Shin, H.Y.; Park, K.H. Outcomes of third-generation cephalosporin plus ciprofloxacin or doxycycline therapy in patients with *Vibrio vulnificus* septicemia: A propensity score-matched analysis. *PLoS Negl. Trop. Dis.* **2019**, *13*, e0007478. [CrossRef]
39. Davidson, N.; Edwards, F.; Harris, P.N.A.; Laupland, K.B. *Vibrio* species bloodstream infections in Queensland, Australia. *Intern. Med. J.* **2024**, *54*, 157–163. [CrossRef]
40. Chen, Y.T.; Tang, H.J.; Chao, C.M.; Lai, C.C. Clinical manifestations of non-O1 *Vibrio cholerae* infections. *PLoS ONE* **2015**, *10*, e0116904. [CrossRef]
41. Ruangsomboon, O.; Boonmee, P.; Limsuwat, C.; Chakorn, T.; Monsomboon, A. The utility of the rapid emergency medicine score (REMS) compared with SIRS, qSOFA and NEWS for Predicting in-hospital Mortality among Patients with suspicion of Sepsis in an emergency department. *BMC Emerg. Med.* **2021**, *21*, 2. [CrossRef] [PubMed]
42. Shapiro, N.I.; Wolfe, R.E.; Moore, R.B.; Smith, E.; Burdick, E.; Bates, D.W. Mortality in Emergency Department Sepsis (MEDS) score: A prospectively derived and validated clinical prediction rule. *Crit. Care Med.* **2003**, *31*, 670–675. [CrossRef] [PubMed]
43. Zhang, G.; Zhang, K.; Zheng, X.; Cui, W.; Hong, Y.; Zhang, Z. Performance of the MEDS score in predicting mortality among emergency department patients with a suspected infection: A meta-analysis. *Emerg. Med. J.* **2020**, *37*, 232–239. [CrossRef] [PubMed]
44. Hsieh, C.C.; Yang, C.Y.; Lee, C.H.; Chi, C.H.; Lee, C.C. Validation of MEDS score in predicting short-term mortality of adults with community-onset bacteremia. *Am. J. Emerg. Med.* **2020**, *38*, 282–287. [CrossRef] [PubMed]
45. Zou, X.L.; Feng, D.Y.; Wu, W.B.; Yang, H.L.; Zhang, T.T. Blood urea nitrogen to serum albumin ratio independently predicts 30-day mortality and severity in patients with *Escherichia coli* bacteraemia. *Med. Clin.* **2021**, *157*, 219–225. [CrossRef] [PubMed]
46. Chiang, H.Y.; Chen, T.C.; Lin, C.C.; Ho, L.C.; Kuo, C.C.; Chi, C.Y. Trend and Predictors of Short-term Mortality of Adult Bacteremia at Emergency Departments: A14-Year Cohort Study of 14625 Patients. *Open Forum Infect. Dis.* **2021**, *8*, ofab485. [CrossRef] [PubMed]
47. Li, X.; Zheng, R.; Zhang, T.; Zeng, Z.; Li, H.; Liu, J. Association between blood urea nitrogen and 30-day mortality in patients with sepsis: A retrospective analysis. *Ann. Palliat. Med.* **2021**, *10*, 11653–11663. [CrossRef] [PubMed]
48. Yun, N.R.; Kim, D.M.; Lee, J.; Han, M.A. pH level as a marker for predicting death among patients with *Vibrio vulnificus* infection, South Korea, 2000–2011. *Emerg. Infect. Dis.* **2015**, *21*, 259–264. [CrossRef] [PubMed]
49. Chen, Y.H.; Hsieh, M.S.; Hu, S.Y.; Huang, S.C.; Tsai, C.A.; Tsai, Y.C. Scoring Systems to Evaluate the Mortality Risk of Patients with Emphysematous Cystitis: A Retrospective Observational Study. *J. Pers. Med.* **2023**, *13*, 318. [CrossRef]

50. Seymour, C.W.; Liu, V.X.; Iwashyna, T.J.; Brunkhorst, F.M.; Rea, T.D.; Scherag, A.; Rubenfeld, G.; Kahn, J.M.; Shankar-Hari, M.; Singer, M.; et al. Assessment of clinical criteria for sepsis: For the Third International Consensus Definitions for Sepsis and Septic Shock (Sepsis-3). *JAMA* **2016**, *315*, 762–774. [CrossRef]
51. vanderWulp, I.; Rullmann, H.A.; Leenen, L.P.; vanStel, H.F. Associations of the Emergency Severity Index triage categories with patients'; vital signs at triage: A prospective observational study. *Emerg. Med. J.* **2011**, *28*, 1032–1035. [CrossRef] [PubMed]

Journal of
Personalized Medicine

MDPI

Article

A Clinical Prediction Model for Personalised Emergency Department Discharge Decisions for Residential Care Facility Residents Post-Fall

Gigi Guan [1,*], Kadison Michel [2], Charlie Corke [3,4] and Geetha Ranmuthugala [1,5]

1 Department of Rural Health, Melbourne Medical School, The University of Melbourne, Shepparton, VIC 3630, Australia; granmuth@une.edu.au
2 Critical Care Unit, Goulburn Valley Health, Shepparton, VIC 3630, Australia; kadison.michel1@gvhealth.org.au
3 School of Medicine, Deakin University, Geelong, VIC 3220, Australia; charlie.corke@deakin.edu.au
4 Critical Care Units, Barwon Health, Geelong, VIC 3220, Australia
5 School of Rural Medicine, University of New England, Armidale, NSW 2350, Australia
* Correspondence: gigiaus@gmail.com; Tel.: +61-(03)-5823-4500

Abstract

Introduction: Falls are the leading cause of Emergency Department (ED) presentations among residents from residential aged care facilities (RACFs). While most current studies focus on post-fall evaluations and fall prevention, limited research has been conducted on decision-making in post-fall management. **Objective**: To develop and internally validate a model that can predict the likelihood of RACF residents being discharged from the ED after being presented for a fall. **Methods**: The study sample was obtained from a previous study conducted in Shepparton, Victoria, Australia. Consecutive samples were selected from January 2023 to November 2023. Participants aged 65 and over were included in this study. **Results**: A total of 261 fall presentations were initially identified. One patient with Australasian Triage Scale category 1 was excluded to avoid overfitting, leaving 260 presentations for analysis. Two logistic regression models were developed using prehospital and ED variables. The ED predictor model variables included duration of ED stay, injury severity, and the presence of an advance care directive (ACD). It demonstrated excellent discrimination (AUROC = 0.83; 95% CI: 0.79–0.89) compared to the prehospital model (AUROC = 0.77, 95% CI: 0.72–0.83). A simplified four-variable Discharge Eligibility after Fall in Elderly Residents (DEFER) score was derived from the prehospital model. The score achieved an AUROC of 0.76 (95% CI: 0.71–0.82). At a cut-off score of $\geq$5, the DEFER score exhibited a sensitivity of 79.7%, a specificity of 60.3%, a diagnostic odds ratio of 5.96, and a positive predictive value of 85.0%. **Conclusions**: The DEFER score is the first validated discharge prediction model for residents of RACFs who present to the ED after a fall. Importantly, the DEFER score advances personalised medicine in emergency care by integrating patient-specific factors, such as ACDs, to guide individualised discharge decisions for post-fall residents from RACFs.

Keywords: Advance Care Directive (ACD); detection; emergency department (ED); falls; prehospital care; nursing home; personalised medicine; prediction; residential aged care facilities (RACF)

1. Introduction

Falls are the most common reason for residents of residential aged care facilities (RACFs) to be transferred to the emergency department (ED) [1]. Residents who experience a fall are often transferred to the ED for assessment and monitoring. However, such transfers do not always reveal significant medical issues, and many individuals are discharged from the ED and returned to the RACF [2].

Routine transfer of post-fall patients to the ED can have significant consequences, including deterioration and delirium, thus worsening patient outcomes [3]. Additionally, such transfers increase healthcare utilisation and strain the healthcare system, leading to ED overcrowding and ambulance ramping [4]. The decision to transfer post-fall patients to the ED also arises from the absence of effective decision-making models that can guide the process regarding individuals who experience a fall in RACFs [5].

Existing models, such as the Morse Fall Scale and STRATIFY, are designed to identify the risk of falls and help prevent them [6]. They are not designed to facilitate decision-making about discharging post-fall patients from the ED. Models such as the Identification of Seniors at Risk and the Triage Risk Screening Tool assess the long-term vulnerability of post-fall patients but do not guide in deciding whether post-fall patients should remain in the ED or be discharged [7]. Furthermore, early warning system (EWS) scores that utilise physiological parameters, such as the National Early Warning System 2 (NEWS2) and the Modified Early Warning System (MEWS), lack specificity for this cohort of patients and often focus on short-term deterioration rather than facilitating discharge decisions [8,9].

To date, no validated model exists to facilitate decision-making regarding the discharge of RACF residents from the ED after they have been presented for a fall. Such models are essential, as they may assist RACF nursing staff members in managing post-fall patients within RACFs, as well as paramedics and ED staff members in making rapid discharge decisions. They may also reduce healthcare utilisation and admission-related complications and improve patient-centred care.

Furthermore, the current practice of transferring all post-fall patients to the ED does not provide personalised care in RACFs for geriatric patients [2,10]. Tailoring healthcare decisions to individual patient characteristics, is particularly crucial in managing fall-related injuries among RACF residents due to their diverse health profiles and care needs [2].

To address these needs, this study aimed to develop and internally validate a prediction model to determine the likelihood of RACF residents being discharged from the ED after presenting for a fall. This study also developed a simplified scoring system, known as the Discharge Eligibility after Fall in Elderly Residents (DEFER) score, to assess the likelihood of discharge for post-fall patients from the ED. The DEFER score aims to provide a tool that facilitates shared clinical decision-making among RACF nursing staff members, paramedics, and ED teams.

2. Methods

2.1. Design and Data Source

The study sample comprised the full dataset from a previous study conducted at Goulburn Valley Health (GVH) [10]. All patient information was obtained from GVH's digital medical records (DMR). GVH is a rural hospital in Shepparton, 180 km north of Melbourne, Victoria, Australia. The study period was from 1 January 2023, to 19 November 2023.

During data collection, one case was excluded because of incomplete data. This exclusion was deemed to have a negligible impact on the study's validity or findings, and there were no missing data in the analysis dataset. This secondary analysis was conducted with the same ethical approval as the original study, which was retrospectively approved by the GVH Human Research Ethics Committee in 2024 before data collection and analysis. The risk to patients is minimal as this study used a retrospective review of de-identified patient data, with a waiver of consent granted (Approval number: GVH 25-24).

2.2. Population

This study collected data from individuals aged 65 or older who lived in RACFs and had presented to the ED due to fall-related presentations during the study period. Individuals were selected using triage notes, ICD-10 codes, and injury classifications. (Appendix A) This study excluded cases in which the patient died on arrival, the fall occurred outside the RACF (e.g., in the hospital or community), or an external cause (such as a motor vehicle accident) precipitated the fall. (Figure 1. Patient flow) A 10% random data audit showed an inter-rater agreement rate of 99.6%, indicating a robust data extraction process. The sample size was deemed to be sufficient based on the previous study.

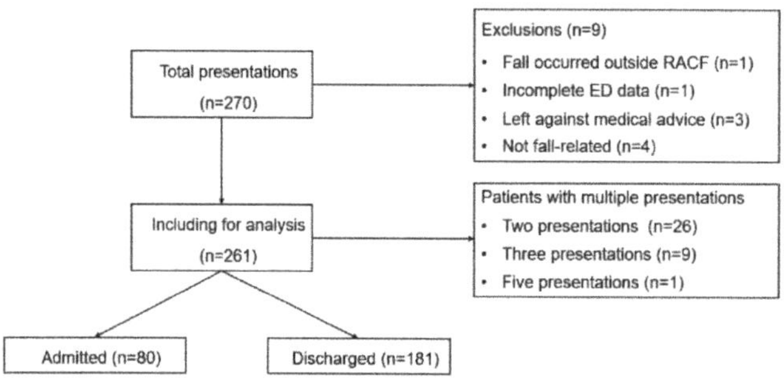

Figure 1. Flow chart of study sample selection.

2.3. Variables

The dependent variable was ED disposition, which was defined as whether the patient was admitted to the ED or discharged. If patients were admitted during an ED stay, the final disposition was from the ED or short-stay unit (an observation unit located within the ED). The key independent variables were injury severity, injury region, presence of an obvious injury, presence of pain, presence of an advance care directive (ACD), and duration of ED stay. In addition, the triage category was collected using the Australian Triage Scale (ATS, which ranges from 1 to 5, where 1 is the most urgent).

Independent variables included: Injury severity, which was classified as major or minor. Fractures, intracranial injuries, multiple injuries, and dislocations were considered major injuries, whereas superficial lacerations, muscle/tendon injuries, sprains/strains, and isolated open wounds were considered minor injuries. The injury region was classified as central or peripheral based on the anatomical region (Appendices B and C). An obvious injury was deemed to be present if there were any visible injuries, including haematoma, bruising, altered consciousness, inability to bear weight, and joint/bone angulation. The presence of pain was ascertained based on triage notes. The presence of an ACD was determined by reviewing triage notes, the ED discharge summary, and documents related to advance care planning. The duration of ED stay was automatically populated by the DMR and calculated from the time of ED presentation to the time of ED discharge or admission for inpatient care. As GVH is not a tertiary hospital, transfers out of GVH for admission or tertiary ED presentations were also included in the admissions count.

2.4. Data Analysis

All statistical analyses were conducted using Stata version 18 SE. For all inferential tests, statistical significance was set at $\alpha = 0.05$. Patient characteristics, as described in the ED, were compared for model development.

2.5. Model Development and Selection Strategy

Using Transparent reporting of a multivariable prediction model for individual prognosis or diagnosis as a guide, this study constructed prehospital and ED models using the respective variables in each setting. Only one case had an ATS triage level 1; therefore, it was excluded from data analysis to avoid overfitting.

Due to the small sample size and to avoid overfitting, multiple statistical methods were used in the model development. Initially, multivariate logistic regression was conducted to exclude non-significant variables. Then, the selection of remaining variables was refined using multiple complementary methods, including backward, forward, and stepwise selection, as well as likelihood ratio tests ($p < 0.05$), to ensure parsimony and model robustness. LASSO regression, which applies regularisation to shrink noninformative coefficients, was also used. In addition, we limited the number of predictors relative to the number of events and performed ten-fold cross-validation to evaluate model stability and generalisability. These steps were explicitly undertaken to minimise overfitting given the modest sample size.

Furthermore, a block-wise nested model testing approach was used to assess the incremental contributions of added variable blocks to the model's performance. For each modelling strategy, discrimination and model fit were compared using the area under the receiver operating characteristic curve (AUROC), the Akaike information criterion (AIC), and the Bayesian information criterion (BIC). The final model for each setting was selected based on discrimination, simplicity, and internal stability. In this study, AUROC values between 0.60 and 0.69, 0.70 and 0.79, 0.80 and 0.89, and 0.90 and 1.0 indicated poor, acceptable, good, and excellent discriminatory powers of the outcome, respectively [8].

2.6. Model Evaluation and Internal Validation

Model discrimination was assessed using AUROC with 95% confidence intervals (CIs). The DeLong test was used to compare the significance of the two models [11]. Model calibration was evaluated using the Hosmer–Lemeshow goodness-of-fit test and by visually inspecting calibration plots that compared predicted and observed discharge rates across deciles. The predictive accuracy was further assessed using the Brier score, which was decomposed into components of reliability, resolution, and uncertainty. Classification metrics based on a 0.5 threshold were used to evaluate model performance, including sensitivity, specificity, positive and negative likelihood ratios (LR^+, LR^-), and diagnostic odds ratios (DORs). Ten-fold cross-validation was conducted to estimate the internal validity of the models. Odds ratios (ORs) were monitored for consistency, and multicollinearity was assessed using variance inflation factors (VIFs) to ensure model stability. Model sensitivity, specificity, and positive and negative predictive value (PPV, NPV) were also reported. To reduce the risk of overfitting with the modest sample size, we performed internal validation using 1,000 bootstrap replications. Model performance (AUROC) from each resample was compared with the original sample to calculate optimism-corrected AUROC and 95% CI. Finally, clinical utility was examined using decision curve analysis (DCA), which quantified the net benefit across varying decision thresholds.

2.7. Derivation of the DEFER Score

After validating the prehospital model, the final prehospital logistic regression model was converted into a four-variable scoring system for its application in clinical practice. The variable selection process is the same as that for the ED/prehospital model selection, including backward, forward, stepwise selection, and LASSO regression. The predictor variables retained in the final prehospital model were converted into integer-point values by scaling and rounding the original logistic regression coefficients. Higher DEFER scores are intentionally aligned with a greater likelihood of safe discharge.

This transformation preserved each variable's relative predictive contribution while enabling easy calculation in a clinical setting. It also led to the creation of the DEFER score, which ranges from 2 to 9. The point allocation reflects reduced clinical severity and fewer significant findings (e.g., minor injuries, absence of obvious injuries, or the presence of an ACD), which collectively indicate that the patient is more likely to be managed within RACF settings.

2.8. Evaluation of the Performance of the DEFER Score

The DEFER score was subjected to the same tests as the original ED/prehospital model to assess its discriminatory performance, calibration, and clinical utility. The AUROC, Brier score, Hosmer–Lemeshow goodness-of-fit, ten-fold cross-validation, DCA, and DOR were redetermined for the DEFER score. Although the Liu method identifies a cut-off point of 5.5, we selected a threshold of $\geq$5 for the DEFER score due to its clinical interpretability and superior predictive value in identifying patients suitable for discharge from the ED [12]. Consequently, the patients were divided into two groups based on the total score calculated from specific variables: low discharge-likelihood group (<5) and high discharge-likelihood group ($\geq$5).

3. Results

A total of 261 RACF presentations occurred during the study period. 69.4% were discharged from ED (n = 181) and 30.6% were admitted for inpatient care (n = 80). The discharged patients were more likely to have ACD, minor injuries, peripheral injuries, and lower ATS triage levels ($p < 0.05$ for all variables). Other factors, such as the use of anticoagulants ($p = 0.75$) and computer tomography brain imaging ($p = 0.14$), did not vary significantly between the two groups (Table 1).

3.1. Model Development and Discriminative Performance

After removing one case with triage level 1, 260 presentations were analysed. The ED and prehospital models were developed using logistic regression and multiple variable selection processes. Using variables exclusively available at first clinical contact, the prehospital model retained four predictors: injury severity, presence of an obvious injury, presence of an ACD, and presence of pain. The ED model incorporated information available after in-hospital assessment and included three predictors: duration of ED stays (a post hoc predictor), injury severity, and presence of an ACD (Table 2).

Table 1. Characteristics of ED presentations following falls in RACFs by discharge status (n = 261).

Characteristics of ED Presentations				
	Total	Discharged	Admitted	p Value
	261	**181 (69.4%)**	**80 (30.6%)**	
Age, median (max-min)	87 (66–101)	87 (68–101)	86 (66–101)	0.538 †
Prior medical review	50	37 (74.0%)	13 (26.0%)	0.428
First Nations status	9	6 (66.7%)	3 (33.3%)	0.819
Duration of ED stay (mean minutes, SD)	629.8 (450.7)	485.1 (368.2)	956.9 (450.9)	**<0.001**
Use of anticoagulant or antiplatelet agents	156	107 (68.6%)	49 (31.4%)	0.746
Female	166	115 (69.3%)	51 (30.7%)	0.974
Mode of Presentation, *n* (%)				
Ambulance	250	172 (68.8%)	78 (31.2%)	0.359
Private vehicle	11	9 (81.82%)	2 (18.18%)	
ATS, *n* (%)				
ATS-1 Immediate	1	1 (100%)	0 (0%)	
ATS-2 Time-Critical	17	8 (47.1%)	9 (52.9%)	
ATS-3 Urgent	216	149 (69.0%)	67 (31.0%)	**0.028**
ATS-4 Potential	27	23 (85.2%)	4 (14.8%)	
Injury Severity, *n* (%)				
Major	132	73 (55.3%)	59 (44.7%)	**<0.001**
Minor	129	108 (83.7%)	21(16.3%)	
Body Injury Region, *n* (%)				
Central	180	48 (26.7%)	132 (73.3%)	**<0.001**
Peripheral	81	49 (60.5%)	32 (39.5%)	
ACD, *n* (%)				
Presence of ACD	115	91 (79.1%)	24 (20.9%)	**<0.001**
Advised transfer to ED	53	9 (17.0%)	44 (83.0%)	0.719 ‡
Against transfer to ED	15	3 (20.0%)	12 (80.0%)	
ED Triage Notes, *n* (%)				
Fall	257	177 (68.9%)	80 (31.1%)	0.316 ‡
Obvious injuries	140	85 (60.7%)	55 (39.3%)	**<0.001**
Head strike	71	52 (73.2%)	19 (26.8%)	0.405
CTB, *n* (%)				
Had CTB	192	138 (71.9%)	54 (28.1%)	0.140
Normal CTB results	180	133 (73.9%)	47 (26.1%)	**<0.001 ‡**
Abnormal CTB results	11	4 (36.4%)	7 (63.6%)	

Bold text in the p values indicates $p < 0.05$. † Mann–Whitney U-test; ‡ Fisher's exact test. All other p-values were calculated using the chi-square test. $p < 0.05$ was considered statistically significant. Abbreviations: ACD = Advance Care Directive; CTB = computerised tomography brain scan; ATS = Australasian Triage Scale.

Table 2. Multivariate logistic regression analysis of factors associated with emergency department discharge following fall-related presentations from residential aged care facilities (n = 260) p value in bold indicates $p < 0.05$.

Variable	Adjusted Odds Ratio	95% CI (Lower-Upper)	p Value
Presence of ACD	2.8877	**1.3773–6.0543**	**0.005**
ATS	2.6892	**1.0634–6.8008**	**0.037**
CTB performed	2.1835	0.9149–5.2114	0.078
Body injury region (Central vs. Peripheral)	1.5383	0.6699–3.5328	0.310
Sex (Male vs. Female)	1.2519	0.5914–2.6501	0.557
Fall was documented in the triage notes	1.1072	0.5694–2.1530	0.764
Age	1.0130	0.9637–1.0649	0.611
Prior medical review	0.9013	0.3597–2.2582	0.824
First Nations status	0.7013	0.2493–1.9728	0.501
Anticoagulant/antiplatelet use	0.6380	0.3079–1.3222	0.227
Head strike in triage notes	0.8394	0.3586–1.9644	0.686
Pain was documented in the triage notes	0.4802	0.2079–1.1091	0.086
ED duration (minutes)	0.9974	**0.9966–0.9983**	**<0.001**
Obvious injury	0.2393	**0.1022–0.5603**	**0.001**
Injury severity	0.2004	**0.0941–0.4270**	**<0.001**

Outcome variable: ED disposition (vs. admission). Abbreviations: ACD = Advance Care Directive; CTB = computerised tomography brain; CI = Confidence Interval; ATS = Australian Triage Scale. The model was adjusted for age, sex, injury severity, CTB findings, ACD presence, and other covariates as listed. Values represent adjusted odds ratios from a multivariate logistic regression model. Bold text in 95% CI (Lower-Upper) indicates aOR did not cross 1.

The ED model (AUROC = 0.83; 95% CI: 0.79–0.89) and the prehospital model (AUROC = 0.77; 95% CI: 0.72–0.83) demonstrated acceptable to excellent discrimination. A comparative analysis using the DeLong test confirmed that the ED model significantly outperformed the prehospital model in distinguishing discharge outcomes ($p = 0.04$) (Figure 2).

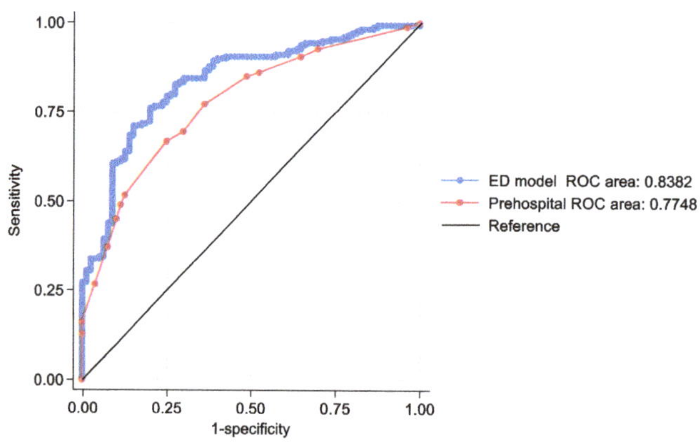

Figure 2. The area under the Receiver operating characteristic (AUROC) curve compares the ED-based model (Blue colour, AUROC 0.83) with the prehospital model (Red colour, AUROC 0.77) in predicting discharge. The ED model curve is above the prehospital model curve, indicating better discrimination.

3.2. Evaluation of Model Performance and Validation

The calibration of both models was acceptable. The Hosmer–Lemeshow goodness-of-fit test showed a non-significant result for both models, indicating the absence of miscalibration. Specifically, the ED model showed χ^2 (8) = 12.21, $p = 0.14$, while the prehospital model showed χ^2 (7) = 2.23, $p = 0.95$. Visual inspection of the calibration plots revealed close agreement between the predicted and observed probabilities in the ED model, whereas the prehospital model showed a modest overprediction (Appendix D).

According to the Brier scores, the predictive accuracy was better in the ED model (0.15) than in the prehospital model (0.17). The decomposition of this score showed greater resolution (0.06 vs. 0.04) and higher reliability (0.006 vs. 0.001) in the ED model, as well as equivalent uncertainty (0.21) across both models. Classification metrics based on a 0.5 threshold further highlighted the differences in the performance of the two models. The ED model showed a sensitivity of 90.6%, specificity of 56.3%, LR^+ of 2.07, LR^- of 0.17, and DOR of 12.33. Meanwhile, the prehospital model showed a sensitivity of 86.1%, specificity of 47.5%, LR^+ of 1.64, LR^- of 0.29, and DOR of 5.61.

Ten-fold cross-validation revealed good results for both models. The ED model exhibited a mean AUROC of 0.84, whereas the prehospital model showed a mean AUROC of 0.73. The predictor coefficients remained stable across folds, and no evidence of multicollinearity was detected. Internal validation using 1,000 non-parametric bootstrap methods showed the AUROC of the ED model was 0.84 (95% CI: 0.79–0.89; bootstrap standard error 0.03, $p < 0.001$), while the prehospital model had an AUROC of 0.78 (95% CI: 0.71–0.84; bootstrap standard error 0.0309, $p < 0.001$). The DCA demonstrated that both models provided greater net benefits than default strategies ('treat all' or 'treat none') across clinically relevant thresholds. The ED model performed marginally better than the prehospital model (Appendix E).

3.3. Derivation and Performance of the DEFER Score

The final prehospital model was translated into a simplified scoring system to support clinical implementation. This system comprised the DEFER score, which was calculated based on four predictors: injury severity, presence of an obvious injury, presence of an ACD, and presence of pain at the time of examination. Each assigned weighted-point value was based on the scaled regression coefficients.

The scoring algorithm and component weights are listed in Table 3. We assigned 2 points for a minor injury, 0 points for a major injury, 2 points for the absence of an obvious injury, 0 points for the presence of an obvious injury, 2 points for the absence of pain, 1 point for the presence of pain, 3 points for the presence of an ACD, and 1 point for the absence of an ACD. Consequently, the total score ranged from 2 to 9 (Table 3), and higher scores indicated an increased likelihood of ED discharge.

Patients were divided into two groups based on their discharge likelihood scores. The observed discharge rates for the low and high discharge-likelihood groups were 39.7% and 79.7%, respectively, reflecting clinically meaningful differences in discharge probability. For example, consider a 75-year-old RACF resident who presents after a fall with a minor lower limb laceration only (+2 points), no obvious external injuries such as fractures (+2 points), an existing advance care directive in place (+3 points), and reports pain on the laceration site only (+1 point). The total DEFER score would be 2 + 2 + 3 + 1 = 8 points. A score of 8 is $\geq$5, indicating a high likelihood of safe discharge, which means the patient can typically be managed in the RACF setting with appropriate follow-up rather than requiring hospital admission.

Table 3. Variables and points allocation in the DEFER score.

Variable	Condition	Points
Injury severity	Minor injury	+2
	Major injury	0
Obvious injury	No obvious injury	+2
	Obvious injury	0
Advance Care Directive	Present	+3
	Absent	+1
Pain on examination	Absent	+2
	Present	+1
	Total DEFER Score (Range: 2 to 9)	
Interpretation	Score ≥5	Increased likelihood of safe discharge
	Score <5	Consider further evaluation or admission

Post DEFER score testing, an AUROC of 0.76 (95% CI: 0.71–0.82) was achieved. The Hosmer–Lemeshow goodness-of-fit test showed non-significant results (χ^2 (5) = 2.44, p = 0.79), indicating the absence of miscalibration between the predicted and observed discharge outcomes. With a cross-validated AUROC of 0.74 (95% CI: 0.68–0.81), the DEFER score showed robust internal validity and confirmed good discriminative performance across subsamples. The DEFER score also demonstrated good calibration with a cross-validated Brier score of 0.18. A calibration plot based on the decile grouping of the predicted probabilities revealed a close alignment between the predicted and observed discharge rates, indicating reliable probabilistic performance across risk strata (Appendix F). Furthermore, the DeLong test demonstrated that the DEFER score achieved comparable discrimination to the prehospital model (χ^2 (1) = 1.38, p = 0.24).

Although Liu's method identified a mathematically optimal cut-off score of 5.5, the DEFER score is an integer-based tool. Thus, a sensitivity analysis was conducted at these thresholds, including cut-off scores of ≥5 and ≥6, and using Liu's method at a cut-off score of 5.5. At cut-off score ≥5, the DEFER score achieved a sensitivity of 79.7% (95% CI: 73.3–85.1%), specificity of 60.3% (95% CI: 47.7–72.0%), PPV of 85.0% (95% CI: 78.9–89.9%), and NPV of 51.2% (95% CI: 39.8–62.6%). This threshold provided the best balance for identifying patients suitable for discharge.

At cut-off score ≥6, sensitivity increased to 87.5% (95% CI: 79.9–93.0%) but specificity dropped to 44.6% (95% CI: 36.4–53.0%), with PPV declining to 54.4% (95% CI: 46.9–61.9%) and NPV improving to 82.5% (95% CI: 72.4–90.1%). This lower specificity results in more false positives at the cut-off score of ≥6. This indicates that patients who score high on the DEFER may still require hospital admission. In this context, false positives are less desirable than false negatives, as failing to provide ED-level care to patients who require inpatient care could result in missed treatment opportunities or delayed detection of deterioration.

The Liu method's cut-off score of 5.5 achieved a specificity of 82% and a sensitivity of 54%, but PPV and NPV were not reported. This threshold would miss nearly half of the true discharges, limiting the tool's usefulness. For the above reasons, the cut-off score ≥5 was selected as a clinically practical cut-off score, optimised as a rule-in tool that balances sensitivity and specificity while minimising the risk of inappropriate discharge. At the cut-off score ≥5, the DEFER score crosses a broad range of threshold probabilities (0.4–0.7) (Appendix G).

4. Discussion

4.1. Key Findings

The prediction model developed from ED and prehospital settings can be used to determine the likelihood of an RACF resident being discharged from the ED after a fall-related presentation. When comparing the two models, the prehospital model demonstrated a lower AUROC (0.77) than the ED model (0.83). Variables such as frailty, comorbidities, and cognitive status—known to influence fall outcomes—were omitted because they were not available in the dataset. This absence likely reflects that such assessments are not consistently documented in RACF records or prehospital settings, which may limit the generalisability of the prehospital model.

The newly developed and internally valid DEFER score is novel and innovative. The four-variable aggregate score ensures user friendliness while demonstrating good predictive power. The DEFER score supports more efficient resource allocation and improves patient-centred care by accurately identifying patients who may be rapidly discharged from the ED or managed within the RACF. Before this study, no validated tool existed to guide ED discharge decisions for RACF residents transferred to the ED after a fall.

The variables included in the DEFER score facilitate rapid decision-making in environments where access to physiological data is limited or absent. The discovery of ACD as a predictor for discharge decision-making highlights the importance of patients' wishes in medical care. Incorporating patients' wishes enables patient-centred care and may drive system-wide improvements in healthcare efficiency for RACF residents experiencing falls.

4.2. Clinical Utility of the DEFER Score

Unlike other EWS scores, such as NEWS2 or MEWS, the DEFER score uses non-physiological parameters [9]. The variables included in this score are often accessible during decision-making, making the DEFER score a pragmatic solution for discharge decision-making in settings where diagnostic infrastructure is unavailable or limited. This score may streamline ED disposition decisions and help prevent avoidable admissions, offering significant value to resource-constrained rural hospitals.

The DEFER score may be integrated into inter-professional communication to ensure the best outcomes for RACF residents who experience a fall. Integrating the handover process among RACF nursing staff members, paramedics, and the ED team can facilitate a shared decision-making process that aligns with patients' wishes. When the DEFER score $\geq$5, it supports the decision to discharge; such patients may be safely cared for within the RACFs.

However, to manage residents within the RACF, facilities must ensure appropriate medical follow-up (for instance, by using telehealth consultations or medical reviews) and monitor the patients for delayed complications [13]. Implementing our model in practice would entail strengthening the care capabilities of RACFs and improving communication with ED and ambulance services.

In practice, a DEFER score of $\geq$5 indicates approximately an 80% chance that the patient can be discharged safely, whereas a score of $<$5 suggests caution and likely admission. However, integrating key clinical exclusions, such as unstable vital signs or concerning injuries, may enhance safety and sensitivity, especially for paramedics or RACF staff deciding whether an ED transfer is required. This is because the DEFER score was optimised for specificity and PPV and intended to function as a rule-in tool for discharge rather than as a broad screening instrument.

4.3. Other Factors Influencing Discharge

Discharge decisions, the management of patients within RACFs, and long-term fall outcomes are often complex in RACF settings [14]. Moreover, several complex conditions must be considered among RACF residents, such as existing comorbidities, frailty, cognitive changes, and, more importantly, post-fall physiological changes [15,16]. Thus, like any other EWS score, the DEFER score alone cannot predict post-fall outcomes in a real clinical context.

Variables in the DEFER score, such as pain and injury severity, may indirectly reflect a resident's physiological reserve or frailty [17]. When in doubt, a lower score should be assigned, particularly in the presence of pain. ACDs often reflect care preferences linked to cognitive or functional decline [18]. While the DEFER score prioritises feasibility, essential in fast-paced or resource-limited settings, this focus limits its ability to address more complex cases.

Like all other predictive scores, the DEFER score should complement clinical judgement, not replace it. The DEFER score is designed not to reassure clinicians but to improve decision-making by highlighting cases where discharge is highly likely and further ED care may not be needed. Current post-fall protocols often reassure clinicians by over-investigating rather than improving patient outcomes by providing patient-centred care [19]. Importantly, the DEFER score is intended to be integrated within multidisciplinary workflows involving RACF staff, paramedics, and ED clinicians, rather than applied in isolation. It is designed to inform, not replace, clinical judgement—particularly in cases where abnormal vital signs, clinical instability, or other red-flag features are present. In such situations, clinical teams should prioritise comprehensive assessment and individualised decision-making, using the DEFER score as a supportive guide rather than a sole determinant.

While including ACDs in the DEFER score supports alignment with documented preferences, variability in ACD documentation and interpretation presents an ongoing challenge [18]. Documentation of ACDs can vary between RACFs, pre-hospital records, and ED settings, potentially limiting the reliability of this predictor. Strategies to address this include standardising ACD forms across services, implementing electronic health record integration so that ACDs are accessible in real time, and providing staff training on routine ACD verification and recording during transfers. Such measures could improve consistency and further enhance the applicability of the DEFER score across various settings. Clinicians should be aware that broader systemic or behavioural factors, including clinician risk tolerance, institutional policies, and family expectations, may influence discharge decisions in such models.

4.4. Advancing Personalised Medicine in Emergency Care with the DEFER Score

With the development of the DEFER score, along with recent advancements in personalised medicine, this study emphasises that the "one size fits all" approach should not be applied in healthcare.

Recognising that individuals, particularly geriatric patients, have differences in genetics, lifestyle, and, more importantly, individuals' preferences, which all have an impact on health outcomes [20]. Standardised protocols often failed to address the diverse needs of patients, particularly patients from RACFs who had fallen. The DEFER score is a pioneering tool designed to predict the likelihood of safe discharge for these patients by incorporating non-physiological parameters, such as ACD. By integrating ACDs, the DEFER score ensures that discharge decisions align with patients' values and wishes, fostering a patient-centred approach that respects individual preferences. This personalised strategy has the potential to reduce unnecessary hospitalisations, which can be costly and exacerbate health decline in frail elderly patients.

Current research has demonstrated that personalised geriatric medicine can reduce hospitalisation, which in turn, improves health outcomes [21]. Similarly, the DEFER score aims to optimise resource use and enhance patient outcomes by facilitating timely, individualised discharge decisions. The score's simplicity and practicality make it particularly suited for the fast-paced ED environment, where time constraints and high patient volumes often hinder the implementation of personalised care. In addition, in resource-limited settings, such as prehospital and within RACFs, the DEFER score serves a crucial and valuable purpose in facilitating the decision-making process.

By providing a quick, straightforward method to incorporate patient-specific information, the DEFER score enables clinicians to make informed, efficient, and personalised decisions, addressing a critical gap in emergency care for vulnerable populations.

4.5. Implementation Pathway and Future Research

Future research should focus on external and prospective validation of the DEFER score in diverse settings. This includes other rural, regional, and metropolitan healthcare settings, particularly those with limited access to out-of-hospital care. Additionally, various state-wide and local post-fall protocols require interstate validation studies. This will help assess generalisability and refine the model's performance. Prospective studies must also address other downstream factors of RACF outcomes, such as readmission, mortality, and patient or family satisfaction.

Integrating existing triage models, paramedic assessment tools, ED decision-making models, and the RACF post-fall screening protocols may enhance the implementation of the DEFER score. In the ED, the DEFER score may facilitate rapid triage decisions and assist junior clinicians and discharge planners by providing structured, evidence-informed support for complex discharge decisions. In prehospital settings, paramedics may use the DEFER score to facilitate more detailed clinical examinations and observations, thereby informing discharge decisions. In RACF settings, nursing staff members can apply the DEFER score after a fall and use the results to guide consultations with general practitioners and ambulance services.

The successful uptake of the DEFER score requires interprofessional education, alignment with existing protocols, and integration with the healthcare system. Future research should explore optimal ways for integrating the DEFER score into clinical workflows, such as incorporating it into ambulance assessment checklists or RACF nursing protocols. It should also measure outcomes, such as reduced transfer rates and patient safety.

5. Strengths and Limitations

The DEFER score is a novel and clinically useful model for predicting discharge outcomes among RACF residents presented to the ED after a fall. This score includes a minimal set of variables—four non-physiological factors—readily available at the bedside, thus facilitating rapid decision-making. Furthermore, the incorporation of ACDs in the score ensures patient-centred care. However, several limitations exist before the widespread application of the DEFER score.

First, this study's inherent retrospective, single-centred design may have limited the generalisability of its findings. While the DEFER score performed well in a rural Australian cohort, external and prospective validation in metropolitan EDs and other rural regions will help determine whether the model is accurate, especially when there are different admission thresholds or RACF resources.

Second, the dataset included only fall-related presentations that were brought to the local ED. Data on patients managed within the RACF or bypassed the local ED was unavailable. Thus, introducing a selection bias may reduce the overall performance of the DEFER score.

Third, 'safe discharge' is a context-sensitive concept influenced by local factors, such as RACF staffing, the availability of medical reviews, risk-averse practices within RACFs, local admission norms, and diagnostic capacity. Consequently, the model's recommendations may not translate uniformly across settings with different care infrastructures.

In addition, our analysis assumed that factors such as pain and obvious injuries were accurately documented. However, in practice, under-documentation may have affected the model's performance. Nevertheless, our comprehensive data extraction process ensured that no missing data was present, which mitigates this concern.

Finally, despite rigorous model selection and validation, the small sample size may have led to overfitting of the model, as other important factors such as comorbidities, frailty, or cognitive status were not included in the subgroup analysis. As a result, the DEFER score may be less applicable in residents with more complex clinical profiles, such as patients with significant comorbidities, marked frailty, or cognitive impairment. In these cases, additional clinical assessment and multidisciplinary input remain essential, and the score should be interpreted with caution.

6. Conclusions

The prediction model developed from prehospital and ED settings effectively guides ED discharge decisions for RACF residents presented to the ED after a fall. Such models can also determine whether a patient can be managed within RACFs. Using four easily obtainable variables, the newly developed DEFER score has a good discriminative effect on decision-making. Notably, the inclusion of ACD ensures that discharge decisions are aligned with each patient's unique preferences and values, thereby advancing personalised medicine in emergency care settings. This patient-centred approach is particularly crucial for elderly patients, who often have complex care needs and specific wishes regarding treatments, fostering respect for patients' autonomy and enhancing care quality. However, prospective studies are needed to confirm these results. Future studies should focus on the external validation of the DEFER score and its integration into clinical workflows to maximise its impact on RACFs and policies. The broader implementation of the DEFER score has the potential to deliver system-level benefits, including reducing unnecessary hospital admissions, optimising the use of limited healthcare resources, and enhancing patient and family satisfaction with care.

Author Contributions: Conceptualization: G.G.; Methodology: G.G. and G.R.; Data curation: G.G. and K.M.; Formal analysis: G.G. and G.R.; Investigation: G.G. and K.M.; Validation: G.G. and K.M.; Project administration: G.G. and C.C.; Writing—original draft preparation: G.G.; Writing—review and editing: G.G., C.C. and G.R.; Supervision: C.C. and G.R. All authors have read and agreed to the published version of the manuscript.

Funding: This research received no external funding.

Institutional Review Board Statement: The study was conducted in accordance with the Declaration of Helsinki, and approved by the Goulburn Valley Health Human Research Ethics Committee (Approval number: GVH 25-24; 9 August 2024).

Informed Consent Statement: The Goulburn Valley Health Human Research Ethics Committee granted a waiver of consent for this study.

Data Availability Statement: Data is available upon reasonable request to the corresponding author.

Acknowledgments: We would like to acknowledge the Goulburn Valley Health for the ongoing contribution to this research.

Conflicts of Interest: The authors declare no conflicts of interest for this paper.

Appendix A. Inclusion Criteria

1. ICD-10 with a fall-related presentation in either primary or secondary diagnosis.

- W00-W19: Falls.
- R29.6: Tendency to fall, not elsewhere classified.
- X59: Exposure to unspecified factor causing other and unspecified injury.
- R26: Abnormalities of gait and mobility.
- R42: Dizziness and giddiness.
- H81: Disorders of vestibular function.
- R55: Syncope and collapse.
- W25: Contact with sharp glass fall involving glass.

2. If, based on documentation from the ED notes, the injury's cause was due to a fall.

Appendix B. Injury Severity

Major Injuries:

- Fracture
- Intracranial Injury
- Multiple Injuries
- Dislocation
- Crushing Injury

Minor Injuries:

- Superficial
- Laceration
- Muscle/Tendon Injury
- Sprain/Strain
- Open Wound

Appendix C. Body Injury Location (Central vs. Peripheral)

Based on the criteria below and anatomical location, the body injury locations were classified as central or peripheral. Patients with central and peripheral injuries were classified as having a central injury.

Central classification:

- Hip;
- Back, lower (includes loin);
- Face;
- Neck;
- Abdomen;
- Pelvis (includes anogenital, perineum);
- Thorax;
- Head.

Peripheral body region:

- Knee;
- Ankle;
- Leg, lower;
- Shoulder;

- Forearm;
- Hand (includes fingers);
- Elbow;
- Foot (includes toes);
- Wrist;
- Thigh;
- Upper arm

Appendix D. Calibration Plots for the ED and Prehospital Models

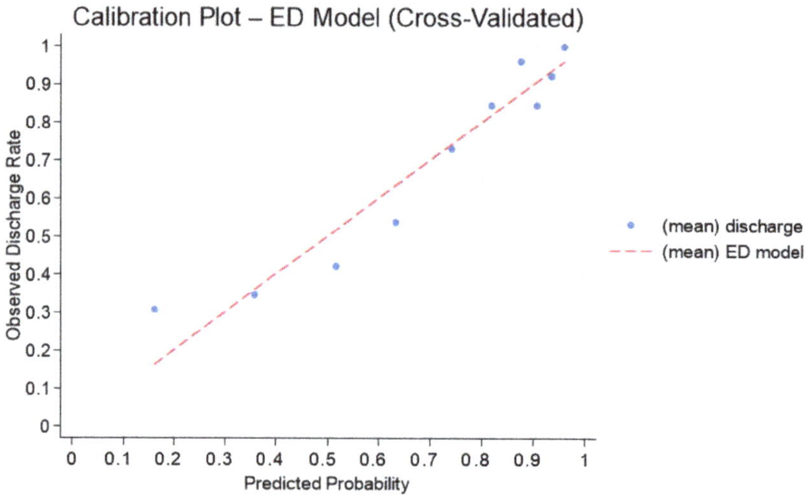

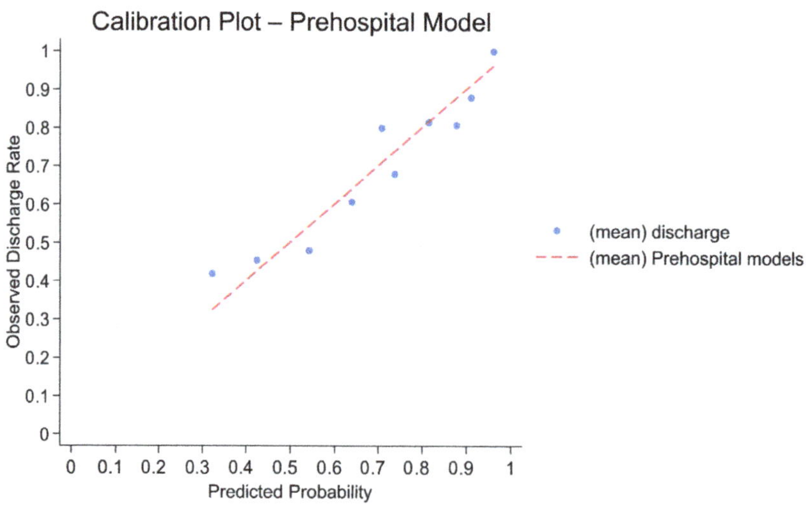

Appendix E. Decision Curve Analysis Plot for the ED Model and Prehospital Model

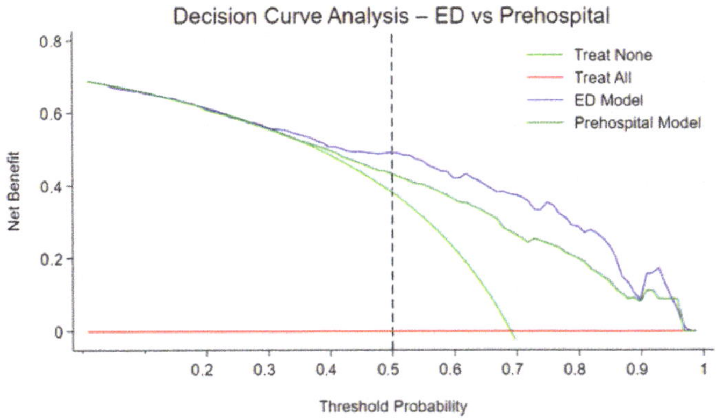

Appendix F. Calibration Plots for the DEFER and Prehospital Models

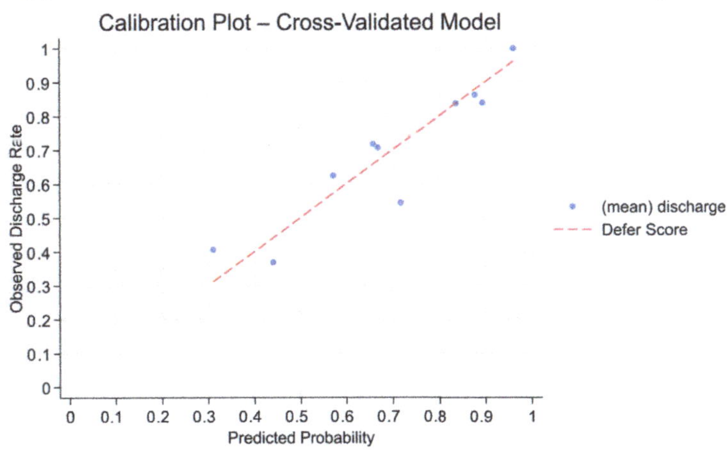

Appendix G. Decision Curve Analysis Plot for DEFER Score at a Cut-Off of 5

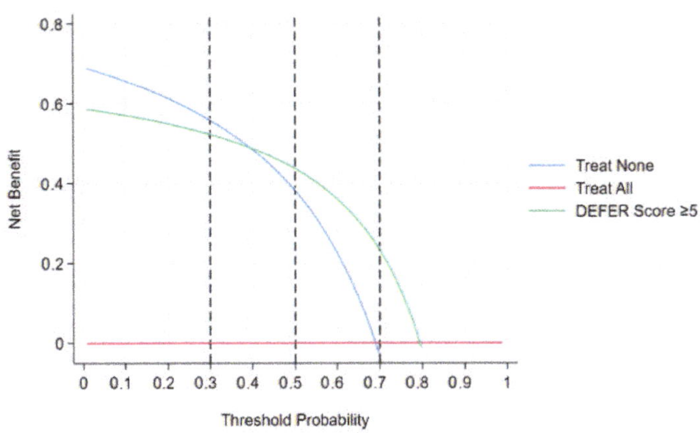

References

1. Wabe, N.; Seaman, K.L.; Nguyen, A.D.; Siette, J.; Raban, M.Z.; Hibbert, P.; Close, J.C.T.; Lord, S.R.; Westbrook, J.I. Epidemiology of falls in 25 Australian residential aged care facilities: A retrospective longitudinal cohort study using routinely collected data. *Int. J. Qual. Health Care* **2022**, *34*, mzac050. [CrossRef]
2. Gullick, D.; Islam, M.R. Exploring avoidable presentations from residential aged care facilities to the emergency department of a large regional Australian hospital. *Aust. J. Rural Health* **2023**, *31*, 514–521. [CrossRef]
3. Li, K.Y.; Gore, J.L.; Phelan, E.A.; Hall, J.; Gunaje, N.; Sabbatini, A.K. Potentially avoidable emergency department transfers among Medicare beneficiaries. *Am. J. Emerg. Med.* **2025**, *88*, 145–151. [CrossRef] [PubMed]
4. Goldberg, E.M.; Marks, S.J.; Resnik, L.J.; Long, S.; Mellott, H.; Merchant, R.C. Can an Emergency Department-Initiated Intervention Prevent Subsequent Falls and Health Care Use in Older Adults? A Randomized Controlled Trial. *Ann. Emerg. Med.* **2020**, *76*, 739–750. [CrossRef]
5. Gurung, A.; Sendall, M.C.; Barnard, A. To transfer or not to transfer: Aged care nurses' decision-making in transferring residents to the emergency department. *Collegian* **2021**, *28*, 162–170. [CrossRef]
6. Strini, V.; Schiavolin, R.; Prendin, A. Fall Risk Assessment Scales: A Systematic Literature Review. *Nurs. Rep.* **2021**, *11*, 430–443. [CrossRef] [PubMed]
7. Gretarsdottir, E.; Jonsdottir, A.B.; Sigurthorsdottir, I.; Gudmundsdottir, E.E.; Hjaltadottir, I.; Jakobsdottir, I.B.; Tomasson, G.; Jonsson, P.V.; Thorsteinsdottir, T. Patients in need of comprehensive geriatric assessment: The utility of the InterRAI emergency department screener. *Int. Emerg. Nurs.* **2021**, *54*, 100943. [CrossRef] [PubMed]
8. Guan, G.; Lee, C.M.Y.; Begg, S.; Crombie, A.; Mnatzaganian, G. Performance of 21 Early Warning System scores in predicting in-hospital deterioration among undifferentiated admitted patients managed by ambulance services. *Emerg. Med. J.* **2024**, *41*, 481–487. [CrossRef] [PubMed]
9. Guan, G.; Lee, C.M.Y.; Begg, S.; Crombie, A.; Mnatzaganian, G. The use of early warning system scores in prehospital and emergency department settings to predict clinical deterioration: A systematic review and meta-analysis. *PLoS ONE* **2022**, *17*, e0265559. [CrossRef] [PubMed]
10. Guan, G.; Ranmuthugala, G.; Michel, K.; Corke, C. Factors Associated with Emergency Department Discharge After Falls in Residential Aged Care Facilities: A Rural Australian Observational Study. *J. Clin. Med.* **2025**, *14*, 3893. [CrossRef] [PubMed]
11. DeLong, E.R.; DeLong, D.M.; Clarke-Pearson, D.L. Comparing the areas under two or more correlated receiver operating characteristic curves: A nonparametric approach. *Biometrics* **1988**, *44*, 837–845. [CrossRef] [PubMed]
12. Liu, H.; Tang, Y.; Zhang, H.H. A new chi-square approximation to the distribution of non-negative definite quadratic forms in non-central normal variables. *Comput. Stat. Data Anal.* **2009**, *53*, 853–856. [CrossRef]
13. Amadoru, S.; Rayner, J.A.; Joseph, R.; Yates, P. Factors influencing decision-making processes for unwell residents in residential aged care: Hospital transfer or Residential InReach referral? *Australas. J. Ageing* **2018**, *37*, E61–E67. [CrossRef] [PubMed]
14. Rameli, P.M.; Rajendran, N. Outcomes of complex discharge planning in older adults with complex needs: A scoping review. *J. Int. Med. Res.* **2022**, *50*, 3000605221110511. [CrossRef] [PubMed]
15. Wilson, N.; Hilmer, S.; March, L.; Cameron, I.; Lord, S.; Mason, R.; Sambrook, P. Physical functioning measures and risk of falling in older people living in residential aged care facilities. *Ther. Adv. Musculoskelet. Dis.* **2011**, *3*, 9–15. [CrossRef] [PubMed]
16. Lee, C.-H.; Chen, Y.-A.; Yang, C.-M.; Huang, K.-H.; Tsai, T.-H.; Chang, Y.; Shieh, S.-H. Risk Factors Associated with Unplanned Hospitalization Among Long-Term Care Facility Residents: A Retrospective Study in Central Taiwan. *Healthcare* **2024**, *12*, 2069. [CrossRef] [PubMed]
17. Pecheva, M.; Phillips, M.; Hull, P.; Carrothers A, O.L.R.; Queally, J.M. The impact of frailty in major trauma in older patients. *Injury* **2020**, *51*, 1536–1542. [CrossRef] [PubMed]
18. Bryant, J.; Sellars, M.; Sinclair, C.; Detering, K.; Buck, K.; Waller, A.; White, B.; Nolte, L. Inadequate completion of advance care directives by individuals with dementia: National audit of health and aged care facilities. *BMJ Support. Palliat. Care* **2021**, *12*, e319–e328. [CrossRef] [PubMed]
19. Lee, C.; Beavers, J.; Pham, J.; Hackett, L.; Miller, J.; Buntine, P. Impact of the Canadian CT head rule supplemented by the original published minimum inclusion criteria to assist emergency department clinicians' assessment of patients presenting post fall from residential aged care: A retrospective audit. *BMC Geriatr.* **2022**, *22*, 607. [CrossRef] [PubMed]

20. Australian Institute of Health and Welfare. The ongoing challenge of chronic conditions in Australia. In *Australia's Health 2024: Data Insights*; Australian Institute of Health and Welfare: Canberra, Australia, 2024.
21. Kotsani, M.; Kravvariti, E.; Avgerinou, C.; Panagiotakis, S.; Bograkou Tzanetakou, K.; Antoniadou, E.; Karamanof, G.; Karampeazis, A.; Koutsouri, A.; Panagiotopoulou, K.; et al. The Relevance and Added Value of Geriatric Medicine (GM): Introducing GM to Non-Geriatricians. *J. Clin. Med.* **2021**, *10*, 3018. [CrossRef] [PubMed]

Journal of *Personalized Medicine*

MDPI

Article

Geriatric Population Triage: The Risk of Real-Life Over- and Under-Triage in an Overcrowded ED: 4- and 5-Level Triage Systems Compared: The CREONTE (Crowding and R E Organization National TriagE) Study

Gabriele Savioli [1,*], Iride Francesca Ceresa [2], Maria Antonietta Bressan [1], Gaia Bavestrello Piccini [3], Viola Novelli [4], Sara Cutti [4], Giovanni Ricevuti [5], Ciro Esposito [6], Yaroslava Longhitano [7], Andrea Piccioni [8], Zoubir Boudi [9], Alessandro Venturi [10,11], Damiano Fuschi [12], Antonio Voza [2], Roberto Leo [13], Abdelouahab Bellou [14,15,16,*] and Enrico Oddone [17,18]

1 Department of Emergency Medicine and Surgery, IRCCS Fondanzione Policlinico San Matteo, 27100 Pavia, Italy; mita.bressan@gmail.com
2 Emergency Department, IRCCS Humanitas Research Hospital, Via Manzoni 56, Rozzano, 20089 Milan, Italy; irideceresa@gmail.com (I.F.C.); antonio.voza@humanitas.it (A.V.)
3 Emergency Medicine, Université Libre de Bruxelles (ULB), 1050 Brussels, Belgium; gaia.bavestrellopic01@universitadipavia.it
4 Medical Direction, IRCCS Fondanzione Policlinico San Matteo, 27100 Pavia, Italy; v.novelli@smatteo.pv.it (V.N.); s.cutti@smatteo.pv.it (S.C.)
5 Department of Drug Science, University of Pavia, 27100 Pavia, Italy; giovanni.ricevuti@unipv.it
6 Nephrology and Dialysis Unit, ICS Maugeri, University of Pavia, 27100 Pavia, Italy; ciro.esposito@unipv.it
7 Residency Program in Emergency Medicine, Department of Emergency Medicine, IRCCS Humanitas Research Hospital, Rozzano, 20089 Milan, Italy; lon.yaro@gmail.com
8 Emergency Department, Fondazione Policlinico Universitario A. Gemelli, IRCCS, 00168 Rome, Italy; andrea.piccioni@policlinicogemelli.it
9 Department of Emergency Medicine, Dr Sulaiman Alhabib Hospital, Dubai 2542, United Arab Emirates; zoubir.boudi@gmail.com
10 Department of Political and Social Sciences, University of Pavia, 27100 Pavia, Italy; alessandro.venturi@unipv.it
11 Bureau of the Presidency, IRCCS Fondanzione Policlinico San Matteo, 27100 Pavia, Italy
12 Department of Italian and Supranational Public Law, Faculty of Law, University of Milan, 20133 Milan, Italy; damiano.fuschi@unimi.it
13 Department of Systems Medicine, University of Rome "Tor Vergata", 00133 Rome, Italy; rtoleo@tiscali.it
14 Global Network on Emergency Medicine, Brookline, MA 02446, USA
15 Department of Emergency Medicine, Wayne State University School of Medicine, Detroit, MI 48201, USA
16 Institute of Sciences in Emergency Medicine, Department of Emergency Medicine, Guangdong Provincial People's Hospital (Guangdong Academy of Medical Sciences), Southern Medical University, Guangzhou 510080, China
17 Department of Public Health, Experimental and Forensic Medicine, University of Pavia, 27100 Pavia, Italy; enrico.oddone@unipv.it
18 Occupational Medicine Unit (UOOML), ICS Maugeri IRCCS, 27100 Pavia, Italy
* Correspondence: gabrielesavioli@gmail.com (G.S.); abellou402@gmail.com (A.B.)

Abstract: Elderly patients, when they present to the emergency department (ED) or are admitted to the hospital, are at higher risk of adverse outcomes such as higher mortality and longer hospital stays. This is mainly due to their age and their increased fragility. In order to minimize this already increased risk, adequate triage is of foremost importance for fragile geriatric (>75 years old) patients who present to the ED. The admissions of elderly patients from 1 January 2014 to 31 December 2020 were examined, taking into consideration the presence of two different triage systems, a 4-level (4LT) and a 5-level (5LT) triage system. This study analyzes the difference in wait times and under- (UT) and over-triage (OT) in geriatric and general populations with two different triage models. Another outcome of this study was the analysis of the impact of crowding and its variables on the triage system during the COVID-19 pandemic. A total of 423,257 ED presentations were included. An increase in admissions of geriatric, more fragile, and seriously ill individuals was observed, and a progressive increase in crowding was simultaneously detected. Geriatric patients, when presenting to the emergency department, are subject to the problems of UT and OT in both a 4LT system and a 5LT system. Several indicators and variables of crowding increased, with a net increase in throughput and output factors, notably the length of stay (LOS), exit block, boarding, and processing times. This in turn led to an increase in wait times and an increase in UT in the geriatric population. It has indeed been shown that an increase in crowding results in an increased risk of UT, and this is especially true for 4LT compared to 5LT systems. When observing the pandemic period, an increase in admissions of older and more serious patients was observed. However, in the pandemic period, a general reduction in waiting times was observed, as well as an increase in crowding indices and intrahospital mortality. This study demonstrates how introducing a 5LT system enables better flow and patient care in an ED. Avoiding UT of geriatric patients, however, remains a challenge in EDs.

Keywords: triage; emergency service; hospital; crowding; triage (under-triage); triage (over-triage); geriatric emergencies; overcrowding and access block; overcrowding detection; overcrowding effect; overcrowding; ED management

1. Introduction

Triage for geriatric patients is an open challenge for emergency physicians, especially in increasingly overcrowded EDs [1–4]. In this Special Issue, we focus on the effects of re-thinking the triage system in the geriatric population (>75 years) pertaining to our ED.

Due to an aging population, visits to emergency departments (EDs) by geriatric patients are increasing worldwide. With increasing age, frailty is defined by multiple aspects: among geriatric ED patients, a high proportion have balance difficulties, an unsteady gait, require assistance for mobility, or have decreased muscle strength in their lower limbs. Frail and elderly patients are at risk of adverse outcomes (for example: mortality and prolonged hospital stays). In this respect, suitable triage for fragile geriatric ED patients is a critical healthcare issue.

Waiting times have often been described as improving with the transition to the 5-level triage system [3,4]; however, there is not complete agreement on this in the literature, as on the other hand, a lengthening of waiting times has been described [5]. The various triage systems need to identify and prioritize patients who require an urgent intervention in a short time; therefore, it is important to find solutions with efficacy to reduce waiting times [3–8]. For this reason, we went to see how the transition to the 5-level triage system affected waiting times.

In EDs organized by areas of intensity of care, patients at triage receive a priority code and are channeled toward low- or medium-high-intensity care areas [9,10].

It is the common opinion of the authors that 5LTs, due to their increased accuracy and safety, are better than 3LT or 4LT systems. The fact that this advantage also affects geriatric patients has not yet been widely studied [3,8,11–30].

The triage process is complex, and its complexity is even greater for geriatric patients who are more prone to UT [31–38].

Hence, there is a need to study how UT and OT vary in reality during the transition from a 4LT to a 5LT, especially in geriatric people.

Overcrowding compromises the quality of patient care, not just the quality received. However, the reciprocal effects between crowding and triage are still not widely studied. In particular, the influence of the various factors that determine crowding with triage waiting times and the frequency of UT and OT requires investigation. In addition, the outcomes associated with adopting a 5LT system have been explored in the field only by a few studies, and with low numbers of patients [39–53].

Some real-life studies have focused on only one symptom or have enrolled a low number of patients. Hence, there is a need to study triage with the complexity of real life in a crowded ED with a large population.

For all these reasons, we analyzed the triage efficacy for geriatric people in a real-life ED, both in a four-level triage system (4LT) and in a five-level triage system (5LT). We studied the waiting times (primary objective) and (secondary objectives) over- and under-triage (OT and UT, respectively). Finally, we analyzed the relationships, in real life, between crowding and triage and the functioning of the 5LT, also during the COVID-19 pandemic.

2. Methods

2.1. Study Design

We conducted a retrospective study, which encompassed the admittances to the ED of the Foundation IRCCS Policlinic San Matteo from 1 January 2014 to 31 December 2020. During this period, our ED underwent reorganization with a subdivision into areas of different intensities of care and a shift from a 4LT (from 1 January 2014, to 30 November 2015) to a 5LT (from 30 November 2015, to 31 December 2020). The admissions during the two periods were compared.

A tailored investigation was performed to investigate the data of interest. Anonymization was performed in order to ensure confidentiality. The mandatory consent to data utilization for medical and research purposes as well as health data processing, was obtained at admission from all patients.

2.2. Endpoints

This investigation was conducted considering the number of patients presenting to the ED during a period of time which was then further subdivided into two periods: the 4LT and 5LT periods. The objective was to ascertain the effects that the introduction of a 5LT system would have on wait times in geriatric (>75 years old) and young populations. The secondary objective was to determine whether adopting a 5LT system had any effect on the accuracy level of the triage of geriatric patients. The accuracy of triage in geriatric people has been measured as the percentages of patients undergoing UT and OT, as well as by verifying the correlation between the code attributed at triage by the triage nurse and the severity code attributed at discharge by a physician.

A further outcome is the correlation between triage and crowding indices. The most robust crowding indices in the literature were used, such as the length of ED stay, total access block time, and rate of access block [54–83]. For a detailed definition of the calculation of the same, we referred to our previous publications [84–86]. Finally, we analyzed the proficiency of a 5LT system during the exceptional circumstances of the COVID-19 pandemic.

2.3. Statistics

Continuous variables are expressed as means, medians, and interquartile ranges; qualitative variables are expressed as the number of observations and appropriate proportions. The non-parametric Mann–Whitney test was used to make between-group comparisons for continuous variables, according to their non-normal distributions. The χ^2 test was used to study associations between the qualitative variables. The statistical analysis was performed with pertinent logistic multivariate regression models to assess the correlation between time variables while accounting for crowding, exit block, and the different triage periods. The differences in UT and OT by year of observation were examined using the test of proportions. For each passage, the presence/absence of over-triage and under-triage was modeled as a binary variable, as described in the Methods section, and the risk of undergoing either UT or OT was defined as the odds ratio (OR) resulting from multiple regression analysis adjusted for age, gender, and year of observation. The investigation was performed for all the patients presenting in the selected period, as well as for subgroups in which boarding or exit blocks were present. The significance level was set at alpha 0.05 (statistical significance at $p < 0.05$), and all tests were two-tailed.

The analyses were conducted using STATA software (version 14; Stata Corporation, College Station, TX, USA, 2015). The ethics committee submitted and approved the study (protocol number: 20200114609). The analyses were made using data from the PIESSE software (GBIM, Pavia, 2020).

3. Results

3.1. Overall

Geriatric patients (>75 years) constituted about 24% of the total population taken into consideration, and their number grew over the years (from 21% to 24%) (Table 1). As can be seen in the table below, the patients became increasingly complex, as can be seen from the triage priority code, priority code at discharge, the need for high care intensity, and outcomes (Table 1).

Table 1. Principal personal and ED presentation features of patients included in the study, by period of observation.

	Period		
	4LT N (%)	5LT N (%)	p [a]
Sex			
Male	59,432 (51.2)	158,914 (51.7)	
Female	56,628 (48.8)	148,283 (48.3)	0.002
Age			
<75	91,102 (78.5)	234,512 (76.3)	
75+	24,968 (21.5)	72,686 (23.7)	<0.001
Triage priority code			
Code 5	13,443 (11.6)	25,748 (8.4)	
Code 4	78,777 (67.9)	191,981 (62.5)	
Code 3	0 (-)	17,297 (5.6)	
Code 2	22,711 (19.6)	67,688 (22.0)	
Code 1	1129 (0.9)	4484 (1.5)	<0.001
Priority code at discharge			
Code 5	29,240 (25.2)	43,141 (14.0)	
Code 4	73,995 (63.8)	224,039 (72.9)	
Code 3	0 (-)	425 (0.1)	
Code 2	11,952 (10.3)	36,341 (11.8)	
Code 1	873 (0.7)	3252 (1.2)	<0.001
Care intensity			
Low	92,220 (79.5)	235,026 (76.5)	
Medium-to-high	23,840 (20.5)	72,172 (23.5)	<0.001
Outcome			
Discharge	94,701 (81.6)	246,413 (80.2)	
Hospitalization	17,347 (14.9)	51,043 (16.6)	
Transfer	2166 (1.9)	5746 (1.9)	
Left without being seen	1385 (1.2)	2933 (0.9)	
Other	461 (0.4)	1063 (0.4)	<0.001

The 4LT period (T4) spanned from 1 January 2014 to 30 November 2015; the 5LT period (T5) spanned from 1 December 2015 to 31 December 2020; [a]: χ^2 test.

3.2. Wait Time for Geriatric Compared to Younger Patients

The differences between the wait times of geriatric (>75 years of age) and younger patients had little statistical significance when considering Code 4 and Code 5 (about 1 or 2 min for codes 1, 2, 3, and 5; about 20 min for code 4) (Table 2).

Table 2. Wait time by period, code at presentation, and age.

		Age < 75 Years				Age ≥ 75 Years			
	Period	N	Median (min)	Interquartile Range (min)	p [a]	N	Median (min)	Interquartile Range (min)	p [a]
Wait time									
Non-urgency									
Code 4	4LT	12,335	51.6	17.9–108.3		1108	57.4	21.4–116.5	
Code 5	5LT	23,379	48.3	17.5–103.8	0.001	2369	50.0	18.2–109.0	0.037
Minor urgency									
Code 3	4LT	64,636	48.4	19.0–102.9		14,141	71.2	30.6–134.1	
Code 4	5LT	156,088	53.1	20.6–115.9	<0.001	35,893	79.4	32.5–151.6	<0.001
Deferrable urgency									
Code 3	5LT	13,403	23.4	12.4–43.9	-	3894	26.9	14.5–48.3	-
High urgency									
Code 2	4LT	13,535	22.5	10.7–47.9		9176	24.7	12.3–51.2	
Code 2	5LT	39,098	31.7	13.4–73.9	<0.001	28,590	33.4	15.1–73.3	<0.001
Emergency									
Code 1	4LT	596	4.6	2.4–9.3		533	5.3	2.6–10.8	
Code 1	5LT	2544	3.6	1.9–7.1	<0.001	1940	5.2	2.6–10.1	0.369

The 4LT period spanned from 1 January 2014 to 30 November 2015; the 5LT period spanned from 1 December 2015 to 31 December 2020. [a]: Kruskal–Wallis test.

In contrast, with the introduction of 5LT, a constant (even though not statistically significant) increase in wait times of ~3–4 min per year was observed for the patients who were assigned Code 2 at triage (Table 2). This was likely dependent on the increased number of patients receiving a priority Code 2 at triage and crowding at our hospital.

Patients who were assigned Code 3 in the 5LT system period had similar wait times to patients who were assigned a Code 2 in the 4LT system period, with equal tendency for both geriatric patients (26.9 vs. 24.7 min) and younger patients (23.4 vs. 22.5 min) (Table 2). Patients who were assigned Code 4 and 5 in the 5LT system period had wait times which were comparable to those of patients who were assigned Codes 3 and 4 during the 4LT system period (Table 2).

3.3. UT and OT in the Geriatric Population

The risk of UT is slightly greater in geriatric patients than in the general population (OR = 2.22; $p < 0.001$). (Table 3). However, when separately analyzing the areas of low intensity of care (OR = 0.85; $p < 0.001$) and those of medium-high intensity of care (OR = 0.56; $p < 0.001$), this trend was found to be reverted (Tables 3 and 4). The top three complaints of geriatric patients at triage were minor signs and symptoms (27.3%), abdominal pain (13.1%), and dyspnea (10.5%). These symptoms alone accounted for >50% of admissions. Minor trauma (7.3%) and neurological disorders (6.5%) were less frequently observed (Table 3).

Table 3. Distribution of undertriage (UT) and overtriage (OT) percentages during 4LT and 5LT periods, in geriatric and younger patients.

Variable		Period		
		4-Level Triage N (%)	**5-Level Triage N (%)**	p [a]
Age < 75 years				
	OT			
	No	81,483 (89.4%)	205,378 (87.6%)	
	Yes	9619 (10.6%)	29,134 (12.4%)	<0.001
	UT			
	No	83,837 (92.0%)	215,494 (91.9%)	
	Yes	7265 (8.0%)	19,018 (8.1%)	0.204
Age ≥ 75 years				
	OT			
	No	19,705 (79.0%)	55,553 (76.4%)	
	Yes	5253 (21.0%)	17,133 (23.6%)	<0.001
	UT			
	No	22,898 (91.8%)	66,104 (90.9%)	
	Yes	2060 (8.2%)	6582 (9.1%)	<0.001

The 4LT period (T4) spanned from 1 January 2014 to 30 November 2015; the 5LT period (T5) spanned from 1 December 2015 to 31 December 2020; [a]: χ^2 test, UT: under-triage; OT: over-triage.

Table 4. Risk of under-triage (UT), by age, triage level period, and presence of access block.

Period	Age	Intensity of Care	Access Block	OR [a]	95% Confidence Interval	p
4-level triage	<75	Low	No	1.00 (ref.)	-	
			Yes	4.37	3.75–5.10	<0.001
		Moderate-to-high	No	1.00 (ref.)	-	
			Yes	1.12	0.35–3.60	0.847
	≥75	Low	No	1.00 (ref.)	-	
			Yes	4.53	3.79–5.43	<0.001
		Moderate-to-high	No	1.00 (ref.)	-	
			Yes	1.18	0.47–2.95	0.724
5-level triage	<75	Low	No	1.00 (ref.)	-	
			Yes	6.92	6.47–7.39	<0.001
		Moderate-to-high	No	1.00 (ref.)	-	
			Yes	0.94	0.63–1.41	0.761
	≥75	Low	No	1.00 (ref.)	-	
			Yes	6.09	5.63–6.59	<0.001
		Moderate-to-high	No	1.00 (ref.)	-	
			Yes	1.82	1.43–2.32	<0.001

[a]: Odds ratios (ORs) estimated by multiple regression analysis adjusted for age and sex.

The elderly patients underwent over-triage more often than the general population, and this occurred in both the 4LT and the 5LT system periods, with no difference according to areas of intensity of care (Tables 3 and 5).

Table 5. Risk of over-triage (OT), by age, triage level period, and presence of access block.

Period	Age	Intensity of Care	Access Block	OR [a]	95% Confidence Interval	p
4-level triage	<75	Moderate-to-high	No	1.00 (ref.)	-	
			Yes	0.23	0.16–0.31	<0.001
	≥75	Moderate-to-high	No	1.00 (ref.)	-	
			Yes	0.34	0.27–0.45	<0.001
5-level triage	**<75**	Low	No	1.00 (ref.)	-	
			Yes	0.05	0.01–0.36	0.003
		Moderate-to-high	No	1.00 (ref.)	-	
			Yes	0.16	0.15–0.18	<0.001
	≥75	Moderate-to-high	No	1.00 (ref.)	-	
			Yes	0.21	0.19–0.23	<0.001

[a]: Odds ratios (OR) estimated by multiple regression analysis, adjusted for age and sex. No presence of OT was observed for low intensity of care during the 4-level triage period or the 5-level triage period for patients ≥75 years of age.

3.4. Crowding

The phenomenon of crowding was aggravated over the years following the progressive increase in boarding and exit blocks observed from 2014 to 2020 (Table 6). The total number of ED admissions rose gradually up to 2018, with the exception of a period of decrease in 2015, and then lowered again in 2019 and 2020 (Table 6). The wait times for patients in low and medium-high-intensity care areas (Table 7; $p < 0.001$) increased, as shown by the indices of the boarding and exit blocks. These indices of crowding were chosen due to their higher reproducibility with automated data extraction [84–86]. In the 4LT system, boarding substantially correlates with a slight reduction in the rate of under-triage in the low-intensity care area, but with a reversed tendency of increased risk of UT in geriatric patients in medium-high-intensity care areas. When considering the period with a 5LT system, on the other hand, boarding was no longer correlated with a greater risk of UT in elderly patients, and similarly, the probability of UT was also reduced for young people in medium-high-intensity care areas. There is, therefore, a correlation between the phenomenon of boarding, a greater risk of OT in young people, and a lower risk of OT in the elderly. In the 5LT system, this risk of OT in the younger patients was, however, found to be lower, and the risk of OT for elderly patients was also greatly reduced, as shown in Table 8. The exit block correlated with an increase in the rate of under-triage in both 4LT and 5LT. However, switching to 5LT in the medium-high-intensity care area did not increase the risk of UT for young people. During the exit block, there was a clear reduction in the number of over-triage cases, which was an even more marked reduction in the period of 5LT, as shown in Table 9.

Table 6. Trend of crowding indices over the years.

	2014	2015	2016	2017	2018	2019	2020	p for Trend
Boarding #	926 9.0%	1010 10.1%	1241 11.4%	1431 12.8%	1475 12.8%	2033 18.8%	4230 36.7%	<0.001
Access block #	786 7.6%	951 9.5%	1141 10.5%	1289 11.5%	1368 11.9%	2022 18.7%	3833 33.3%	<0.001
Accesses per day	165.8	165.3	170.8	174.4	176.8	175.8	129.8	
Number of accesses	60,512	60,336	62,527	63,662	64,540	64,181	47,500	

Boarding and access blocks were calculated only for hospitalized patients.

Table 7. Selected time variables accounting for crowding, by age and intensity of care.

Wait Time		Age < 75				Age 75+			
		Observations (N)	Median (min)	Interquartile Range (min)	p [a]	Observations (N)	Median (min)	Interquartile Range (min)	p [a]
Low-intensity care									
	No boarding *	18,128	46.5	18.4–104.4		10,603	64.3	27.4–131.1	
	Boarding #	4579	55.6	22.5–129.7	<0.001	2837	75.5	29.5–156.6	<0.001
Medium-to-high care intensity									
	No boarding *	16,716	15.9	6.5–39.3		18,509	21.3	9.5–48.5	
	Boarding #	2100	24.5	10.3–56.0	<0.001	2830	22.0	9.5–53.9	0.041
Low-intensity c are									
	No access block °	265,186	48.4	18.9–106.4		53,915	67.5	27.6–134.4	
	Access block °°	4655	92.7	34.0–182.4	<0.001	3490	113.7	43.8–205.5	<0.001
Medium-to-high care intensity									
	No access block °	46,443	27.2	11.0–27.2		32,584	29.2	12.7–65.3	
	Access block °°	1998	32.0	12.9–85.3	<0.001	2912	29.6	11.4–80.2	0.122

[a]: Kruskal–Wallis test. No boarding. * = Mean number and percentage of patients who did not go to boarding (for example, patients who did not have to wait for a bed). Boarding # = mean number and percentage of patients who underwent boarding. ° No access block: mean number and percentage of patients who did not go to access block. °° Access block: mean number and percentage of patients who experienced boarding.

Table 8. Risk of under-triage (UT), by age, triage level period, and presence of boarding.

Period	Age	Intensity of Care	Boarding	OR [a]	95% Confidence Interval	p
4-level triage	<75	Low	No	1.00 (ref.)	-	
			Yes	0.70	0.59–0.83	<0.001
		Moderate-to-high	No	1.00 (ref.)	-	
			Yes	0.99	0.53–1.86	0.987
	≥75	Low	No	1.00 (ref.)	-	
			Yes	0.75	0.60–0.94	0.014
		Moderate-to-high	No	1.00 (ref.)	-	
			Yes	1.38	0.77–2.48	0.279
5-level triage	<75	Low	No	1.00 (ref.)	-	
			Yes	1.01	0.94–1.09	0.753
		Moderate-to-high	No	1.00 (ref.)	-	
			Yes	0.49	0.34–0.69	<0.001
	≥75	Low	No	1.00 (ref.)	-	
			Yes	1.03	0.94–1.12	0.570
		Moderate-to-high	No	1.00 (ref.)	-	
			Yes	1.02	0.81–1.30	0.849

[a]: Odds ratios (ORs) estimated by multiple regression analysis adjusted for age and sex.

Table 9. Risk of over-triage (OT), by age, triage level period, and presence of boarding.

Period	Age	Intensity of Care	Boarding	OR [a]	95% Confidence Interval	p
4-level triage	<75	Moderate-to-high	No	1.00 (ref.)	-	
			Yes	1.27	1.01–1.61	0.044
	≥75	Moderate-to-high	No	1.00 (ref.)	-	
			Yes	0.96	0.77–1.19	0.711
5-level triage	<75	Moderate-to-high	No	1.00 (ref.)	-	
			Yes	1.12	0.99–1.26	0.06
	≥75	Low	No	1.00 (ref.)	-	
			Yes	1.03	0.94–1.12	0.570
		Moderate-to-high	No	1.00 (ref.)	-	
			Yes	0.75	0.68–0.84	<0.001

[a]: Odds ratios (ORs) estimated by multiple regression analysis and adjusted for age and sex. No presence of OT was observed for low intensity of care during the 4-levels triage period or in 5-level triage period for patients <75 years of age.

When we examined individual triage priority codes for the intensity of the medical examinations and areas of care, we found no statistically significant differences between geriatric (>75 years of age) and younger patients.

3.5. LT of COVID Patients

In the period characterized by the COVID pandemic, 3826 patients presented to our ED. 125 patients were assigned a triage Code 5, 2789 a Code 4, 169 a Code 3, 810 a Code 2, and 86 were assigned a triage Code 1. A total of 159 patients tested positive for COVID-19, and 78 infected patients died in the ED. The wait times for patients in the area dedicated to COVID patients were 48 min for Code 5, 47 min for Code 4, 48 min for Code 3, 27 min for Code 2, and 10 min for Code 1.

4. Discussion

4.1. Overall

The age of patients admitted to the ED has constantly risen through the years. The number of patients presenting to the ED has progressively increased, and patients are currently older, more fragile, and sicker. This trend is in turn reflected by a decrease in spontaneous accesses, a higher number of admissions through the territorial emergency service or on a gurney, and the percentage of more severe priority codes assigned at triage and higher severity codes assigned at discharge. This trend has already been extensively described in the literature [54–66,74,75,83,84,87,88] and has been negatively influenced by the COVID-19 pandemic, with a greater number of patients requiring hospitalization [85,86]. As a consequence, exit blocks and boarding have increased as well, and together with the progressive reduction in beds, this has led to a worsening of crowding.

All these changes in the population and the flow in the ED have led to a change in the work of ED physicians, transforming their practice from "admit-to-care" to "care-to-admit" [85,86]. This change has resulted in a gradual extension of LOS and processing times. It has already been demonstrated that the increase in crowding has negative effects on patient outcomes and satisfaction; however, until now, the effects of overcrowding on triage—particularly on wait times and on the risk of UT and OT—have not been thoroughly analyzed. The 5LT system has proven itself more accurate, with better correspondence between the code assigned at triage and the severity code assigned at discharge. This therefore suggests that 5LT system triage codes reflect, in a more precise way, the actual acuity of the patient in comparison to 4LT systems. This evidence, together with the data that show a global decrease in the risk of UT, demonstrates that a system that allows a lower risk of UT has clear benefits for the patients in the ED, and especially for those patients who are sicker and more fragile, with a subsequent improvement in the outcome.

4.2. Wait Time

Age does not seem to play a significant role in waiting issues. When we corrected age data according to triage code and area of care intensity, our results were in line with what was expected. Some studies correctly described increases in ED crowding due to increases in geriatric access to EDs. As is similar to our findings, Kawano et al. noted that the geriatric population tended to consist of more complex patients who presented more frequently in ambulances. The geriatric frequently required medium-high care intensity and higher triage codes. Therefore, our study is in line with the literature and underscores the finding that age itself does not cause crowding; however, age is a factor related to frailty in compromised patients [89–92]. The general fragility of geriatric patients increases crowding and wait times. Once age is corrected according to the need for more intense care and faster medical examination, it no longer appears to affect crowding. However, these findings require verification within the context of multicenter studies.

Additional focus should be put on the effects of having both doctors and nurses working at triage. The presence of dedicated doctors at triage allows for a quicker examination of patients coming for less severe problems. This also allows for a prompter evaluation of more-complex patients, helping to reduce the impact that crowding has on ED functioning. The presence of a senior doctor, meaning a medical doctor having obtained the title of specialist in emergency medicine, alongside the triage nurse at the triage station, has positive effects, with reductions in wait time, LOS, LWBS rates, and the percentage of patients leaving without having had a complete workup and treatment. Additionally, triage teams consisting of a doctor and a nurse can also be beneficial for a more rapid admission of more fragile patients (such as geriatric patients) who are not required to stay in the emergency department for further investigations or time-sensitive interventions, but would benefit more from prompt hospitalization. This type of triage team can therefore exert positive effects by reducing overcrowding [93–95].

Exit blocks and boarding often influence the wait times of patients who require hospitalization or a secondary transfer, and this phenomenon is prevalent in ED areas with higher care intensity [9,10]. The medium-high-intensity patient requires a set of tools for their care (such as oxygen, non-invasive ventilation, telemetry, and monitoring of vital parameters), and these are dependent on structural limits (i.e., the number of oxygen outlets, ventilators, and monitors). The fact that more and more patients need to be placed in areas of medium-high intensity of care, and the concurrent increase in the phenomenon of exit blocks, result in a saturation of the resources which are available, with a consequent increase in the time needed for patient management.

Increased LOS could also be due to other changes in the internal departmental organization (such as doctor and nurse turn-over, differences in the organization of shifts, etc.). The relationship that exists between boarding times in the ED and patients' outcomes is still being analyzed. There is a need for larger studies to better analyze the influence that boarding and exit blocks have on adverse ED outcomes [96].

4.3. UT and OT in the Geriatric Population

The geriatric population was found to be at increased risk of UT in this study. This tendency remained constant during the 4LT and 5LT system periods, regardless of the area of care intensity to which the patients were allocated [37,97–100]. This phenomenon may be due to physiological changes during senescence, pain habits, and the inability to communicate [101–120].

The geriatric population is expected to represent ~20% of the overall population by 2030. Importantly, geriatric patients are more complex, require more resources, and have higher admission rates. Geriatric triage is more complex for various reasons. The interpretation of vital signs in the geriatric is more challenging due to homeostatic mechanisms. For example, when considering the respiratory system of an aging individual, the lungs will have less elastic recoil, and there will be increased dead space and a decreased physiologic reserve. Therefore, a respiratory rate >27 breaths/minute in the elderly is an accurate predictor of adverse events and can help to identify the critical patients. When considering the cardiovascular system in the elderly, it is important to note that the combination of myocardial thickening, arterial wall stiffness, and hypertension will result in an increase in the workload of the heart. Elderly patients are more prone to events of orthostatic hypotension due to larger pulse pressures and a reduced effect of circulating catecholamines. A systolic blood pressure <110 mmHg often represents hypotension in geriatric patients, especially among those with traumatic injuries. Resting heart rate also increases with age [101–104]. Analogous homeostatic changes also occur with the body's temperature. Elderly patients are also less likely to present with fever because of several factors, such as the presence of a weaker immune system, a decreased cardiac output, and diminished muscle mass. Consequently, slight temperature changes, as well as hypothermia, may represent severe infection in this category of patients [105,121].

In addition to homeostatic changes, several factors that complicate pain assessment should be considered. Elderly people may indeed have altered pain perception; an increased risk of persistent pain; and, when cognitive impairment is present, they might have difficulty in assessing pain and its location [106,107,122–124].

Other domains also require special consideration, such as the atypical presentations of common diseases. For example, in geriatric patients, acute coronary syndromes are more likely to present without chest pain. Meanwhile, patients with sepsis may have unaltered parameters and symptoms which are not specific for the identification of the source of the infection. Elderly people with pneumonia often present to the ED without respiratory symptoms, and might not have any chest pain or fever. Some geriatric patients with acute surgical abdomens report only mild pain [108,109].

These data agree with our results. We found that dyspnea and abdominal pain were common in cases of UT. The atypical presentation and communication difficulties can be responsible for a high UT symptomology classified as "minor signs and symptoms".

Cognitive impairment in this population is also important to consider. Prospective ED studies of patients older than 65 and 70 have evidenced delirium rates of 9.6% and 10%, respectively. Sixteen percent of patients older than 70 years demonstrated an impairment of their mental status, and six percent were found to meet the criteria for both delirium and dementia. A great percentage of patients in the geriatric populations who were affected by delirium were not correctly diagnosed, and several geriatric patients were discharged. Early detection of acute changes in the cognitive behavior at triage and timely transmission of this information to the remaining care team are extremely important [10,85,110,125]. These factors were likely at play among patients who experienced UT in our study.

Polypharmacy in the aged population should also be considered: 44% of US males and 57% of US females older than 65 take 5 or more medications per week. These patients are particularly susceptible to adverse drug events (ADEs). Notably, ADEs account for up to 10% of geriatric ED presentations. Cardiovascular, diuretic, antibiotic, hypoglycemic, sedative, opioid analgesic, anticholinergic, and anti-inflammatory medications are commonly implicated in ADEs [126].

Finally, there is a constant increase in ED visits attributable to falls and trauma among the elderly, with significant morbidity and mortality. However, unlike the younger cohorts, falls are the major trauma mechanism and often occur as a consequence of decreased autonomy, increased fragility, modifications in vision acuity, impaired muscle strength with altered gait and balance issues, an acute medical event, or the introduction of a new medication. In these patients, UT is potentially more frequent due to underestimation of the gravity of the injury as well as of the impact of the comorbidities on the clinical picture [111,126,127]. We found that patients with trauma and minor dynamics often experienced UT. It is important to reduce UT in this category of fragile patients, thereby improving recognition of critical situations. Further studies are needed to investigate possible ways to counteract the increase in OT while keeping the risk of UT to a minimum. Correct triage of geriatric patients, even when adopting 5LT systems, remains an extremely complicated task for triage teams. The implementation of triage algorithms through artificial intelligence could help in overcoming age-related specificities.

4.4. Crowding Indices

The increase in LOS, exit blocks, boarding, and processing times provoked a net increase in throughput and output factors, which, in consequence, caused an increase in wait times, both in geriatric people and in young people. This trend was especially observed with exit blocks, more than boarding, in low-intensity areas and for less-urgent triage codes. In these conditions, the presence of an exit block resulted in a wait time which was almost doubled. Additionally, the lengths of wait times for patients who required prompt medical examination and who were assigned high priority codes (triage Codes 1 or 2) increased by approximately 25–30%.

These results confirm the effect of output factors on the flow in the ED. Processing and LOS times are increased due to an increase in the phenomenon of exit blocks, and this in turns influences all ED processes and flows, with a lengthening of wait and handling times.

Exit block allows for a reduction in the risk of OT for those patients assigned to low-intensity care areas and who are given lower priority triage codes, and boarding reduces OT in medium-high intensity care areas. Regarding, O.T.; in both cases, triage is more accurate for patients, for both young and geriatric ones. This may be a consequence of increased vigilance of the triage nurses during crowding. Nevertheless, this increased specificity may be dependent on the fact that during prolonged wait times, patients can undergo re-evaluations more often. The OT reduction is greater in areas of medium-high intensity of care because it is likely that, in these patients, the attention of triage nurses is concentrated in cases of crowding.

During crowding represented by boarding and, even more, by exit blocks, the under-triage worsens: the situation of overcrowding caused by the output factors therefore causes a reduced accuracy of the triage with regard to the under-triage. This reduction in accuracy is probably also due to the lengthening of waiting times in the context of increased crowding. It is interesting to note that 5LT proved to be more effective at minimizing UT risk in the medium-high intensity area where, for young people, there is even a reduction in the risk of UT. It is, therefore, the opinion of the authors that the increased risk of UT is not only due to a lengthening of waiting times with a consequent increase in the stress of triage nurses, but could also be due to an attitude of greater attention paid to the most acute patients in crowding conditions, those destined for areas of medium-high intensity of care. This attitude is more pronounced in younger patients and much reduced in elderly patients, perhaps because of the greater insidiousness of the acute manifestation of geriatric patients. The reasons for a more insidious manifestation in geriatric patients were reviewed in the previous paragraph (change in homeostatic processes, lower reliability of some vital parameters, difficulty in expressing symptoms by the geriatric patient, presence of dementia, etc.).

The study, therefore, shows a greater susceptibility of geriatric patients during crowding. The use of artificial intelligence algorithms could reduce this risk, thus outlining a need for studies in this sense for the future.

Finally, it should be noted that the doubling of crowding represented in Table 4 was simultaneous to the beginning of the COVID-19 epidemic (2020), therefore putting a further strain on the system. Thus, the 5LT system also confirmed the aforementioned advantages in extreme conditions, such as those of the pandemic.

4.5. 5-Level Triage in COVID Patients

In the areas dedicated to COVID-19 patients, the waiting times were analogous to the wait times of the general population. During the COVID-19 pandemic, the ED of our hospital had to be deeply reorganized in order to reduce the risk of transmission of the infection as much as possible, and to better direct the flow of patients. During the first phase of the pandemic in 2020, the positive COVID patients were admitted to a specific area that had been created in the Infectious Disease department. The COVID patients who were in need of hospital admission were subsequently referred to specialty inpatient wards which were reserved for positive patients. Further on, when the pressure of the pandemic decreased, the need to create separate flows of patients persisted, and a separated area inside the general ED was rearranged. Simultaneously, the restrictions on visitors and companions (except for special circumstances) were kept in place in order to minimize the potential risk of contagion and retransmission. Screenings with rapid SARS-CoV-2 nasal swabs, which allowed the results to be seen within 6 h, were performed upon presentation to the hospital, and the results were of the utmost importance for identifying and redirecting COVID-positive patients. Despite having process times which were comparable to those of the general population, these patients were subjected to a higher mortality rate.

4.6. Strengths and Limitations of the Study

One of the main strengths of this study is the size of the cohort analyzed. Others strong points consist of the fact are that it includes all the causes of access to triage in real life and that it investigates the effects of crowding on the triage system by examining in detail all the variables of crowding, as well as wait times and over- and under-triage. The results of simulations that can be conducted to better manage the flow of patients in the ED are of course important; however, even studies that are carefully tailored will eventually not be representative of the "real life" scenarios when considering data that are obtained over a longer period. This study, conducted on-site, permits the analysis of the events that characterize a "real" clinical cohort, composed of geriatric patients as well as more complex and fragile patients. However, it should be underlined that the study in question has two main major limitations. It is, in fact, a retrospective study, with all the resulting limitations: first of all, the impossibility of selecting patients a posteriori and, therefore, the possibility that the result of the study is modulated by variables that the experimenter cannot control. Furthermore, it is a single-center study, which therefore analyzes the catchment area of our hospital. It will be necessary to carry out multicenter and prospective studies that validate these data.

4.7. Future Directions

Our study demonstrates the superiority of the 5-level triage system in our reality. We also underline the importance of multicenter studies representative of the various Italian realities in order to be able to more strongly recommend the use of a 5-level triage system as the standard in the Italian country.

Triage in geriatric people remains a real-life challenge. It is the opinion of the authors that an improvement is possible through the use of artificial intelligence, thus opening up a new field of research.

5. Conclusions

The waiting times for geriatric patients, when corrected for triage code, overlap with those of younger patients. With the introduction of the 5-level triage system, geriatric patients, as well as younger patients who required urgent medical examination but did not require high care intensity, have seen reductions in waiting time.

Triage in the geriatric population remains an open challenge for the emergency physician, as these patients are at increased risk of UT and OT.

Increased waiting times have an influence on crowding indices, such as boarding and exit blocks. The worsening of crowding output factors is accompanied by an increased risk of UT. The 5LT already seems to improve the risks of UT and OT triage in crowding conditions.

During the pandemic, and at the same time as a reduction in ED visits, we experienced reduced wait times and increased UT. At the same time, exit blocks and boarding worsened.

Author Contributions: Conceptualization, G.S., I.F.C. and M.A.B.; methodology, G.S., M.A.B., C.E., A.B. and E.O.; validation, G.S., I.F.C., M.A.B., G.R., C.E., A.P., Z.B., A.V. (Alessandro Venturi), A.V. (Antonio Voza) and A.B.; formal analysis, E.O.; investigation, G.S., I.F.C. and M.A.B.; data curation, G.S. and E.O.; writing—original draft, G.S. and E.O.; writing—review and editing, G.S., G.B.P. and A.B.; visualization, I.F.C., M.A.B., G.B.P., V.N., S.C., R.L.; G.R., C.E., Y.L., A.P., Z.B., A.V. (Alessandro Venturi), D.F. and A.B.; supervision, I.F.C., M.A.B., G.R., C.E., Z.B. and A.B.; project administration, G.S. and I.F.C. All authors have read and agreed to the published version of the manuscript.

Funding: This research received no external funding.

Institutional Review Board Statement: The studies involving human participants were reviewed and approved by the San Matteo Hospital IRCCS Ethics Committee (protocol number: 20200114609, approved on 14 June 2021).

Informed Consent Statement: No potentially identifiable human images or data are presented in this study. According to national legislation and institutional requirements, this study did not require informed consent for participation.

Data Availability Statement: The raw data supporting the conclusions of this article will be made available by the authors upon reasonable request.

Conflicts of Interest: The authors declare no conflicts of interest.

References

1. Chaou, C.H.; Chiu, T.F.; Pan, S.L.; Yen, A.M.; Chang, S.H.; Tang, P.; Lai, C.C.; Wang, R.F.; Chen, H.H. Quantifying Dynamic Flow of Emergency Department (ED) Patient Managements: A Multistate Model Approach. *Emerg. Med. Int.* **2020**, *2020*, 2059379. [CrossRef]
2. Hamamoto, J.; Yamase, H.; Yamase, Y. Impacts of the introduction of a triage system in Japan: A time series study. *Int. Emerg. Nurs.* **2014**, *22*, 153–158. [CrossRef]
3. Ng, D.; Vail, G.; Thomas, S.; Schmidt, N. Applying the Lean principles of the Toyota Production System to reduce wait times in the emergency department. *Can. J. Emerg. Med.* **2010**, *12*, 50–57. [CrossRef]
4. McGillicuddy, D.C.; O'Connell, F.J.; Shapiro, N.I.; Calder, S.A.; Mottley, L.J.; Roberts, J.C.; Sanchez, L.D. Emergency department abnormal vital sign "triggers" program improves time to therapy. *Acad. Emerg. Med.* **2011**, *18*, 483–487. [CrossRef]
5. Maleki, M.; Fallah, R.; Riahi, L.; Delavari, S.; Rezaei, S. Effectiveness of Five-Level Emergency Severity Index Triage System Compared with Three-Level Spot Check: An Iranian Experience. *Arch. Trauma Res.* **2015**, *4*, e29214. [CrossRef]
6. Christian, M.D. Triage. *Crit. Care Clin.* **2019**, *35*, 575–589. [CrossRef] [PubMed]
7. Weerasinghe, S.S.; Campbell, S.G. Homelessness and Emergency Department Use: Wait Time Disparities Across Triage Acuity Levels. *Cureus* **2023**, *15*, e49520. [CrossRef] [PubMed]
8. Yuzeng, S.; Hui, L.L. Improving the wait time to triage at the emergency department. *BMJ Open Qual.* **2020**, *9*, e000708. [CrossRef]
9. Savioli, G.; Ceresa, I.F.; Maggioni, P.; Lava, M.; Ricevuti, G.; Manzoni, F.; Oddone, E.; Bressan, M.A. Impact of ED Organization with a Holding Area and a Dedicated Team on the Adherence to International Guidelines for Patients with Acute Pulmonary Embolism: Experience of an Emergency Department Organized in Areas of Intensity of Care. *Medicines* **2020**, *7*, 60. [CrossRef]
10. Savioli, G.; Ceresa, I.F.; Manzoni, F.; Ricevuti, G.; Bressan, M.A.; Oddone, E. Role of a Brief Intensive Observation Area with a Dedicated Team of Doctors in the Management of Acute Heart Failure Patients: A Retrospective Observational Study. *Medicina* **2020**, *56*, 251. [CrossRef] [PubMed]
11. Alquraini, M.; Awad, E.; Hijazi, R. Reliability of Canadian Emergency Department Triage and Acuity Scale (CTAS) in Saudi Arabia. *Int. J. Emerg. Med.* **2015**, *8*, 80. [CrossRef]
12. Considine, J.; Lucas, E.; Payne, R.; Kropman, M.; Stergiou, H.E.; Chiu, H. Analysis of three advanced practice roles in emergency nursing. *Australas. Emerg. Nurs. J.* **2012**, *15*, 219–228. [CrossRef]
13. Gómez-Angelats, E.; Miró, Ò.; Bragulat Baur, E.; Antolín Santaliestra, A.; Sánchez Sánchez, M. Triage level assignment and nurse characteristics and experience. *Emergencias* **2018**, *30*, 163–168, English, Spanish.
14. Rivers, E.P.; Katranji, M.; Jaehne, K.A.; Brown, S.; Abou Dagher, G.; Cannon, C.; Coba, V. Early interventions in severe sepsis and septic shock: A review of the evidence one decade later. *Minerva Anestesiol.* **2012**, *78*, 712–724.
15. Savioli, G.; Ceresa, I.F.; Bressan, M.A.; Piccini, G.B.; Varesi, A.; Novelli, V.; Muzzi, A.; Cutti, S.; Ricevuti, G.; Esposito, C.; et al. Five Level Triage vs. Four Level Triage in a Quaternary Emergency Department: National Analysis on Waiting Time, Validity, and Crowding-The CREONTE (Crowding and RE-Organization National TriagE) Study Group. *Medicina* **2023**, *59*, 781. [CrossRef]
16. Kim, J.H.; Kim, S.K.; Choi, J.; Lee, Y. Reliability of ChatGPT for performing triage task in the emergency department using the Korean Triage and Acuity Scale. *Digit. Health* **2024**, *10*, 20552076241227132. [CrossRef] [PubMed]
17. Høyvik, H.E.; Straume, V.; Østerås, Ø.; Engan, M. Triaging of acutely ill children transported by ambulance. *Tidsskr Nor Laegeforen* **2024**, *144*. [CrossRef] [PubMed]

18. Yamamoto, A.; Kuriyama, A.; Ikegami, T. Validity of a five-level prehospital triage system in Japan: A cohort study. *Am. J. Emerg. Med.* **2021**, *45*, 329–334. [CrossRef] [PubMed]
19. Liu, T.T.; Cheng, C.T.; Hsu, C.P.; Chaou, C.H.; Ng, C.J.; Jeng, M.J.; Chang, Y.C. Validation of a five-level triage system in pediatric trauma and the effectiveness of triage nurse modification: A multi-center cohort analysis. *Front. Med.* **2022**, *9*, 947501. [CrossRef] [PubMed]
20. Kuriyama, A.; Urushidani, S.; Nakayama, T. Five-level emergency triage systems: Variation in assessment of validity. *Emerg. Med. J.* **2017**, *34*, 703–710. [CrossRef] [PubMed]
21. Chakraborty, R.; Achour, N. Setting Up a Just and Fair ICU Triage Process during a Pandemic: A Systematic Review. *Healthcare* **2024**, *12*, 146. [CrossRef]
22. Chien, C.Y.; Chaou, C.H.; Yeh, C.C.; Hsu, K.H.; Gao, S.Y.; Ng, C.J. Using mobility status as a frailty indicator to improve the accuracy of a computerised five-level triage system among older patients in the emergency department. *BMC Emerg. Med.* **2022**, *22*, 86. [CrossRef]
23. Zachariasse, J.M.; van der Hagen, V.; Seiger, N.; Mackway-Jones, K.; van Veen, M.; Moll, H.A. Performance of triage systems in emergency care: A systematic review and meta-analysis. *BMJ Open* **2019**, *9*, e026471. [CrossRef]
24. Davis, S.; Ju, C.; Marchandise, P.; Diagne, M.; Grant, L. Impact of Pain Assessment on Canadian Triage and Acuity Scale Prediction of Patient Outcomes. *Ann. Emerg. Med.* **2022**, *79*, 433–440. [CrossRef]
25. Shi, H.X.; Wu, J.Z.; Chen, G.B.; Zhu, B.Z.; Yan, W.Y.; Chen, L.; Xiao, Y.J.; Zhang, L.Y. Application of the five-level pediatric emergency triage system: A single center study. *Zhonghua Er Ke Za Zhi* **2018**, *56*, 933–938. (In Chinese) [CrossRef] [PubMed]
26. Chmielewski, N.; Moretz, J. ESI Triage Distribution in U.S. Emergency Departments. *Adv. Emerg. Nurs. J.* **2022**, *44*, 46–53. [CrossRef]
27. Jesus, A.P.S.; Okuno, M.F.P.; Campanharo, C.R.V.; Lopes, M.C.B.T.; Batista, R.E.A. Manchester Triage System: Assessment in an emergency hospital service. *Rev. Bras. Enferm.* **2021**, *74*, e20201361. [CrossRef]
28. Peta, D.; Day, A.; Lugari, W.S.; Gorman, V.; Ahayalimudin, N.; Pajo, V.M.T. Triage: A Global Perspective. *J. Emerg. Nurs.* **2023**, *49*, 814–825. [CrossRef] [PubMed]
29. Marincowitz, C.; Hasan, M.; Omer, Y.; Hodkinson, P.; McAlpine, D.; Goodacre, S.; Bath, P.A.; Fuller, G.; Sbaffi, L.; Wallis, L. Prognostic accuracy of eight triage scores in suspected COVID-19 in an Emergency Department low-income setting: An observational cohort study. *Afr. J. Emerg. Med.* **2024**, *14*, 51–57. [CrossRef] [PubMed]
30. Davis, S.; Ju, C.; Marchandise, P.; Diagne, M.; Grant, L. The Effect of Human Supervision on an Electronic Implementation of the Canadian Triage Acuity Scale (CTAS). *J. Emerg. Med.* **2022**, *63*, 498–506. [CrossRef] [PubMed]
31. Pham, K.D.; Lim, F.A. The Impact of Geriatric-Specific Triage Tools Among Older Adults in the Emergency Department. *Crit. Care Nurs. Q.* **2020**, *43*, 39–57. [CrossRef]
32. Tejero, I.; Amor, E.; Vázquez-Ibar, O. Virtual geriatric and frailty assessment for older adults with cancer. *Curr. Opin. Support. Palliat. Care* **2024**, *18*, 16–21. [CrossRef]
33. Blomaard, L.C.; Speksnijder, C.; Lucke, J.A.; de Gelder, J.; Anten, S.; Schuit, S.C.E.; Steyerberg, E.W.; Gussekloo, J.; de Groot, B.; Mooijaart, S.P. Geriatric Screening, Triage Urgency, and 30-Day Mortality in Older Emergency Department Patients. *J. Am. Geriatr. Soc.* **2020**, *68*, 1755–1762. [CrossRef] [PubMed]
34. de Groot, A.J.; Wattel, E.M.; van Dam, C.S.; van Balen, R.; van der Wouden, J.C.; Hertogh, C.M.P.M. Referral to geriatric rehabilitation: A scoping review of triage factors in acutely hospitalised older patients. *Age Ageing* **2022**, *51*, afac015. [CrossRef] [PubMed]
35. Groening, M.; Wilke, P. Triage, Screening und Assessment des alten Menschen in der Notaufnahme [Triage, screening, and assessment of geriatric patients in the emergency department]. *Med. Klin. Intensivmed. Notfmed.* **2020**, *115*, 8–15. (In German) [CrossRef] [PubMed]
36. Alshibani, A.; Alharbi, M.; Conroy, S. Under-triage of older trauma patients in prehospital care: A systematic review. *Eur. Geriatr. Med.* **2021**, *12*, 903–919. [CrossRef] [PubMed]
37. Hoyle, A.C.; Biant, L.C.; Young, M. Undertriage of the elderly major trauma patient continues in major trauma centre care: A retrospective cohort review. *Emerg. Med. J.* **2020**, *37*, 508–514. [CrossRef] [PubMed]
38. Bullard, M.J.; Melady, D.; Emond, M.; members of the CTAS National working group; Musgrave, E.; Unger, B.; van der Linde, E.; Grierson, R.; Skeldon, T.; Warren, D.; et al. Guidance when Applying the Canadian Triage and Acuity Scale (CTAS) to the Geriatric Patient: Executive Summary. *Can. J. Emerg. Med.* **2017**, *19* (Suppl. S2), S28–S37, Erratum in *Can. J. Emerg. Med.* **2017**, *19*, 415. [CrossRef] [PubMed]
39. Javidi, S.; Movahedi, M.; Honarmand, A.; Mirafzal, A. Emergency Severity Index Triage in Iran: A Comparison between Age Groups in a Trauma Center. *Adv. Emerg. Nurs. J.* **2023**, *45*, 145–153. [CrossRef]
40. Savioli, G.; Bressan, M.; Ceresa, I. How Many Patients Are Triaged Using Five-Level Triage Scales Compared to Any Other Triage Acuity System in Italy? A SIMEU (Italian Scientific Society of Emergency Medicine) Faculty Triage Survey. In Proceedings of the European Emergency Medicine Congress, Lisbon, Portugal, 27–31 October 2021.
41. Bullard, M.J.; Musgrave, E.; Warren, D.; Unger, B.; Skeldon, T.; Grierson, R.; van der Linde, E.; Swain, J. Revisions to the Canadian Emergency Department Triage and Acuity Scale (CTAS) Guidelines 2016. *Can. J. Emerg. Med.* **2017**, *19* (Suppl. S2), S18–S27. [CrossRef]

42. Available online: https://www.parliament.vic.gov.au/images/stories/documents/council/scfpa/hospitals/submissions/scfpa_hospitals_06_app.pdf (accessed on 3 January 2020).
43. Vermeulen, M.J.; Guttmann, A.; Stukel, T.A.; Kachra, A.; Sivilotti, M.L.; Rowe, B.H.; Dreyer, J.; Bell, R.; Schull, M. Are reductions in emergency department length of stay associated with improvements in quality of care? A difference-in-differences analysis. *BMJ Qual. Saf.* **2016**, *25*, 489–498. [CrossRef] [PubMed]
44. Wu, L.; Chen, X.; Khalemsky, A.; Li, D.; Zoubeidi, T.; Lauque, D.; Alsabri, M.; Boudi, Z.; Kumar, V.A.; Paxton, J.; et al. The Association between Emergency Department Length of Stay and In-Hospital Mortality in Older Patients Using Machine Learning: An Observational Cohort Study. *J. Clin. Med.* **2023**, *12*, 4750. [CrossRef]
45. Lauque, D.; Khalemsky, A.; Boudi, Z.; Östlundh, L.; Xu, C.; Alsabri, M.; Onyeji, C.; Cellini, J.; Intas, G.; Soni, K.D.; et al. Length-of-Stay in the Emergency Department and In-Hospital Mortality: A Systematic Review and Meta-Analysis. *J. Clin. Med.* **2022**, *12*, 32. [CrossRef] [PubMed]
46. Elrod, J.K.; Fortenberry, J.L., Jr. The hub-and-spoke organization design: An avenue for serving patients well. *BMC Health Serv. Res.* **2017**, *17* (Suppl. S1), 457. [CrossRef]
47. Fernandes, C.M.; Tanabe, P.; Gilboy, N.; Johnson, L.A.; McNair, R.S.; Rosenau, A.M.; Sawchuk, P.; Thompson, D.A.; Travers, D.A.; Bonalumi, N.; et al. Five-level triage: A report from the ACEP/ENA Five-level Triage Task Force. *J. Emerg. Nurs.* **2005**, *31*, 39–118. [CrossRef]
48. Chin, B.; Alter, N.; Wright, D.D.; Arif, H.; Haddadi, M.; OLeary, J.; Elkbuli, A. Assessing Effectiveness and Efficiency of Need for Trauma Intervention (NFTI) and Modified NFTI in Identifying Overtriage and Undertriage Rates and Associated Outcomes. *Am. Surg.* **2023**, *89*, 6181–6189. [CrossRef]
49. Jones, E.K.; Tignanelli, C.J. Postoperative Intensive Care Unit Overtriage: An Application of Machine Learning. *Ann. Surg.* **2023**, *277*, 186–187. [CrossRef] [PubMed]
50. Olofsson, P.; Gellerstedt, M.; Carlström, E.D. Manchester Triage in Sweden—Interrater reliability and accuracy. *Int. Emerg. Nurs.* **2009**, *17*, 143–148. [CrossRef]
51. Hernández Ruipérez, T.; Leal Costa, C.; Adánez Martínez, M.G.; García Pérez, B.; Nova López, D.; Díaz Agea, J.L. Evidencias de validez del sistema de triaje Emergency Severity Index en un servicio de urgencias de un hospital general [Evidence of the validity of the Emergency Severity Index for triage in a general hospital emergency department]. *Emergencias* **2015**, *27*, 301–306.
52. Hansoti, B.; Jenson, A.; Keefe, D.; De Ramirez, S.S.; Anest, T.; Twomey, M.; Lobner, K.; Kelen, G.; Wallis, L. Reliability and validity of pediatric triage tools evaluated in Low resource settings: A systematic review. *BMC Pediatr.* **2017**, *17*, 37. [CrossRef]
53. Simon, H., Jr.; Schvartsman, C.; Sukys, G.A.; Farhat, S.C.L. Pediatric emergency triage systems. *Rev. Paul. Pediatr.* **2022**, *41*, e2021038. [CrossRef]
54. Jones, P.; Wells, S.; Ameratunga, S. Towards a best measure of emergency department crowding: Lessons from current Australasian practice. *Emerg. Med. Australas.* **2018**, *30*, 214–221. [CrossRef] [PubMed]
55. Kenny, J.F.; Chang, B.C.; Hemmert, K.C. Factors Affecting Emergency Department Crowding. *Emerg. Med. Clin. N. Am.* **2020**, *38*, 573–587. [CrossRef]
56. Franklin, B.J.; Vakili, S.; Huckman, R.S.; Hosein, S.; Falk, N.; Cheng, K.; Murray, M.; Harris, S.; Morris, C.A.; Goralnick, E. The Inpatient Discharge Lounge as a Potential Mechanism to Mitigate Emergency Department Boarding and Crowding. *Ann. Emerg. Med.* **2020**, *75*, 704–714. [CrossRef] [PubMed]
57. Morley, C.; Unwin, M.; Peterson, G.M.; Stankovich, J.; Kinsman, L. Emergency department crowding: A systematic review of causes, consequences and solutions. *PLoS ONE* **2018**, *13*, e0203316. [CrossRef] [PubMed]
58. Gross, T.K.; Lane, N.E.; Timm, N.L.; Committee on Pediatric Emergency Medicine. Crowding in the Emergency Department: Challenges and Recommendations for the Care of Children. *Pediatrics* **2023**, *151*, e2022060971. [CrossRef] [PubMed]
59. Brasseur, E.; Gilbert, A.; Servotte, J.C.; Donneau, A.F.; D'Orio, V.; Ghuysen, A. Emergency department crowding: Why do patients walk-in? *Acta Clin. Belg.* **2021**, *76*, 217–223. [CrossRef]
60. Wretborn, J.; Wilhelms, D.B.; Ekelund, U. Emergency department crowding and mortality: An observational multicenter study in Sweden. *Front. Public Health* **2023**, *11*, 1198188. [CrossRef]
61. Voaklander, B.; Gaudet, L.A.; Kirkland, S.W.; Keto-Lambert, D.; Villa-Roel, C.; Rowe, B.H. Interventions to improve consultations in the emergency department: A systematic review. *Acad. Emerg. Med.* **2022**, *29*, 1475–1495. [CrossRef]
62. Gross, T.K.; Lane, N.E.; Timm, N.L.; Committee on Pediatric Emergency Medicine. Crowding in the Emergency Department: Challenges and Best Practices for the Care of Children. *Pediatrics* **2023**, *151*, e2022060972. [CrossRef]
63. McNeilly, B.P.; Lawner, B.J.; Chizmar, T.P. The Chronicity of Emergency Department Crowding and Rethinking the Temporal Boundaries of Disaster Medicine. *Ann. Emerg. Med.* **2023**, *81*, 282–285. [CrossRef]
64. Scott, B.S.; Fahimi, J.; Mourad, M. Addressing the Emergency Department Crowding Crisis: Is Discharge by Noon Really the Answer? *Jt. Comm. J. Qual. Patient Saf.* **2023**, *49*, 179–180. [CrossRef]
65. Soriano, P.; Kanis, J.; Abulebda, K.; Schwab, S.; Coffee, R.L., Jr.; Wagers, B. Determining the Association Between Emergency Department Crowding and Debriefing After Pediatric Trauma Resuscitations. *Pediatr. Emerg. Care* **2023**, *39*, 848–852. [CrossRef] [PubMed]
66. Lindner, G.; Woitok, B.K. Emergency department overcrowding: Analysis and strategies to manage an international phenomenon. *Wien Klin. Wochenschr.* **2021**, *133*, 229–233. [CrossRef]

67. Schmitz, G.R.; Viccellio, P.; Litvak, E. Emergency Department Crowding after Coronavirus Disease 2019: Time to Change the Hospital Paradigm. *Ann. Emerg. Med.* **2023**, *82*, 661–663. [CrossRef]
68. Moskop, J.C.; Geiderman, J.M.; Marshall, K.D.; McGreevy, J.; Derse, A.R.; Bookman, K.; McGrath, N.; Iserson, K.V. Another Look at the Persistent Moral Problem of Emergency Department Crowding. *Ann. Emerg. Med.* **2019**, *74*, 357–364. [CrossRef] [PubMed]
69. Carter, E.J.; Pouch, S.M.; Larson, E.L. The relationship between emergency department crowding and patient outcomes: A systematic review. *J. Nurs. Scholarsh.* **2014**, *46*, 106–115. [CrossRef] [PubMed]
70. Liston, P.; Conyngham, G.; Brady, M.; Byrne, P.J.; Gilligan, P. Growing Old in the Emergency Department. *Ir. Med. J.* **2017**, *110*, 621.
71. De Freitas, L.; Goodacre, S.; O'Hara, R.; Thokala, P.; Hariharan, S. Interventions to improve patient flow in emergency departments: An umbrella review. *Emerg. Med. J.* **2018**, *35*, 626–637. [CrossRef]
72. Wartelle, A.; Mourad-Chehade, F.; Yalaoui, F.; Laplanche, D.; Sanchez, S. Analysis of Saturation in the Emergency Department: A Data-Driven Queuing Model Using Machine Learning. *Stud. Health Technol. Inform.* **2022**, *294*, 88–92. [CrossRef]
73. Javidan, A.P.; Hansen, K.; Higginson, I.; Jones, P.; Lang, E.; IFEM Task Force on Emergency Department Crowding, Access Block. The International Federation for Emergency Medicine report on emergency department crowding and access block: A brief summary. *Can. J. Emerg. Med.* **2021**, *23*, 26–28. [CrossRef] [PubMed]
74. Chiu, I.M.; Lin, Y.R.; Syue, Y.J.; Kung, C.T.; Wu, K.H.; Li, C.J. The influence of crowding on clinical practice in the emergency department. *Am. J. Emerg. Med.* **2018**, *36*, 56–60. [CrossRef] [PubMed]
75. Baugh, C.W.; Freund, Y.; Steg, P.G.; Body, R.; Maron, D.J.; Yiadom, M.Y.A.B. Strategies to mitigate emergency department crowding and its impact on cardiovascular patients. *Eur. Heart J. Acute Cardiovasc. Care* **2023**, *12*, 633–643. [CrossRef] [PubMed]
76. Eiset, A.H.; Kirkegaard, H.; Erlandsen, M. Crowding in the emergency department in the absence of boarding—A transition regression model to predict departures and waiting time. *BMC Med. Res. Methodol.* **2019**, *19*, 68. [CrossRef] [PubMed]
77. Chan, S.S.; Cheung, N.K.; Graham, C.A.; Rainer, T.H. Strategies and solutions to alleviate access block and overcrowding in emergency departments. *Hong Kong Med. J.* **2015**, *21*, 345–352. [CrossRef] [PubMed]
78. Smith, A.J.; Patterson, B.W.; Pulia, M.S.; Mayer, J.; Schwei, R.J.; Nagarajan, R.; Liao, F.; Shah, M.N.; Boutilier, J.J. Multisite evaluation of prediction models for emergency department crowding before and during the COVID-19 pandemic. *J. Am. Med. Inform. Assoc.* **2023**, *30*, 292–300. [CrossRef] [PubMed]
79. Pearce, S.; Marchand, T.; Shannon, T.; Ganshorn, H.; Lang, E. Emergency department crowding: An overview of reviews describing measures causes, and harms. *Intern. Emerg. Med.* **2023**, *18*, 1137–1158. [CrossRef]
80. Al-Qahtani, S.; Alsultan, A.; Haddad, S.; Alsaawi, A.; Alshehri, M.; Alsolamy, S.; Felebaman, A.; Tamim, H.M.; Aljerian, N.; Al-Dawood, A.; et al. The association of duration of boarding in the emergency room and the outcome of patients admitted to the intensive care unit. *BMC Emerg. Med.* **2017**, *17*, 34. [CrossRef]
81. Cha, W.C.; Cho, J.S.; Shin, S.D.; Lee, E.J.; Ro, Y.S. The impact of prolonged boarding of successfully resuscitated out-of-hospital cardiac arrest patients on survival-to-discharge rates. *Resuscitation* **2015**, *90*, 25–29. [CrossRef]
82. Eiset, A.H.; Erlandsen, M.; Møllekær, A.B.; Mackenhauer, J.; Kirkegaard, H. A generic method for evaluating crowding in the emergency department. *BMC Emerg. Med.* **2016**, *16*, 21. [CrossRef]
83. Noel, G.; Drigues, C.; Viudes, G.; Fedoru Crowding Working Group. Which indicators to include in a crowding scale in an emergency department? A national French Delphi study. *Eur. J. Emerg. Med.* **2018**, *25*, 257–263. [CrossRef]
84. Savioli, G.; Ceresa, I.F.; Gri, N.; Bavestrello Piccini, G.; Longhitano, Y.; Zanza, C.; Piccioni, A.; Esposito, C.; Ricevuti, G.; Bressan, M.A. Emergency Department Overcrowding: Understanding the Factors to Find Corresponding Solutions. *J. Pers. Med.* **2022**, *12*, 279. [CrossRef]
85. Savioli, G.; Ceresa, I.F.; Novelli, V.; Ricevuti, G.; Bressan, M.A.; Oddone, E. How the coronavirus disease 2019 pandemic changed the patterns of healthcare utilization by geriatric patients and the crowding: A call to action for effective solutions to the access block. *Intern. Emerg. Med.* **2022**, *17*, 503–514. [CrossRef] [PubMed]
86. Savioli, G.; Ceresa, I.F.; Guarnone, R.; Muzzi, A.; Novelli, V.; Ricevuti, G.; Iotti, G.A.; Bressan, M.A.; Oddone, E. Impact of Coronavirus Disease 2019 Pandemic on Crowding: A Call to Action for Effective Solutions to "Access Block". *West J. Emerg. Med.* **2021**, *22*, 860–870. [CrossRef] [PubMed]
87. Jaboyedoff, M.; Starvaggi, C.; Suris, J.C.; Kuehni, C.E.; Gehri, M.; Keitel, K. Drivers for low-acuity pediatric emergency department visits in two tertiary hospitals in Switzerland: A cross-sectional, questionnaire-based study. *BMC Health Serv. Res.* **2024**, *24*, 103. [CrossRef]
88. Lahiri, K.; Indrasena, B.S.H.; Aylott, J. Unprecedented times in the emergency department: Are "board rounds" and leadership the missing links to improve patient flow? *Leadersh. Health Serv.* **2021**, *35*, 74–90. [CrossRef]
89. Savioli, G.; Ceresa, I.F.; Novara, E.; Persiano, T.; Grulli, F.; Ricevuti., G.; Bressan, M.A.; Oddone, E. Brief Intensive Observation areas in the management of acute heart failure in elderly patients leading to high stabilisation rate and less admissions. *J. Gerontol. Geriatr.* **2021**, *69*, 87–97. [CrossRef]
90. Wolf, L.A.; Lo, A.X.; Serina, P.; Chary, A.; Sri-On, J.; Shankar, K.; Sano, E.; Liu, S.W. Frailty assessment tools in the emergency department: A geriatric emergency department guidelines 2.0 scoping review. *J. Am. Coll. Emerg Physicians Open* **2023**, *5*, e13084. [CrossRef]
91. Bonfichi, A.; Ceresa, I.F.; Piccioni, A.; Zanza, C.; Longhitano, Y.; Boudi, Z.; Esposito, C.; Savioli, G. A Lethal Combination of Delirium and Overcrowding in the Emergency Department. *J. Clin. Med.* **2023**, *12*, 6587. [CrossRef]

92. Wilkins, T.; Shiver, S.; Butler, C.; Corcoran, L.; Marshall, R.; Brody, C.; Cliett, K.; Nolan, M.A.; Sowinski, T.; Schreiber, M. Development of an Emergency Department Surge Plan Based on the NEDOCS score. *Ann. Fam. Med.* **2024**, *21* (Suppl. S3), 4789. [CrossRef]
93. Vlodaver, Z.K.; Anderson, J.P.; Brown, B.E.; Zwank, M.D. Emergency medicine physicians' ability to predict hospital admission at the time of triage. *Am. J. Emerg. Med.* **2019**, *37*, 478–481. [CrossRef]
94. Herzog, S.M.; Jenny, M.A.; Nickel, C.H.; Nieves Ortega, R.; Bingisser, R. Emergency department patients with weakness or fatigue: Can physicians predict their outcomes at the front door? A prospective observational study. *PLoS ONE* **2020**, *15*, e0239902. [CrossRef]
95. Zwank, M.D.; Koops, J.J.; Adams, N.R. Provider-in-triage prediction of hospital admission after brief patient interaction. *Am. J. Emerg. Med.* **2021**, *40*, 60–63. [CrossRef] [PubMed]
96. Boudi, Z.; Lauque, D.; Alsabri, M.; Östlundh, L.; Oneyji, C.; Khalemsky, A.; Rial, C.L.; Liu, S.W.; Camargo, C.A.; Aburawi, E.; et al. Association between boarding in the emergency department and in-hospital mortality: A systematic review. *PLoS ONE* **2020**, *15*, e0231253. [CrossRef] [PubMed]
97. Chang, Y.C.; Ng, C.J.; Wu, C.T.; Chen, L.C.; Chen, J.C.; Hsu, K.H. Effectiveness of a five-level Paediatric Triage System: An analysis of resource utilisation in the emergency department in Taiwan. *Emerg. Med. J.* **2013**, *30*, 735–739. [CrossRef]
98. Morris, R.S.; Karam, B.S.; Murphy, P.B.; Jenkins, P.; Milia, D.J.; Hemmila, M.R.; Haines, K.L.; Puzio, T.J.; de Moya, M.A.; Tignanelli, C.J. Field-Triage, Hospital-Triage and Triage-Assessment: A Literature Review of the Current Phases of Adult Trauma Triage. *J. Trauma Acute Care Surg.* **2021**, *90*, e138–e145. [CrossRef] [PubMed]
99. Lerner, E.B.; Cushman, J.T.; Drendel, A.L.; Badawy, M.; Shah, M.N.; Guse, C.E.; Cooper, A. Effect of the 2011 Revisions to the Field Triage Guidelines on Under- and Over-Triage Rates for Pediatric Trauma Patients. *Prehosp. Emerg. Care* **2017**, *21*, 456–460. [CrossRef] [PubMed]
100. Ellebrecht, N. Why Is Treatment Urgency Often Overestimated? An Experimental Study on the Phenomenon of Over-triage. *Disaster Med. Public Health Prep.* **2020**, *14*, 563–567. [CrossRef]
101. Zhang, D.Y.; Shy, B.; Genes, N. Early Rooming Triage: Accuracy and Demographic Factors Associated with Clinical Acuity. *West J. Emerg. Med.* **2022**, *23*, 145–151. [CrossRef]
102. Dani, M.; Dirksen, A.; Taraborrelli, P.; Panagopolous, D.; Torocastro, M.; Sutton, R.; Lim, P.B. Orthostatic hypotension in older people: Considerations, diagnosis and management. *Clin. Med.* **2021**, *21*, e275–e282. [CrossRef]
103. Brown, J.B.; Gestring, M.L.; Forsythe, R.M.; Stassen, N.A.; Billiar, T.R.; Peitzman, A.B.; Sperry, J.L. Systolic blood pressure criteria in the National Trauma Triage Protocol for geriatric trauma: 110 is the new 90. *J. Trauma Acute Care Surg.* **2015**, *78*, 352–359. [CrossRef] [PubMed]
104. Wod, M.; Jensen, M.T.; Galatius, S.; Hjelmborg, J.B.; Jensen, G.B.; Christensen, K. Resting heart rate and mortality in the very old. *Scand. J. Clin. Lab. Investig.* **2019**, *79*, 566–571. [CrossRef] [PubMed]
105. Shimazui, T.; Nakada, T.A.; Walley, K.R.; Oshima, T.; Abe, T.; Ogura, H.; Shiraishi, A.; Kushimoto, S.; Saitoh, D.; Fujishima, S.; et al. Significance of body temperature in elderly patients with sepsis. *Crit. Care* **2020**, *24*, 387. [CrossRef] [PubMed]
106. Soler-Sanchis, A.; Martínez-Arnau, F.M.; Sánchez-Frutos, J.; Pérez-Ros, P. Clinical Risk Group as a predictor of mortality in delirious older adults in the emergency department. *Exp. Gerontol.* **2023**, *174*, 112129. [CrossRef] [PubMed]
107. Rajput, K.; Ng, J.; Zwolinski, N.; Chow, R.M. Pain Management in the Elderly: A Narrative Review. *Anesthesiol. Clin.* **2023**, *41*, 671–691. [CrossRef] [PubMed]
108. Davis, P.; Evans, D.D. The Undertriage of Older Adults in the Emergency Department: A Review of Interventions. *Adv. Emerg. Nurs. J.* **2021**, *43*, 178–185. [CrossRef] [PubMed]
109. Schöll, N.; Rohde, G.G.U. Ambulant erworbene Pneumonie bei älteren Menschen [Community-acquired Pneumonia in the Elderly]. *Pneumologie* **2019**, *73*, 605–616. Erratum in *Pneumologie* **2019**, *73*, e3. (In German) [CrossRef]
110. Tran, J.; Nimojan, T.; Saripella, A.; Tang-Wai, D.F.; Butris, N.; Kapoor, P.; Berezin, L.; Englesakis, M.; Chung, F. Rapid cognitive assessment tools for screening of mild cognitive impairment in the preoperative setting: A systematic review and meta-analysis. *J. Clin. Anesth.* **2022**, *78*, 110682. [CrossRef]
111. Weber, C.; Millen, J.C.; Liu, H.; Clark, J.; Ferber, L.; Richards, W.; Ang, D. Undertriage of Geriatric Trauma Patients in Florida. *J. Surg. Res.* **2022**, *279*, 427–435. [CrossRef]
112. Grossmann, F.F.; Zumbrunn, T.; Ciprian, S.; Stephan, F.P.; Woy, N.; Bingisser, R.; Nickel, C.H. Undertriage in older emergency department patients--tilting against windmills? *PLoS ONE* **2014**, *9*, e106203. [CrossRef]
113. Savioli, G.; Ceresa, I.F.; Macedonio, S.; Gerosa, S.; Belliato, M.; Luzzi, S.; Lucifero, A.G.; Manzoni, F.; Ricevuti, G.; Bressan, M.A. Major Trauma in Elderly Patients: Worse Mortality and Outcomes in an Italian Trauma Center. *J. Emerg. Trauma Shock* **2021**, *14*, 98–103. [CrossRef]
114. Savioli, G.; Ceresa, I.F.; Giordano, M.; Ferrari, I.; Varesi, A.; Floris, V.; Esposito, C.; Croesi, B.; Ricevuti, G.; Calvi, M.; et al. The Reliability of Anamnestic Data in the Management of Clostridium Tetani Infection in Elderly. *Front. Med.* **2021**, *8*, 684594. [CrossRef]
115. Grossmann, F.F.; Zumbrunn, T.; Frauchiger, A.; Delport, K.; Bingisser, R.; Nickel, C.H. At risk of undertriage? Testing the performance and accuracy of the emergency severity index in older emergency department patients. *Ann. Emerg. Med.* **2012**, *60*, 317–325.e3. [CrossRef] [PubMed]

116. Savioli, G.; Ceresa, I.F.; Luzzi, S.; Giotta Lucifero, A.; Pioli Di Marco, M.S.; Manzoni, F.; Preda, L.; Ricevuti, G.; Bressan, M.A. Mild Head Trauma: Is Antiplatelet Therapy a Risk Factor for Hemorrhagic Complications? *Medicina* **2021**, *57*, 357. [CrossRef] [PubMed]
117. Savioli, G.; Ceresa, I.F.; Macedonio, S.; Gerosa, S.; Belliato, M.; Iotti, G.A.; Luzzi, S.; Del Maestro, M.; Mezzini, G.; Giotta Lucifero, A. Trauma Coagulopathy and Its Outcomes. *Medicina* **2020**, *56*, 205. [CrossRef] [PubMed]
118. Savioli, G.; Ceresa, I.F.; Luzzi, S.; Giotta Lucifero, A.; Cambiè, G.; Manzoni, F.; Preda, L.; Ricevuti, G.; Bressan, M.A. Mild Head Trauma (MHT) and Antiplatelet Therapy. Reply to Lorenzati et al. Comment on "Savioli et al. Mild Head Trauma: Is Antiplatelet Therapy a Risk Factor for Hemorrhagic Complications? *Medicina* **2021**, *57*, 357". *Medicina* **2021**, *57*, 889. [CrossRef] [PubMed]
119. Savioli, G.; Ceresa, I.F.; Luzzi, S.; Gragnaniello, C.; Giotta Lucifero, A.; Del Maestro, M.; Marasco, S.; Manzoni, F.; Ciceri, L.; Gelfi, E.; et al. Rates of Intracranial Hemorrhage in Mild Head Trauma Patients Presenting to Emergency Department and Their Management: A Comparison of Direct Oral Anticoagulant Drugs with Vitamin K Antagonists. *Medicina* **2020**, *56*, 308. [CrossRef] [PubMed]
120. Savioli, G.; Ceresa, I.F.; Ciceri, L.; Sciutti, F.; Belliato, M.; Iotti, G.A.; Luzzi, S.; Del Maestro, M.; Mezzini, G.; Lafe, E.; et al. Mild head trauma in elderly patients: Experience of an emergency department. *Heliyon* **2020**, *6*, e04226. [CrossRef]
121. Cristofaro, P.A. Infection and fever in the elderly. *J. Am. Podiatr. Med. Assoc.* **2004**, *94*, 126–134. [CrossRef] [PubMed]
122. Phongtankuel, V.; Amorapanth, P.X.; Siegler, E.L. Pain in the Geriatric Patient with Advanced Chronic Disease. *Clin. Geriatr. Med.* **2016**, *32*, 651–661. [CrossRef]
123. Varesi, A.; Carrara, A.; Pires, V.G.; Floris, V.; Pierella, E.; Savioli, G.; Prasad, S.; Esposito, C.; Ricevuti, G.; Chirumbolo, S.; et al. Blood-Based Biomarkers for Alzheimer's Disease Diagnosis and Progression: An Overview. *Cells* **2022**, *11*, 1367. [CrossRef] [PubMed]
124. Deumer, U.S.; Varesi, A.; Floris, V.; Savioli, G.; Mantovani, E.; López-Carrasco, P.; Rosati, G.M.; Prasad, S.; Ricevuti, G. Myalgic Encephalomyelitis/Chronic Fatigue Syndrome (ME/CFS): An Overview. *J. Clin. Med.* **2021**, *10*, 4786. [CrossRef]
125. Arneson, M.L.; Oliveira JE Silva, L.; Stanich, J.A.; Jeffery, M.M.; Lindroth, H.L.; Ginsburg, A.D.; Bower, S.M.; Mullan, A.F.; Bellolio, F. Association of delirium with increased short-term mortality among older emergency department patients: A cohort study. *Am. J. Emerg. Med.* **2023**, *66*, 105–110. [CrossRef] [PubMed]
126. Martinelli, A.N. Rapid Fire: Polypharmacy in the Geriatric Patient. *Emerg. Med. Clin. N. Am.* **2021**, *39*, 395–404. [CrossRef]
127. Clare, D.; Zink, K.L. Geriatric Trauma. *Emerg. Med. Clin. N. Am.* **2021**, *39*, 257–271. [CrossRef] [PubMed]

Journal of *Personalized Medicine*

MDPI

Review

Drinking from the Holy Grail—Does a Perfect Triage System Exist? And Where to Look for It?

Anna Ingielewicz [1,2,*], Piotr Rychlik [2] and Mariusz Sieminski [1]

1 Department of Emergency Medicine, Faculty of Health Science, Medical University of Gdansk, Mariana Smoluchowskiego Street 17, 80-214 Gdansk, Poland; sieminski@gumed.edu.pl
2 Emergency Department, Copernicus Hospital, Nowe Ogrody Street 1-6, 80-203 Gdansk, Poland
* Correspondence: anna.ingielewicz@gumed.edu.pl; Tel.: +48-512434828

Abstract: The Emergency Department (ED) is a facility meant to treat patients in need of medical assistance. The choice of triage system hugely impactsed the organization of any given ED and it is important to analyze them for their effectiveness. The goal of this review is to briefly describe selected triage systems in an attempt to find the perfect one. Papers published in PubMed from 1990 to 2022 were reviewed. The following terms were used for comparison: "ED" and "triage system". The papers contained data on the design and function of the triage system, its validation, and its performance. After studies comparing the distinct means of patient selection were reviewed, they were meant to be classified as either flawed or non-ideal. The validity of all the comparable segregation systems was similar. A possible solution would be to search for a new, measurable parameter for a more accurate risk estimation, which could be a game changer in terms of triage assessment. The dynamic development of artificial intelligence (AI) technologies has recently been observed. The authors of this study believe that the future segregation system should be a combination of the experience and intuition of trained healthcare professionals and modern technology (artificial intelligence).

Keywords: triage system comparison; in-hospital triage; medical segregation; emergency severity index; Manchester triage system

1. Introduction

The Emergency Department (ED) is dedicated to patients requiring urgent medical assistance. Globally, EDs are faced with an inflow of patients who outnumber their capacity. Moreover, a consequent year-to-year increase in the number of patients visiting EDs has been observed globally [1,2]. ED patients are not only growing in number but are also growing older. Approximately 30% of the visitors to EDs are above 65 years old with medical consequences of advanced age, such as the fragility syndrome, multiple comorbidities, and a higher risk of life-threatening conditions [3,4]. This overcrowding in EDs results in an increase in burden on the medical staff, need for resources, boarding time, and time to treatment [5,6]. A crucial organizational need in EDs is the proper allocation of resources to provide medical services to patients on time, adjusted to the urgency of their condition. One of the tools for solving this challenge is the medical triage.

The in-hospital medical triage is aimed at the prioritization of patients to determine the time during which physicians should assess them. It facilitates the flow of patients within the ED [1,3,5,6]. The emergency room triage is usually performed by a trained nurse or paramedic who assesses patients' signs and symptoms as well as vital signs. Additionally, the in-hospital triage aims to determine the amount and type of resources required for patients as well as allocation of these resources to provide care in time to patients according to their severity [1,3,6]. Experiments were conducted to assess the effect of replacing nurse-performed triage systems with AI-run triage systems [7,8], or by the patients themselves, but results have not been clear [9].

On the other hand, prehospital triage has also been postulated and assessed in scientific projects [10–13], as well as using machine learning models to optimize care in emergency services e.g., chest pain, trauma brain injuries, or ophthalmic problems [14–16]. The results of the mentioned solutions have increasingly strong evidence based in science, but further studies are required [17].

The purpose of this study is to review the literature on the topic of triage to find an answer to the question of whether an ideal segregation system currently exists, and if not, where to look for it. In this paper, we briefly characterize the selected triage systems in an attempt to describe an ideal triage system and review the results of comparisons among the studies on the various triage systems. The authors know that other systems of medical triage with proven usefulness exist; however, the choice of systems compared in this article resulted from the fact that they are a reference point for most of the world's publications [18–21]. To select sources for this review, PubMed search was performed from 1990 to April 2024. The following terms were used for comparison: "ED", "triage system", "triage system comparison", and "artificial intelligence". Publications available in English were selected for analysis. The first search identified 700 publications. After reading the abstracts, 126 were singled out and were then read in full. After a comprehensive study of the publications, 66 articles were selected for final analysis.

The papers contain data about the following:

(a) The design and function of a triage system
(b) Its validation
(c) Its performance
(d) The comparison between the two triage systems

The use of machine-learning methods in the triage process was first analyzed, and the final reference list was created based on the relevance to the topic of the review.

Many triage systems have been created and used in hospitals worldwide, such as the Manchester Triage System (MTS) [5,22], Emergency Severity Index (ESI) [23–25], Canadian Triage and Acuity Scale (CTAS) [26], and Australian Triage Scale (ATS) [27]. Triage systems based on a five-grade scale are the most common, with scientifically proven superiority to the three-grade solutions [28–30].

The patient's urgency is coded by the color or the digit, descending from the most urgent cases (e.g., red—1; orange—2; Yellow—3; green—4. Blue—5). While the two top grades represent a minority of patients and are served immediately in most cases, the most common are the three lowest categories. This is a confusion-generating disadvantage of the triage systems, because of which the ED staff face a high number of patients with similar priorities, among whom patients still require urgent help [4,31]. The latter is another problem of the triage system in terms of sensitivity and specificity.

The triage system used plays a pivotal role in the organization of the ED's functions. Therefore, the criteria which is useful in the assessment of triage systems, and for comparative studies focused on the analysis of the specificity and sensitivity of triage systems, is required in the context of the effective screening of patients at risk of death, cardiac arrest, immediate intervention (e.g., the percutaneous coronary intervention—PCI), and hospitalization in the Intensive Care Unit (ICU). This article deals with issues rarely discussed on this topic, such as the ease of use of the triage system, the time needed to learn it, and the diversity of triage use in different groups of patients. The authors did not find any papers addressing all the issues discussed in this article.

2. Ideal Triage System

As mentioned above, triage systems presently used worldwide are five-degree scales in most cases. The most common systems that were created in the last decade of the previous century have undergone constant optimization until now. Since their creation, their authors have been making efforts to analyze whether the triage systems meet the needs of patients and ED staff, and the results of studies in that area have been used to improve the systems. This has been carried out to design a system characterized as follows (Figure 1):

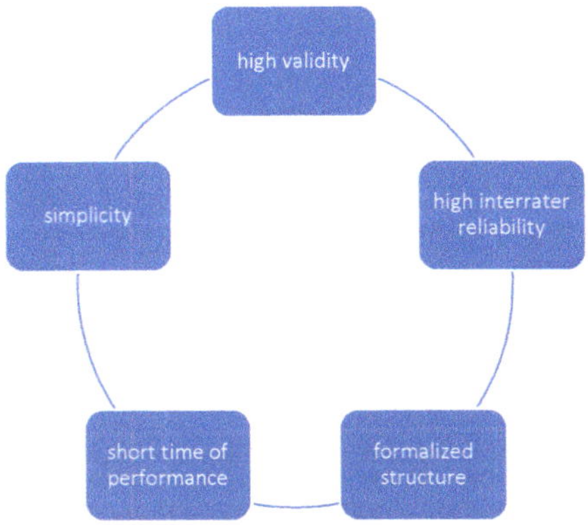

Figure 1. Features of an ideal in-hospital triage system.

High validity is defined as the ability of a system to prioritize patients concordantly with their actual conditions. The difficulty achieving this goal lies in the lack of an ideal benchmark (a "gold standard") to which the priority established during triage could have been compared.

High interrater reliability means the repeatability of the results regardless of the person performing the triage. It is expressed by Cohen's kappa coefficient, taking values from 0.0 to 1.0—the closer to 1.0, the larger the agreement between the raters' results.

Simplicity is understood as the ease of proceeding with the triage. This can be measured using users' satisfaction. This parameter may impact the kappa coefficient described above and is related to the time required for training during triage.

Short time of performance means the time taken for diagnosis and treatment—the actual aims behind visiting the ED. The authors of the systems of triage focus on time, for example, assuming that it is supposed to last no longer than two minutes.

Formalized structure is important because using the system is described by an algorithm of triage that influences the kappa coefficient and improves staff training.

Combining all the above elements presently seems impossible therefore, systems that compromise these expectations are used at the ED.

3. Most Common Triage Systems

To discuss all medical segregation systems in the world is impossible, and a few of the most common systems will be highlighted here. Because of the higher reliability proven in many studies, only five-step systems [2] will be presented in the alphabetical order:

I. ATS (Australian Triage Scale)

The system was introduced in the Emergency Departments in Australia in 1994 and was closely related to the patient's waiting time for a medical examination:

- 0 min. for priority 1 (red)
- Up to 10 min for priority 2 (orange)
- Up to 30 min for priority 3 (green)
- Up to 60 min for priority 4 (blue)
- Up to 120 min. for priority 5 (white) [27].

At the same time, it is noted that the system's task is to assess the urgency of providing help, not necessarily the severity of the patient's condition.

The nurse has at his disposal a table presenting five priorities, with the discriminators listed next to them, which are a description of clinical situations, e.g., suspected sepsis (hemodynamically unstable), testicular torsion, severe pain.

The nurse conducting the assessment determined the reason for the report. The triage process is a two-stage process, it begins with an assessment according to the ABCD scheme, with the task of establishing at the outset whether the patient is unstable and requires immediate care. If not, a more complete assessment is made, based on discriminators.

The system includes additional lists of discriminators for patients with mental disorders and for children, vital parameters are checked although they do not directly influence the result of the scale.

II. CTAS (Canadian Triage and Acuity Scale)

The system was developed in the 1990s in Canada, based on the ATS system. It is related to the specific waiting times for the first medical evaluation.

- For priority 1 (blue), assistance must be provided immediately,
- Priority 2 (red) can wait up to 15 min,
- Priority 3 (yellow) waiting time up to 30 min,
- Priority 4 (green) waiting time up to 60 min,
- Priority 5 (white) waiting time up to 120 min [26].

This system also includes the obligation to conduct re-triage in intervals, depending on the priority, which coincides with the patient's time of acceptable expectation.

CTAS is referred to as a four-stage system as follows:

1. "Critical Look"—A short, several-second assessment according to the ABCD scheme, aimed at quick recognition of patients in priorities 1 and 2
2. Assessment for infectious diseases—Aimed at the rapid isolation of potentially dangerous patients or their decontamination
3. Identify the patient's main or major complaints, collect objective data (including, for example, vital signs, injury assessment, bleeding severity), use a list of "modifiers". They are grouped into 17 categories, there are about 177 of them in total, and some of them are additionally graded, so that after confirming a given modifier, the priority can be read from the table
4. The prioritization of the CTAS

An additional advantage is the inclusion of a separate section on children in CTAS.

III. ESI (Emergency Severity Index)

This system was developed in the USA in the 1990s. Unlike the others discussed here, only the first two priorities have the following specific time periods for medical evaluation:

- Immediately for priority 1
- Up to 10 min for priority [25]

It is based on four decision points.

1. Point A—The nurse must assess whether the patient requires life-saving procedures. If so, give priority 1.
2. Point B—Features of a high-risk state for the patient are looked for, the presence of severe pain or disturbances of consciousness—if the result is positive, priority 2 is given.
3. Point C—it is necessary to assess what will be the "consumption" of resources while supplying the patient to the ED. This is a feature that distinguishes the ESI system from others. Patients requiring one or none of the resources receive Priority 4 and 5, respectively. Patients requiring two or more resources go to the next point.
4. Point D—vital parameters are assessed: saturation O_2, pulse rate, respiratory rate, and temperature in children, based on the table, it is determined whether the patient "promotes" to the priority 2 group or receives priority 3. This point is a kind of "Fuse", enabling reconsideration of the prioritization of 2 patients [24].

IV. MTS (Manchester Triage System)

It is a system developed in Great Britain, also in the 1990s. Priority is given to specific times for the first contact with a doctor as follows:

- Priority 1 (red)—immediate aid,
- Priority 2 (orange)—up to 10 min,
- Priority 3 (yellow)—up to 60 min,
- Priority 4 (green)—up to 120 min.
- Priority 5 (blue)—up to 240 min [22].

This system is similar to the ATS, which together with the CTAS, forms them into a group of systems based on "discriminators"/"modifiers", i.e., the confirmation or exclusion of several symptoms or clinical conditions.

What distinguishes it is the presentation of the discriminators in the form of a decision-making algorithm. The nurse initially identifies the patient's main problem and assigns it to one of 52 cards that reflect the most common reasons for a patient's presentation to the ED. Then, following the diagram illustrated on the card, individual discriminators should be excluded, grouped, and ranked according to priorities from 1 to 5, until confirmation of the presence of one of the listed ones and the assigned priority can be read.

The scheme forces the focus to first be on proving that the patient is in priority 1, which reduces the triage time in the group of patients urgently in need of help. Vital signs are necessarily measured only if a discriminator is encountered that determines them.

Based on the methodology, the systems can be divided into two groups: based on discriminators, to the confirmation or exclusion of several symptoms or clinical conditions (ATS, CTAS, and MTS), and based on a decision diagram (ESI).

A natural common feature is the desire to ensure that the segregation of patients in Priorities 1 and 2 does not stop the activities in the case of a patient who needs urgent help; that is, it should be conducted as soon as possible.

Therefore, an ideal system of segregation can only be indicated using the criteria from the previous section as shown in Table 1.

Table 1. Table subjectively comparing the most popular medical triage systems with authors' comments (+ good), (++ very good), (? not specified).

	ATS	CTAS	ESI	MTS
Validity	+/? Little research [2]	+/? Good [2]	+/? [2] Different results analyses in research, though seems more accurate in a group of children and elderly people than MTS [19,21,22]	+/? [2] Contradictory data depending on the study. Probably depending on the age of the patient and distance hospital from place uprising triage system
Reliability Kappa value	0.25 to 0.56, but decreases in the group of patients with mental disorders [2]	Adults 0.68–0.89 Children 0.51–0.72 [2]	Adults 0.46–0.91 Children 0.82 [2]	Adults 0.31–0.62 [2]
Simplicity (subjective evaluation)	++	+	+(+) Seems to depend on the presence of clear guidelines (diagnostic and treatment standards) in the hospital	++
Short time of performance	Time depends on patient priority, the higher the priority the shorter the time	Time depends on patient priority, the higher the priority the shorter the time	Time depends on patient priority, the higher the priority the shorter the time	Time depends on patient priority, the higher the priority the shorter the time
Formalized structure	+	+	+	+

4. Triage System Comparisons

Considering a variety of systems of triage and their diverse distribution among EDs globally, some attempts have been made to compare them. Such comparisons are difficult for several reasons. These systems differ in terms of the quality and quantity of collected data and endpoints of studies (usually various events during hospitalization). The authors of the published papers compared selected aspects of the systems or simply described their characteristic features. This makes the conclusive analysis of such papers difficult. However, current research analyses focus on the support offered by the use of machine-learning methods rather than a direct comparison of triage systems [32].

The most common systems worldwide are the MTS, CTAS, ESI, and ATS. They are well studied, validated and characterized by high inter-rater reliability—good and very good for ESI and CTAS (kappa 0.7–0.95) and moderated in the case of MTS and ATS (kappa 0.3–0.6) [2,18,33]. An interesting observation arose after the analysis of articles that specifically considered ESI systems. Analyses of different results show that ESI systems seem to be more accurate in a group of children and elderly people than MTS [24,34]. However, some studies indicated that the risk of under-triage increases in the group of patients over 65 years [4,31,35], while Saberian et al. suggested, based on the frailty index, the need to lower this limit to 50 years [36].

Some studies have compared widely accepted triage systems with local nonformalized systems. A good example is the comparison made between ESI with the Taiwan Triage System (TTS), which has shown that ESI predicts better TTS usage of ED resources as well as time spent by patients in the ED and the severity of their conditions [37]. Contrastingly, Zakeri et al. [38] compared the ESI and MTS in a group of trauma patients, showing that the use of the ESI system may generate over triage in a group of patients in priority 3.

Another study performed in a single Dutch ED compared the ESI, MTS, and the Informally Structured System (ISS) [39]. The authors reported a lack of significant differences in the prediction of increased consumption of ED resources, percentage of hospitalizations, and length of hospitalization among patients with the two highest priorities (1/Red and 2/Orange, respectively). The only significant difference in specificity between ESI and MTS was found only in priority 4/Green (postponed service). It was also found that with MTS, the lowest priority (code Blue) was given significantly less frequently than with ESI (code 5). Moreover, the authors of this study noticed the lower sensitivity of ESI and MTS than for earlier publications [28]. This may be because in previous studies, only selected groups of patients, such as critically ill participants, were analyzed [40]. Under triage of patients from the two highest categories described in this study may be a consequence of the methods of assessing the results of triage by experts who know the further course of hospitalization of the participants.

One of the most recent comparison among the three commonly used systems (MTS, ESI, and CTAS) published in 2020 revealed similar sensitivity and specificity for each of the systems [41]. Additionally, structured algorithms of triage were shown to define very precisely and concordantly the highest (1 and 2) and the lowest (5) priorities, while assigning priorities to the intermediate categories (3 and 4) was less precise. Consequently, the most critically ill participants received assistance immediately and effectively, but care for patients assigned to intermediate categories was postponed, while patients still needed urgent treatment in these groups. This is of special concern, as intermediate categories are usually the most abundant in EDs [2].

Regarding the pediatric population, unsatisfactory agreement rates were observed as follows: poor for ATS (0.25), moderate for CTAS (0.571), good for ESI (0.81), and MTS (0.755) [42].

However, in some articles, the highest reliability was found for the ESI and the pediatric version of the CTAS (good inter-rater reliability, with a kappa of 0.8–0.9). The ESI also most accurately predicts the need for hospitalization of a pediatric patient (sensitivity 52%; specificity 81%; AUC 0.78) [34]. Regardless of the reliability of the triage, the ESI is considered a useful tool for handling children in the ED [43].

5. Future of Triage

The number of patients seeking help in EDs worldwide is frequently higher than the potential of the EDs themselves. Therefore, a method for improving patient flow is required. Overcrowding of the ED leads to the worsening of the patients' condition, increase in in-hospital mortality, elongation of stay in hospital, and higher cost [44–46]. Immediate knowledge that the patient who is just being admitted to the ED requires a further hospital stay would help to allocate resources in a more optimal way and ensure a more comfortable environment for the patient.

Determining whether ED patients require hospitalization is crucial from both clinical and economic perspectives. To solve this issue, predictive scales based on certain clinical and demographic variables (e.g., age, sex, vital signs, triage priority, etc.) were created [1,47–49]. However, attempts have been made to create computational models to facilitate and accelerate the triage process. The task of such a model would be the instant calculation of the probability of patients' hospitalization [44,46,50]. A perfect situation would be to receive information about the possible or probable hospitalization of patients during triage performed immediately after admission to the ED.

To date, there have been a number of publications with data on the application of machine learning technologies to support segregation processes at different stages. The use of a machine learning algorithm as a predictive model effective in pre-hospital detection of post-traumatic intracerebral hemorrhage (AUC 0.78) based on report data alone is described [13]. In addition, the use of AI-based methods in decision support in the ED is being widely explored. The results of experiments on the ability of machine learning algorithms to predict death in the ED, the need for hospitalization, or ICU admission are promising [51–53].

According to some analyses [44,46], the best algorithms for modelling nonlinear relations between variables in the prediction of the need for hospitalization are XGBoosting and deep neural network (DNN). They are fast (taking less than 10 s) [45] and can precisely analyze available data to predict the probability of hospitalization. However, recent reports suggest that DNNs using textual data contained in the available medical documentation of patients can improve the quality of medical triage [19]. Additionally, some studies suggest that the use of modern technological solutions does not have to be difficult or unavailable with the current level of the computerization of medical records but allows for better results, especially in the case of ESI priority [54–56].

Machine learning models can also accurately predict serious medical events with vital signs and main symptoms being the most important predictive factors [50,57]. Computational models can also predict the risk of death during hospitalization better than triage systems alone [47,50]. According to various researchers, good discriminatory results for sudden cardiac arrest (SCA) in the ED, obtained solely from triage data, were obtained using Random Forest (AUC 0.931) [53], Logistic Regression (AUC 0.925) [15], and Ada Boosting and Light Gradient Boosting machine (AUC 0.997) [58].

An additional advantage of such models is a more exact triage, with a lower percentage of under-triaged patients appearing in priorities 1–3 and over-triage in priorities 3–5 [50].

However, regardless of the type of AI-based algorithm being tested, the most common gold standard was the assessment by an experienced medical professional [8,59,60]. It is worth noting that several papers provide evidence that, although the sensitivity and specificity of the diagnostic assessment is acceptable in predicting hospitalization, the accuracy for mental illness is the lowest [60]. Recently, articles have been published describing the use of AI-based language models to assist in medical segregation in the emergency department. It was found that both the Generative Pre-trained Transformer GPT-4 and Gemini can accurately triage critical and urgent ESI group 1 and 2 patients, suggesting that both models can help accurately segregate these patients in the ED [61].

An important but rarely discussed problem in emergency departments is patients who leave without being seen before medical segregation. It has been shown that AI can be used to predict which patients leave the ED without being seen, which can enable trajectories of their stay to be altered and can influence individual decisions of ED staff [62].

A separate issue being investigated in the survey among emergency physicians is their attitude towards the AI tool. Researchers from Turkey showed that there is a strong conviction among ED staff about the benefits of using AI support to assess a patient during triage; however, concerns about the related ethical aspects of such an intervention are also present among them [63]. Some of the misunderstandings about the idea of machine learning are addressed by the publications discussing the topic in more depth in the emergency medicine group [64].

Summarizing the comparison between computational models and traditional triage systems, the authors state that artificial intelligence is more effective in predicting the main final points (hospitalization, admission to ICU, and death) [15,50–53,57,58]. Moreover, they can improve the quality of care in the ED and reduce the burden on healthcare systems [32].

6. Summary

Nowadays, it is difficult to indicate which of the segregation systems available worldwide is the best. To approximate a remedy to this issue, the authors reviewed several publications, comparing triage systems to select the most optimal system for use in the ED [5,65,66].

The most popular existing triage systems can be divided into diagrams with disease symptoms, containing discriminating criteria (ATS, MTS, CTAS), and using one decision algorithm for all patients (ESI).

The training process of each algorithm appears to be equally important in each triage system. In the available publications, little data are used to compare the training schemes for different segregation systems. Many studies in the methodology state that employees performed the triage after several hours of training in each algorithm. However, in practice, professionals trained over a longer period do seem to use these systems more efficiently.

7. Limitations

A significant limitation of this study is the lack of widespread clinical practice related to the use of machine learning methods, including the disproportion in the number of available reports on the effectiveness of traditional triage systems compared to artificial intelligence techniques. Another important limitation is that in the analyzed publications, the evaluation criteria for the triage systems were not the same or comparable. The incompatibility of the methodologies for describing the segregation schemes in the publications resulted in an imperfect and slightly informative approach to comparing these systems.

8. Conclusions

According to a review of the literature, this study concludes that triage systems existing in the world increase the safety of patients waiting for assistance in the ED. It would seem obvious that any system for segregating patients admitted to the ED is better than none; however, numerous studies have shown the superiority of five-step systems over the three-step systems, mainly in terms of reliability. After nearly 30 years of development, the maximum efficiency of the above-mentioned systems seems to have been achieved. Based on the authors' experience, medical segregation, even when handled professionally and using a certified system, does not guarantee 100% safety in regard to unexpected medical events.

Another issue is the process of evaluating the used system, which is inextricably linked to maintaining the proper quality of the process. To compile the learning time required to effectively use each of these systems would be advised as no in-depth studies have been conducted on this topic.

Each of these systems lacks a parameter/criterion that has not yet been considered. To the question of what this additional value could be, the answer may be the results of work on machine learning systems, which very accurately predict the risk of hospitalization, both in the ward and in the ICU, in a much faster time than a human would do. Based on calculations obtained by the AI method, one could add in the case of diagram-based systems (MTS, CTAS, ATS), a specific differentiation criterion, and in the case of algorithmic systems (ESI), an additional parameter at decision point C.

In summary, the authors in this study did not find an answer to the question of which triage methodic is the best. Currently, machine learning seems to provide more opportunities for the unconventional analysis of data available during medical triage. Possibly, an ideal segregation system, or rather a decision-making process including medical segregation, will be a combination of the experience and intuitions of trained medical personnel and modern technology, including artificial intelligence methods based on the analysis of the large amount of data.

Author Contributions: Conceptualization, M.S. and A.I.; methodology, A.I.; validation P.R.; investigation, A.I. and P.R.; resources, A.I.; data curation, A.I.; writing—original draft preparation, A.I. and P.R.; writing—review and editing, M.S.; visualization, A.I.; supervision, M.S.; funding acquisition, M.S. All authors have read and agreed to the published version of the manuscript.

Funding: This research received no external funding.

Institutional Review Board Statement: Not applicable.

Informed Consent Statement: Not applicable.

Data Availability Statement: The original contributions presented in the study are included in the article, further inquiries can be directed to the corresponding authors.

Conflicts of Interest: The authors declare no conflicts of interest.

References

1. Cameron, A.; Rodgers, K.; Ireland, A.; Jamdar, R.; McKay, G.A. A simple tool to predict admission at the time of triage. *Emerg. Med. J.* **2015**, *32*, 174–179. [CrossRef] [PubMed]
2. Christ, M.; Grossmann, F.; Winter, D.; Bingisser, R.; Platz, E. Modern triage in the emergency department. *Dtsch. Arztebl. Int.* **2010**, *107*, 892–898. [CrossRef]
3. Brouns, S.H.A.; Mignot-Evers, L.; Derkx, F.; Lambooij, S.L.; Dieleman, J.P.; Haak, H.R. Performance of the Manchester triage system in older emergency department patients: A retrospective cohort study. *BMC Emerg. Med.* **2019**, *19*, 3. [CrossRef] [PubMed]
4. Grossmann, F.F.; Zumbrunn, T.; Frauchiger, A.; Delport, K.; Bingisser, R.; Nickel, C.H. At risk of undertriage? Testing the performance and accuracy of the emergency severity index in older emergency department patients. *Ann. Emerg. Med.* **2012**, *60*, 317–325.e3. [CrossRef]
5. Azeredo, T.R.M.; Guedes, H.M.; Rebelo de Almeida, R.A.; Chianca, T.C.M.; Martins, J.C.A. Efficacy of the Manchester Triage System: A systematic review. *Int. Emerg. Nurs.* **2015**, *23*, 47–52. [CrossRef]
6. Barfod, C.; Lauritzen, M.M.P.; Danker, J.K.; Sölétormos, G.; Forberg, J.L.; Berlac, P.A.; Lippert, F.; Lundstrøm, L.H.; Antonsen, K.; Lange, K.H.W. Abnormal vital signs are strong predictors for intensive care unit admission and in-hospital mortality in adults triaged in the emergency department—A prospective cohort study. *Scand. J. Trauma. Resusc. Emerg. Med.* **2012**, *20*, 28. [CrossRef] [PubMed]
7. Artificial Intelligence Algorithm to Predict the Need for Critical Care in Prehospital Emergency Medical Services | Scandinavian Journal of Trauma, Resuscitation and Emergency Medicine | Full Text. Available online: https://sjtrem.biomedcentral.com/articles/10.1186/s13049-020-0713-4 (accessed on 21 May 2024).
8. Karlafti, E.; Anagnostis, A.; Simou, T.; Kollatou, A.S.; Paramythiotis, D.; Kaiafa, G.; Didaggelos, T.; Savvopoulos, C.; Fyntanidou, V. Support Systems of Clinical Decisions in the Triage of the Emergency Department Using Artificial Intelligence: The Efficiency to Support Triage. *Acta Medica Litu.* **2023**, *30*, 19–25. [CrossRef]
9. Ilicki, J. Challenges in evaluating the accuracy of AI-containing digital triage systems: A systematic review. *PLoS ONE* **2022**, *17*, e0279636. [CrossRef] [PubMed]
10. Ng, C.-J.; Chien, C.-Y.; Seak, J.C.-J.; Tsai, S.-L.; Weng, Y.-M.; Chaou, C.-H.; Kuo, C.-W.; Chen, J.-C.; Hsu, K.-H. Validation of the five-tier Taiwan Triage and Acuity Scale for prehospital use by Emergency Medical Technicians. *Emerg. Med. J.* **2019**, *36*, 472–478. [CrossRef]
11. Leeies, M.; Ffrench, C.; Strome, T.; Weldon, E.; Bullard, M.; Grierson, R. Prehospital Application of the Canadian Triage and Acuity Scale by Emergency Medical Services. *Can. J. Emerg. Med.* **2017**, *19*, 26–31. [CrossRef]
12. Emergency Medical Services Triage Using the Emergency Severity Index: Is It Reliable and Valid? Available online: https://pubmed.ncbi.nlm.nih.gov/22244546/ (accessed on 21 May 2024).

13. Abe, D.; Inaji, M.; Hase, T.; Takahashi, S.; Sakai, R.; Ayabe, F.; Tanaka, Y.; Otomo, Y.; Maehara, T. A Prehospital Triage System to Detect Traumatic Intracranial Hemorrhage Using Machine Learning Algorithms. *JAMA Netw. Open* **2022**, *5*, e2216393. [CrossRef] [PubMed]
14. Implementation of an All-Day Artificial Intelligence-Based Triage System to Accelerate Door-to-Balloon Times. Available online: https://pubmed.ncbi.nlm.nih.gov/36336511/ (accessed on 18 May 2024).
15. Tu, K.-C.; Eric Nyam, T.-T.; Wang, C.-C.; Chen, N.-C.; Chen, K.-T.; Chen, C.-J.; Liu, C.-F.; Kuo, J.-R. A Computer-Assisted System for Early Mortality Risk Prediction in Patients with Traumatic Brain Injury Using Artificial Intelligence Algorithms in Emergency Room Triage. *Brain Sci.* **2022**, *12*, 612. [CrossRef] [PubMed]
16. Brandao-de-Resende, C.; Melo, M.; Lee, E.; Jindal, A.; Neo, Y.N.; Sanghi, P.; Freitas, J.R.; Castro, P.V.I.P.; Rosa, V.O.M.; Valentim, G.F.S.; et al. A machine learning system to optimise triage in an adult ophthalmic emergency department: A model development and validation study. *eClinicalMedicine* **2023**, *66*, 102331. [CrossRef] [PubMed]
17. Hunter, O.F.; Perry, F.; Salehi, M.; Bandurski, H.; Hubbard, A.; Ball, C.G.; Morad Hameed, S. Science fiction or clinical reality: A review of the applications of artificial intelligence along the continuum of trauma care. *World J. Emerg. Surg.* **2023**, *18*, 16. [CrossRef] [PubMed]
18. Aubrion, A.; Clanet, R.; Jourdan, J.P.; Creveuil, C.; Roupie, E.; Macrez, R. FRENCH versus ESI: Comparison between two nurse triage emergency scales with referent scenarios. *BMC Emerg. Med.* **2022**, *22*, 201. [CrossRef] [PubMed]
19. Roquette, B.P.; Nagano, H.; Marujo, E.C.; Maiorano, A.C. Prediction of admission in pediatric emergency department with deep neural networks and triage textual data. *Neural Netw.* **2020**, *126*, 170–177. [CrossRef] [PubMed]
20. Lucke, J.A.; Mooijaart, S.P.; Conroy, S.; Blomaard, L.C.; De Groot, B.; Nickel, C.H. Mortality risk for different presenting complaints amongst older patients assessed with the Manchester triage system. *Eur. Geriatr. Med.* **2022**, *123*, 323–328. [CrossRef] [PubMed]
21. Trivedi, S.; Littmann, J.; Stempien, J.; Kapur, P.; Bryce, R.; Betz, M. A Comparison Between Computer-Assisted Self-Triage by Patients and Triage Performed by Nurses in the Emergency Department. *Cureus* **2021**, *13*, e14002. [CrossRef] [PubMed]
22. Emergency Triage: Manchester Triage Group, 3rd Edition (Version 3.8, 2023) | Wiley. Available online: https://www.wiley.com/en-fr/Emergency+Triage:+Manchester+Triage+Group,+3rd+Edition+(Version+3.8,+2023)-p-9781118299067 (accessed on 21 May 2024).
23. Cairós-Ventura, L.M.; de Las Mercedes Novo-Muñoz, M.; Rodríguez-Gómez, J.Á.; Ortega-Benítez, Á.M.; Ortega-Barreda, E.M.; Aguirre-Jaime, A. Validity and Reliability of the Emergency Severity Index in a Spanish Hospital. *Int. J. Environ. Res. Public. Health* **2019**, *16*, 4567. [CrossRef]
24. Baumann, M.R.; Strout, T.D. Triage of geriatric patients in the emergency department: Validity and survival with the Emergency Severity Index. *Ann. Emerg. Med.* **2007**, *49*, 234–240. [CrossRef]
25. Esi-Implementation-Handbook-2020—Implementation Handbook 2020 Edition Esi Emergency Severity Index a Triage Tool for Emergency Department. Available online: https://www.sgnor.ch/fileadmin/user_upload/Dokumente/Downloads/Esi_Handbook.pdf (accessed on 21 May 2024).
26. Murray, M.J. The Canadian Triage and Acuity Scale: A Canadian perspective on emergency department triage. *Emerg. Med. Fremantle WA* **2003**, *15*, 6–10. [CrossRef] [PubMed]
27. ACEM—Triage. Available online: https://acem.org.au/Content-Sources/Advancing-Emergency-Medicine/Better-Outcomes-for-Patients/Triage (accessed on 21 May 2024).
28. Travers, D.A.; Waller, A.E.; Bowling, J.M.; Flowers, D.; Tintinalli, J. Five-level triage system more effective than three-level in tertiary emergency department. *J. Emerg. Nurs.* **2002**, *28*, 395–400. [CrossRef] [PubMed]
29. Jelinek, G.A.; Little, M. Inter-rater reliability of the National Triage Scale over 11,500 simulated occasions of triage. *Emerg. Med.* **1996**, *8*, 226–230. [CrossRef]
30. Beveridge, R.; Ducharme, J.; Janes, L.; Beaulieu, S.; Walter, S. Reliability of the Canadian emergency department triage and acuity scale: Interrater agreement. *Ann. Emerg. Med.* **1999**, *34*, 155–159. [CrossRef] [PubMed]
31. Hinson, J.S.; Martinez, D.A.; Schmitz, P.S.K.; Toerper, M.; Radu, D.; Scheulen, J.; Stewart de Ramirez, S.A.; Levin, S. Accuracy of emergency department triage using the Emergency Severity Index and independent predictors of under-triage and over-triage in Brazil: A retrospective cohort analysis. *Int. J. Emerg. Med.* **2018**, *11*, 3. [CrossRef] [PubMed]
32. Larburu, N.; Azkue, L.; Kerexeta, J. Predicting Hospital Ward Admission from the Emergency Department: A Systematic Review. *J. Pers. Med.* **2023**, *13*, 849. [CrossRef] [PubMed]
33. McLeod, S.L.; McCarron, J.; Ahmed, T.; Grewal, K.; Mittmann, N.; Scott, S.; Ovens, H.; Garay, J.; Bullard, M.; Rowe, B.H.; et al. Interrater Reliability, Accuracy, and Triage Time Pre- and Post-implementation of a Real-Time Electronic Triage Decision-Support Tool. *Ann. Emerg. Med.* **2020**, *75*, 524–531. [CrossRef] [PubMed]
34. Aeimchanbanjong, K.; Pandee, U. Validation of different pediatric triage systems in the emergency department. *World J. Emerg. Med.* **2017**, *8*, 223–227. [CrossRef] [PubMed]
35. Rashid, K.; Ullah, M.; Ahmed, S.T.; Sajid, M.Z.; Hayat, M.A.; Nawaz, B.; Abbas, K. Accuracy of Emergency Room Triage Using Emergency Severity Index (ESI): Independent Predictor of Under and Over Triage. *Cureus* **2021**, *13*, e20229. [CrossRef]
36. Saberian, S.M.; Chester, D.J.; Udobi, K.F.; Childs, E.W.; Danner, O.K.; Sola, R. A Comparative Analysis of Hospital Triage Systems in the Geriatric Adult Trauma Patients: A Quality Improvement Pilot Study. *Am. Surg.* **2023**, *89*, 2300–2305. [CrossRef]
37. Chi, C.-H.; Huang, C.-M. Comparison of the Emergency Severity Index (ESI) and the Taiwan Triage System in predicting resource utilization. *J. Formos. Med. Assoc. Taiwan. Yi Zhi* **2006**, *105*, 617–625. [CrossRef] [PubMed]

38. Zakeri, H.; Afshari Saleh, L.; Niroumand, S.; Ziadi-Lotfabadi, M. Comparison the Emergency Severity Index and Manchester Triage System in Trauma Patients. *Bull. Emerg. Trauma.* **2022**, *10*, 65–70. [CrossRef] [PubMed]
39. Storm-Versloot, M.N.; Ubbink, D.T.; Kappelhof, J.; Luitse, J.S.K. Comparison of an informally structured triage system, the emergency severity index, and the manchester triage system to distinguish patient priority in the emergency department. *Acad. Emerg. Med.* **2011**, *18*, 822–829. [CrossRef] [PubMed]
40. Cooke, M.W.; Jinks, S. Does the Manchester triage system detect the critically ill? *J. Accid. Emerg. Med.* **1999**, *16*, 179–181. [CrossRef]
41. Dippenaar, E. Reliability and validity of three international triage systems within a private health-care group in the Middle East. *Int. Emerg. Nurs.* **2020**, *51*, 100870. [CrossRef]
42. Ebrahimi, M.; Mirhaghi, A.; Najafi, Z.; Shafaee, H.; Hamechizfahm Roudi, M. Are Pediatric Triage Systems Reliable in the Emergency Department? *Emerg. Med. Int.* **2020**, *2020*, 9825730. [CrossRef] [PubMed]
43. Beck, N.; Michel, M.; Binder, E.; Kapelari, K.; Maurer, M.; Lamina, C.; Müller, T.; Karall, D.; Scholl-Bürgi, S. The Manchester Triage System in a Pediatric Emergency Department of an Austrian University Hospital: A Retrospective Analysis of Urgency Levels. *Pediatr. Emerg. Care* **2022**, *38*, e639–e643. [CrossRef]
44. Araz, O.M.; Olson, D.; Ramirez-Nafarrate, A. Predictive analytics for hospital admissions from the emergency department using triage information. *Int. J. Prod. Econ.* **2019**, *208*, 199–207. [CrossRef]
45. Predicting Hospital Admission at Emergency Department Triage Using Machine Learning. Available online: https://journals.plos.org/plosone/article?id=10.1371/journal.pone.0201016 (accessed on 21 May 2024).
46. Parker, C.A.; Liu, N.; Wu, S.X.; Shen, Y.; Lam, S.S.W.; Ong, M.E.H. Predicting hospital admission at the emergency department triage: A novel prediction model. *Am. J. Emerg. Med.* **2019**, *37*, 1498–1504. [CrossRef]
47. Coslovsky, M.; Takala, J.; Exadaktylos, A.K.; Martinolli, L.; Merz, T.M. A clinical prediction model to identify patients at high risk of death in the emergency department. *Intensive Care Med.* **2015**, *41*, 1029–1036. [CrossRef]
48. Dinh, M.M.; Russell, S.B.; Bein, K.J.; Rogers, K.; Muscatello, D.; Paoloni, R.; Hayman, J.; Chalkley, D.R.; Ivers, R. The Sydney Triage to Admission Risk Tool (START) to predict Emergency Department Disposition: A derivation and internal validation study using retrospective state-wide data from New South Wales, Australia. *BMC Emerg. Med.* **2016**, *16*, 46. [CrossRef]
49. Ebker-White, A.A.; Bein, K.J.; Dinh, M.M. The Sydney Triage to Admission Risk Tool (START): A prospective validation study. *Emerg. Med. Australas. EMA* **2018**, *30*, 511–516. [CrossRef]
50. Raita, Y.; Goto, T.; Faridi, M.K.; Brown, D.F.M.; Camargo, C.A.; Hasegawa, K. Emergency department triage prediction of clinical outcomes using machine learning models. *Crit. Care Lond. Engl.* **2019**, *23*, 64. [CrossRef]
51. Sánchez-Salmerón, R.; Gómez-Urquiza, J.L.; Albendín-García, L.; Correa-Rodríguez, M.; Martos-Cabrera, M.B.; Velando-Soriano, A.; Suleiman-Martos, N. Machine learning methods applied to triage in emergency services: A systematic review. *Int. Emerg. Nurs.* **2022**, *60*, 101109. [CrossRef]
52. Hwang, S.; Lee, B. Machine learning-based prediction of critical illness in children visiting the emergency department. *PLoS ONE* **2022**, *17*, e0264184. [CrossRef] [PubMed]
53. Lu, T.-C.; Wang, C.-H.; Chou, F.-Y.; Sun, J.-T.; Chou, E.H.; Huang, E.P.-C.; Tsai, C.-L.; Ma, M.H.-M.; Fang, C.-C.; Huang, C.-H. Machine learning to predict in-hospital cardiac arrest from patients presenting to the emergency department. *Intern. Emerg. Med.* **2023**, *18*, 595–605. [CrossRef] [PubMed]
54. Yao, L.-H.; Leung, K.-C.; Tsai, C.-L.; Huang, C.-H.; Fu, L.-C. A Novel Deep Learning-Based System for Triage in the Emergency Department Using Electronic Medical Records: Retrospective Cohort Study. *J. Med. Internet Res.* **2021**, *23*, e27008. [CrossRef]
55. Miles, J.; Turner, J.; Jacques, R.; Williams, J.; Mason, S. Using machine-learning risk prediction models to triage the acuity of undifferentiated patients entering the emergency care system: A systematic review. *Diagn. Progn. Res.* **2020**, *4*, 16. [CrossRef]
56. Levin, S.; Toerper, M.; Hamrock, E.; Hinson, J.S.; Barnes, S.; Gardner, H.; Dugas, A.; Linton, B.; Kirsch, T.; Kelen, G. Machine-Learning-Based Electronic Triage More Accurately Differentiates Patients With Respect to Clinical Outcomes Compared With the Emergency Severity Index. *Ann. Emerg. Med.* **2018**, *71*, 565–574.e2. [CrossRef]
57. Fernandes, M.; Mendes, R.; Vieira, S.M.; Leite, F.; Palos, C.; Johnson, A.; Finkelstein, S.; Horng, S.; Celi, L.A. Predicting Intensive Care Unit admission among patients presenting to the emergency department using machine learning and natural language processing. *PLoS ONE* **2020**, *15*, e0229331. [CrossRef] [PubMed]
58. Lee, S.; Kang, W.S.; Kim, D.W.; Seo, S.H.; Kim, J.; Jeong, S.T.; Yon, D.K.; Lee, J. An Artificial Intelligence Model for Predicting Trauma Mortality Among Emergency Department Patients in South Korea: Retrospective Cohort Study. *J. Med. Internet Res.* **2023**, *25*, e49283. [CrossRef] [PubMed]
59. Kim, J.H.; Kim, S.K.; Choi, J.; Lee, Y. Reliability of ChatGPT for performing triage task in the emergency department using the Korean Triage and Acuity Scale. *Digit. Health* **2024**, *10*, 1–9. [CrossRef]
60. Akhlaghi, H.; Freeman, S.; Vari, C.; McKenna, B.; Braitberg, G.; Karro, J.; Tahayori, B. Machine learning in clinical practice: Evaluation of an artificial intelligence tool after implementation. *Emerg. Med. Australas. EMA* **2024**, *36*, 118–124. [CrossRef] [PubMed]
61. Meral, G.; Ateş, S.; Günay, S.; Öztürk, A.; Kuşdoğan, M. Comparative analysis of ChatGPT, Gemini and emergency medicine specialist in ESI triage assessment. *Am. J. Emerg. Med.* **2024**, *81*, 146–150. [CrossRef]
62. Sarty, J.; Fitzpatrick, E.A.; Taghavi, M.; VanBerkel, P.T.; Hurley, K.F. Machine learning to identify attributes that predict patients who leave without being seen in a pediatric emergency department. *CJEM* **2023**, *25*, 689–694. [CrossRef] [PubMed]

63. Ahun, E.; Demir, A.; Yiğit, Y.; Tulgar, Y.K.; Doğan, M.; Thomas, D.T.; Tulgar, S. Perceptions and concerns of emergency medicine practitioners about artificial intelligence in emergency triage management during the pandemic: A national survey-based study. *Front. Public Health* **2023**, *11*, 1285390. [CrossRef]
64. Okada, Y.; Ning, Y.; Ong, M.E.H. Explainable artificial intelligence in emergency medicine: An overview. *Clin. Exp. Emerg. Med.* **2023**, *10*, 354–362. [CrossRef]
65. Zachariasse, J.M.; van der Hagen, V.; Seiger, N.; Mackway-Jones, K.; van Veen, M.; Moll, H.A. Performance of triage systems in emergency care: A systematic review and meta-analysis. *BMJ Open* **2019**, *9*, e026471. [CrossRef]
66. Parenti, N.; Reggiani, M.L.B.; Iannone, P.; Percudani, D.; Dowding, D. A systematic review on the validity and reliability of an emergency department triage scale, the Manchester Triage System. *Int. J. Nurs. Stud.* **2014**, *51*, 1062–1069. [CrossRef]

Journal of
Personalized Medicine

MDPI

Article

Artificial Intelligence-Assisted Emergency Department Vertical Patient Flow Optimization

Nicole R. Hodgson [1,*], Soroush Saghafian [2], Wayne A. Martini [1], Arshya Feizi [3] and Agni Orfanoudaki [4]

1 Department of Emergency Medicine, Mayo Clinic Arizona, Phoenix, AZ 85054, USA
2 Harvard Kennedy School, Harvard University, Cambridge, MA 02138, USA; soroush_saghafian@hks.harvard.edu
3 Analysis Group, Boston, MA 02199, USA; arshya.feizi@analysisgroup.com
4 Saïd Business School, University of Oxford, Oxford OX1 1HP, UK; agni.orfanoudaki@sbs.ox.ac.uk
* Correspondence: hodgson.nicole@mayo.edu

Abstract

Background/Objectives: Recent advances in artificial intelligence (AI) and machine learning (ML) enable targeted optimization of emergency department (ED) operations. We examine how reworking an ED's vertical processing pathway (VPP) using AI- and ML-driven recommendations affected patient throughput. **Methods:** We trained a non-linear ML model using triage data from 49,350 ED encounters to generate a personalized risk score that predicted whether an incoming patient is suitable for vertical processing. This model was integrated into a stochastic patient flow framework using queueing theory to derive an optimized VPP design. The resulting protocol prioritized a vertical assessment for patients with Emergency Severity Index (ESI) scores of 4 and 5, as well as 3 when the chief complaints involved skin, urinary, or eye issues. In periods of ED saturation, our data-driven protocol suggested that any waiting room patient should become VPP eligible. We implemented this protocol during a 13-week prospective trial and evaluated its effect on ED performance using before-and-after data. **Results:** Implementation of the optimized VPP protocol reduced the average ED length of stay (LOS) by 10.75 min (4.15%). Adjusted analyses controlling for potential confounders during the study period estimated a LOS reduction between 7.5 and 11.9 min (2.89% and 4.60%, respectively). No adverse effects were observed in the quality metrics, including 72 h ED revisit or hospitalization rates. **Conclusions:** A personalized, data-driven VPP protocol, enabled by ML predictions, significantly improved the ED throughput while preserving care quality. Unlike standard fast-track systems, this approach adapts to ED saturation and patient acuity. The methodology is customizable to patient populations and ED operational characteristics, supporting personalized patient flow optimization across diverse emergency care settings.

Keywords: emergency department; patient flow optimization; vertical processing pathway; machine learning; data-driven patient management; vertical care

1. Introduction

Emergency department (ED) vertical processing pathways (VPPs), in which emergency physicians (EPs) assess and treat patients without assigning them to a traditional ED bed, are increasingly utilized. However, selecting appropriate patients for a VPP remains challenging. Existing studies report varying criteria based on emergency severity index (ESI) levels, but there is minimal literature identifying optimal chief complaints for VPP routing [1]. Ideal patient selection likely depends on institutional ED resources; for example, intravenous line placement may not be possible if patients must return to the waiting room after the initial assessment.

Recent advancements in artificial intelligence (AI) and machine learning (ML) have enabled ED directors to optimize patient flow by devising protocols tailored to their institution's unique ED characteristics [2,3]. To this end, we hypothesized that a ML model could analyze patient triage data to determine a patient's suitability for vertical processing.

We previously reported the characteristics of our ED's VPP, where EPs collaborated with a designated nurse to select patients for assessment while awaiting an assigned ED bed [4]. Eligibility for our VPP was determined at the physician's discretion, and all waiting room patients were considered potential candidates. Seeking to improve ED throughput and reduce the inefficiencies present in our VPP model, we redesigned our VPP selection criteria using recommendations from a ML model trained to predict whether an ED patient would require an ED bed [5]. We then studied the impact of these resource-neutral changes on ED metrics.

In this article, we demonstrate the application of ML recommendations combined with queueing analyses to improve ED operations, resulting in the creation of a flexible vertical unit unique to the published literature, which personalizes patient care dynamically based on triage data and ED saturation metrics. Our study contributes to the literature by describing a novel use of ML techniques to create a new patient flow option that may appeal to ED medical directors working in resource-constrained environments.

2. Materials and Methods

The Mayo Clinic Arizona ED is a tertiary care center located in Phoenix, Arizona, serving approximately 56,000 yearly patients in 56 ED beds. A computerized rotational patient assignment system assigns patients to an EP upon arrival [6]. No triage EP is staffed; instead, the ED relies on EPs to perform chart reviews on waiting patients assigned to them and order the appropriate initial studies to facilitate rapid care. During the pre-trial period, any waiting room patient was eligible for VPP evaluation at the discretion of the assigned EP [4]. After the initial assessment in the VPP, patients would return to the waiting room or a main ED bed once available. Rotating residents participated in approximately 15% of patient encounters in conjunction with an EP. During the study periods, a nurse practitioner or physician's assistant rotating through the ED conducted an initial evaluation of 9% of patients; however, all patients were ultimately seen and managed by their assigned EP.

To guide the VPP eligibility decisions, we first trained a non-linear binary classification ML model using triage data from 49,350 ED encounters to predict the likelihood that an incoming patient would ultimately require an ED bed [5]. We used retrospectively collected electronic health record data from the Mayo Clinic Arizona ED spanning 7 October 2018 to 31 December 2019. Data from 2020 to 2022 were excluded due to the operational disruptions caused by the COVID-19 pandemic. The primary outcome variable was whether a patient's care ultimately required an ED bed, defined through a tiered labeling approach. First, patients who were seen in the VPP and discharged without being assigned a bed were labeled as not requiring a bed. To expand the training set, we used clinically guided rules to generate two sets of synthetic labels: (1) patients with an ESI of 3 who were discharged from the ED without imaging or IV therapy and had a total LOS under two hours and (2) patients with an ESI of 4 or 5 who received no IV medications or fluids. All other patients were labeled as requiring a bed. Preprocessing included the removal of duplicate records, exclusion of encounters with missing triage or outcome data, standardization of vital signs, and grouping of chief complaints into clinically meaningful categories based on physician input.

The model outputs a personalized risk score based on each arriving patient's triage data, including the ESI, chief complaint, age, and vital signs. These predictions were integrated into a stochastic queueing model representing the dynamics of vertical and main ED service processes. Specifically, for the VPP unit, we developed a stylized analytical model using an $M/M/1$ queue with exponential vacations to reflect the intermittent availability of physicians to staff the VPP, while the main ED was modeled as a typical $M/M/1$ queue. The model incorporates both patient arrival rates and service times and accounts for the possibility of misclassification by the ML model, namely, routing a patient to the VPP who ultimately requires a bed (type I error) or sending a patient to the main ED who could have been discharged directly via the VPP (type II error). These misclassification trade-offs are embedded in the cost function, which is minimized to determine the optimal routing threshold. Model parameters such as the arrival rates, service times, and VPP reassignment probabilities were estimated from empirical data, and the analytical results were validated using a discrete-event simulation calibrated to our partner ED's operations. This simulation further compared the VPP design against alternative flow models (e.g., fast-track or physician-in-triage) under varying patient acuity and demand scenarios. The full analytical framework, including queue specifications, parameter estimation, and sensitivity analyses, is detailed in our earlier working paper [5].

Based on the outputs of this framework, we analytically derived the optimal patient routing threshold that minimizes the time inefficiencies in the system. These thresholds vary dynamically with ED conditions, such as arrival rates and service speed. To operationalize this in practice, we used the analytical model to generate optimal routing labels across a range of empirically calibrated ED states, which were then used, in combination with the patient observations and the non-linear machine learning model predictions, to approximate the optimal patient routing policy. The approximation model resulted in a clinically interpretable and yet personalized decision tree protocol to operationalize VPP assignment in practice. Vertical examination priority was recommended for patients with an emergency severity index (ESI) of 4 or 5, as well as an ESI of 3s, with chief complaints involving skin, urinary, or eye issues. In periods of ED saturation—as defined by the institutional thresholds for patient volume and resource availability—the protocol recommended expanding VPP eligibility to all patients in the waiting room. The final protocol was summarized into a decision tree diagram used by EPs and triage staff during the trial (Figure 1) [5].

To evaluate the protocol, we conducted a 13-week prospective study from 1 February to 30 April 2024. The study was divided into three periods: (1) a pre-intervention period (1 February–5 March), in which the existing ad hoc VPP process continued; (2) an educational period (6 March–26 March), during which clinicians received structured training on the new VPP protocol via virtual sessions and email communication; and (3) a post-intervention period (27 March–30 April), during which the optimized VPP protocol was implemented in clinical practice [5].

To evaluate the impact of the VPP protocol on ED LOS, we estimate multivariable linear regression models on a patient encounter level using the natural logarithm of LOS as the outcome variable [5]. The primary exposure variable is a binary indicator for the post-intervention period. To adjust for potential confounding, we included control covariates from three categories: (1) Patient level: age, ESI, and chief complaint category; (2) Operational: attending physician assignment, disposition status (e.g., discharge, admission), and diagnostic procedures performed (CT scan, ultrasound, X-ray, IV medications); and (3) ED saturation and timing: the number of physicians and nurses on duty at the time of patient arrival, the number of patients currently in treatment or waiting, and the hour of the day grouped into three shifts (6 am–12 pm, 12 pm–6 pm, 6 pm–12 am). These controls are selected to isolate the effect of the VPP intervention from concurrent variations in patient complexity, staffing, and ED congestion. Equivalent analyses were conducted to assess the outcomes of the 72 h ED return rate with or without hospitalization and the potential effect of the protocol on quality of care. Due to anonymization constraints under our IRB protocol, we could not include explicit calendar-based variables (e.g., month or day of the week). However, our models account for seasonal and cyclical variations indirectly through detailed operational controls that capture real-time ED congestion and staffing, which are key mediators of the time-based effects. To assess the robustness of the findings, we ran multiple model specifications, varying the included covariate sets and functional forms (e.g., categorical vs. continuous ESI, physician fixed effects vs. random effects).

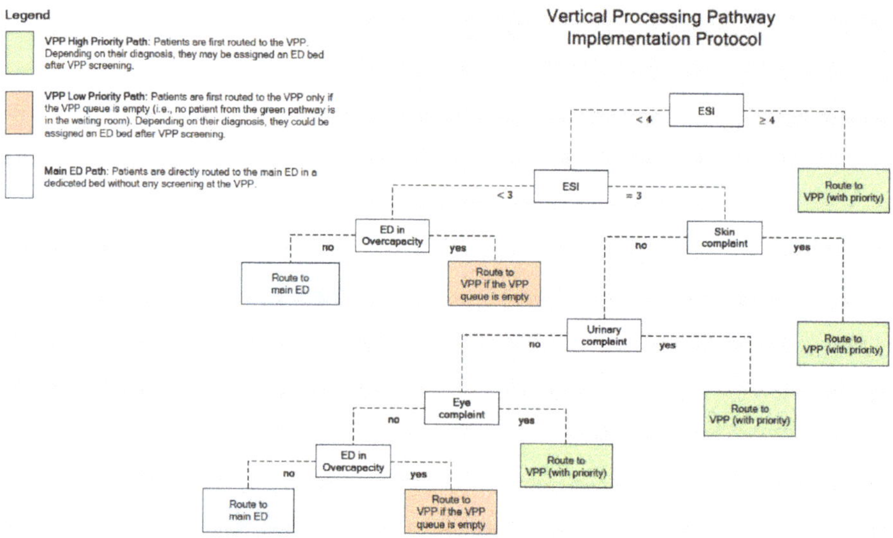

Figure 1. The proposed data-driven VPP implementation protocol [5].

3. Results

The final machine learning model used for VPP eligibility prediction was a random forest classifier [7], which outperformed alternative algorithms across five bootstrap iterations. On the held-out test set—comprising only "gold-standard" cases with a direct VPP discharge—the model achieved an average AUC of 84.6%, with a low variance across splits, indicating strong generalization. Feature importance analysis [8] revealed that lower ESI scores and abnormal vital signs were associated with an increased likelihood of bed need, while skin, eye, and urinary complaints were the most predictive of safe VPP eligibility.

We summarized the encounter characteristics in the pre-intervention and post-intervention periods in Table 1. With post-intervention, we experienced a significant reduction in ED LOS of 10.75 min (4.15%) with no increase in the 72 h returns or 72 h returns with a hospital admission. Although we did not perform statistical testing on our patient satisfaction scores, our post-intervention "top box score" was 86.0 compared to 85.2 pre-intervention, suggesting no deleterious patient satisfaction effects.

Table 1. Encountered characteristics before and after the intervention [5].

	Pre-Intervention (N = 5522)	Post-Intervention (N = 5493)	p-Value
<u>Outcomes</u>			
ED Length of Stay (Minutes [SD])	258.74 (121.88)	247.99 (115.44)	$p < 0.001$
Admission Status Discharged (%)	67.08%	66.96%	$p > 0.05$
ED return within 72 hrs	3.89%	3.84%	$p > 0.05$
ED return within 72 hrs with admit	2.37%	2.17%	$p > 0.05$
<u>Patient Characteristics</u>			
Sex	53.48%	54.31%	$p > 0.05$
Female (%)			
Age	58.92 (20.98)	58.55 (20.92)	$p > 0.05$
Mean Years (SD)			
Race	88.52%	88.15%	$p > 0.05$
White (%)			
ESI (Mean [SD])	2.88 (0.66)	2.90 (0.64)	$p > 0.05$
<u>Procedures Administered</u>			
IV (%)	64.98%	65.83%	$p > 0.05$
CT with IV contrast	24.85%	24.63%	$p > 0.05$
CT without IV contrast	19.76%	19.83%	$p > 0.05$
X-ray	45.60%	44.13%	$p > 0.05$
Ultrasound	11.81%	12.53%	$p > 0.05$

SD = standard deviation; hrs = hours.

The additional regression analyses, adjusting for clinical, operational, and saturation-related variables, confirmed a statistically significant reduction in ED LOS following the implementation of the optimized VPP protocol. Across multiple model specifications, the estimated adjusted reduction in LOS ranged from 7.5 to 11.9 min (2.89% and 4.60%, respectively), which is consistent with the unadjusted mean difference of 10.75 min that was observed in the raw data. This effect remained robust after controlling for variations in acuity (ESI), patient demographics, physician assignment, diagnostic utilization, ED staffing and saturation, and arrival-time crowding conditions. The protocol's effect size suggests that the observed improvement in patient throughput was not driven by changes in the patient mix or staffing patterns but was attributable to the introduction of the data-driven VPP streaming approach. Our analyses did not identify any statistically significant effect on the ED return rate outcomes.

Table 2 displays the ESI breakdowns for patients who were initially assessed inVPP pre- and post-intervention. The total number of patients seen through VPP increased during the post-intervention period, representing increased pathway efficiency.

Table 2. ESI breakdowns for VPP patients pre- and post-intervention.

ESI	Pre-Intervention	Post-Intervention	Statistical Test	p-Value
1	0 (0.0%)	0 (0.0%)	Fisher	$p > 0.05$
2	4 (0.28%)	7 (0.53%)	Fisher	$p > 0.05$
3—Excluding Skin/Urinary/Eye	47 (1.55%)	163 (5.26%)	χ^2	$p < 0.001$
3—Skin/Urinary/Eye	3 (1.23%)	21 (8.64%)	Fisher	$p < 0.001$
4	139 (18.08%)	469 (59.97%)	χ^2	$p < 0.001$
5	7 (20.0%)	19 (82.61%)	Fisher	$p < 0.001$

% represents the percentage of all patients of that ESI during the study period seen in VPP. We used Pearson's chi-square test to compare the pre- and post-intervention VPP routing proportions for each ESI group, applying Fisher's exact test instead for any subpopulation of a size less than 10.

4. Discussion

4.1. Main Discussion

Despite decades of attention [9], "waiting room medicine" remains a reality for overcrowded EDs nationwide [10]. At the heart of the issue, many contributors to ED crowding are not solvable at the individual ED director level, leading to stopgap measures to try to maintain patient care. Most interventions involve manipulating the ED's throughput by flexing resources [11] and redistributing personnel, as the physical construction of new care space takes time and may not have the desired effect of decreasing the LOS [12]. However, common patient flow models have inherent pitfalls. Physician-in-triage, for example, requires an additional staffed physician and may lead to rework if the primary treating physician chooses to deviate from the initial triage-based management plan [4]. Similarly, "fast tracks" are best suited to EDs with high numbers of low acuity patients and may not function well in tertiary facilities specializing in complex care; mistriage of patients to a dedicated fast-track practitioner may lead to both rework when reassigned to a non-fast-track physician and to patient safety issues if the mistriage is not identified.

In contrast, specific patient streaming designs [13,14] have demonstrated an advantage in improving an ED's metrics without additional resource needs or sensitivity to mistriage. The VPP design implemented in our study is a specific patient streaming approach that offers greater flexibility and continuity of care. It allows a single, assigned physician to manage the patient's care from the initial vertical assessment through to the final disposition, reducing unnecessary transitions and rework. Unlike the "physician-in-triage" approach, it does not require additional physician staffing, and unlike fast-track, it does not rely on strict pre-triage rules to segment patients. Leveraging a non-linear ML model, the VPP is inherently adaptable: during periods of ED saturation, our protocol recommends a dynamic expansion of VPP eligibility based on real-time demands—an advantage not offered by the fast-track or physician-in-triage approaches. Combining ease of implementation with flexibility enables the VPP to function effectively in high-acuity environments where patient needs and ED capacity fluctuate rapidly. Moreover, our rotational patient assignment system, combined with the VPP, allows a patient to remain with the same assigned physician throughout their care episode, eliminating handoffs, reducing redundancy, and allowing physicians to rapidly disposition lower acuity patients while still initiating care for more critical patients during times of ED saturation.

By devising a data-driven VPP protocol that couples the output of ML and stochastic queueing models into interpretable decision-tree-based guidelines, we achieved a significant length of stay reduction while seeing an increased number of patients through the pathway. The protocol's recommendation to route all ESI 4s and 5s through the VPP is intuitive and sensible, and although our ED treats fewer of these patients than other EDs, most of our lower acuity patients can be served without an ED bed; thus, requiring them to wait for an ED bed creates a significant bottleneck.

The specific ESI-3 chief complaints recommended for routing to the VPP are also reasonable when considering the patient populations. Ocular complaints (outside of visual field cuts, which were characterized as "Neurological Issues" during the analysis due to stroke potential and would typically be an ESI 2 or 1) often do not require imaging but could occupy an ED bed for some time if awaiting an in-person ophthalmologist consultation. Similarly, more complex skin complaints at our facility may require labs or a virtual dermatology consultation, but will typically not require advanced imaging or continuous intravenous access. We were able to manage many urinary issues through the VPP, as well, since we had access to a private area where foley catheters could be placed or pelvic examinations performed; in some EDs, utilizing non-reclining chairs for vertical patients, including this chief complaint category, may not be practical.

While this study was conducted in a single tertiary academic ED and ideal patient selection for vertical processing may differ based on an individual ED's characteristics, several features of our approach support its broader applicability. First, the protocol relies only on routinely collected triage variables—the ESI, chief complaints, and ED operational status—which are available in most EDs nationwide. Second, the decision tree guidelines were derived based on a site-agnostic stochastic model, matching the theoretical optimal patient routing policy in over 95% of cases, suggesting strong generalizability across the settings. Finally, the implementation did not require dedicated staffing or IT infrastructure changes, further supporting its adoption in resource-constrained environments.

Our implementation of ML-based recommendations to improve VPP patient selection represents a novel use of AI to optimize ED resource allocation. There has been a recent explosion of academic conversation regarding the use of AI to assist EPs with a broad range of tasks. Although many publications present the theoretical benefits of ML protocols based on retrospective data without prospective trials, some recent AI-based inventions are now utilized in cutting-edge EDs. Recognizing the deleterious impacts of the documentation burden on EPs [15], significant investments have focused on tools to summarize portions of the electronic medical record or ambient AI devices to document clinical encounters [16]. Recent publications describe the creation of ML-based predictors of ED patient deterioration that may ultimately improve patient safety; however, most of these systems have yet to be applied in clinical settings [17–19].

AI-based patient flow interventions have been somewhat limited in scope, mainly focused on triage. In conventional ED triage, patient prioritization is based on a combination of ESI and triage nurse gestalts. AI-based triage has the potential to improve patient selection through the awareness of real-time ED resource utilization and dynamic patient flow. It has also been shown to limit biases inherent in a human-based triage model [20]. Some current AI-based triage systems, such as KATE [21], serve to assist triage nurses in assigning a more accurate ESI score, while others seek to replace the ESI entirely with a program running concurrently with the medical record. However, many models remain theoretical and have not been trialed in clinical practice [22,23]. Most interventions have focused on accurately predicting resource utilization during triage for a particular patient and have not examined dedicated streaming pathways based on the AI-assigned score.

Our study, one of the first in the literature to showcase the actual clinical implementation of ML-based ED flow recommendations, displays the clinical practice benefits of combining recommendations from advanced analytics techniques into real-world patient flow protocols. We present our results as a potential option for other EDs struggling with overcrowding, enabling EPs to personalize care pathways for presenting patients.

4.2. Limitations

This study was conducted under real-world clinical conditions and reflects the challenges inherent in implementing protocol-based changes in a high-volume ED. As such, adherence to the optimized VPP protocol was imperfect. Despite instructions to preferentially route skin, urinary, and eye ESI-3 patients through VPP, the triage nurses had greater success routing ESI 4s, 5s, and non-protocol-eligible ESI 3s (presumably during periods of ED saturation). Only 8.64% of skin, urinary, and eye ESI 3s were routed through the VPP post-intervention; although the ML algorithm suggests that increasing this percentage would further benefit the LOS, the actual application of this increase may have unintended effects. Importantly, the protocol relied on manual physician and nurse interpretations rather than automated integration within the electronic medical record. Embedding real-time VPP eligibility recommendations into the triage interface may improve future adherence but would require dedicated IT infrastructure and development timelines that were not feasible within the scope of this study. Finally, like many other before-and-after studies, the Hawthorne effect might have influenced our results. Despite these, our various checks indicated systematic improvements post-implementation, suggesting a useful patient flow redesign approach that could be implemented across a variety of EDs.

5. Conclusions

Using a data-driven quantitative model to personalize the selection of patients seen through a vertical pathway allowed us to treat an increased number of ED patients without the use of an ED bed, reserving these valuable resources for more critical patients and improving the LOS. Beyond demonstrating operational improvements, our study introduces a new, formalized paradigm for VPPs—one that integrates machine learning and stochastic modeling to generate personalized, context-aware streaming decisions. This framework offers a generalizable, scalable, and adaptable approach for EDs seeking to optimize patient flow under resource constraints.

Author Contributions: Conceptualization, N.R.H., S.S., A.F. and A.O.; methodology, N.R.H., S.S., A.F. and A.O.; formal analysis, S.S., A.F. and A.O.; data acquisition, W.A.M.; writing—original draft preparation, N.R.H. and A.O.; writing—review and editing, N.R.H., S.S., W.A.M., A.F. and A.O. All authors have read and agreed to the published version of the manuscript.

Funding: This research received no external funding.

Institutional Review Board Statement: This study was conducted in accordance with the Declaration of Helsinki and approved via expedited review processes with an exemption from a full review by the Institutional Review Board of Mayo Clinic (IRB Study ID: 21-006710, date of approval 9 July 2021).

Informed Consent Statement: Patient consent was waived by the Mayo Clinic Institutional Review Board due to minimal risk.

Data Availability Statement: The original contributions presented in this study are included in the article. Further inquiries can be directed to the corresponding author.

Conflicts of Interest: Arshya Feizi works for the Analysis Group. During his role in the project, he worked at Harvard in the Public Impact Analytics Science Lab of Dr. Soroush Saghafian. The Analysis Group has no knowledge of this project and had no involvement in this project. He has no conflicts of interest to declare.

Abbreviations

The following abbreviations are used in this manuscript:

AI	Artificial Intelligence
ML	Machine Learning
ED	Emergency Department
VPP	Vertical Processing Pathway
ESI	Emergency Severity Index
LOS	Length of Stay
EP	Emergency Physician
IV	Intravenous
IRB	Institutional Review Board
AUC	Area Under the Curve
SD	Standard Deviation
hrs	Hours
IT	Information Technology

References

1. Lowie, B.; Hicks, C.; Falat, C.; Hydorn, S.C.; Windsor, T.A.; Smedley, A.; Fu, Y.; Gatz, J.D. Overcoming stagnant flow: A scoping review of vertical movement in the emergency department. *Acad. Emerg. Med.* **2024**, *31*, 256–262. [CrossRef] [PubMed]
2. Arnaud, E.; Elbattah, M.; Ammirati, C.; Dequen, G.; Ghazali, D.A. Use of Artificial Intelligence to Manage Patient Flow in Emergency Department during the COVID-19 Pandemic: A Prospective, Single-Center Study. *Int. J. Environ. Res. Public Health* **2022**, *19*, 9667. [CrossRef] [PubMed]
3. Aleksandra, S.; Robert, K.; Klaudia, K.; Dawid, L.; Mariusz, S. Artificial Intelligence in Optimizing the Functioning of Emergency Departments; a Systematic Review of Current Solutions. *Arch. Acad. Emerg. Med.* **2024**, *12*, e22.
4. Hodgson, N.R.; Saghafian, S.; Klanderman, M.C.; Urumov, A.; Traub, S.J. Physician-driven early evaluation: Encounters seen in a vertical model. *JEM Rep.* **2023**, *2*, 100028. [CrossRef]
5. Feizi, A.; Orfanoudaki, A.; Saghafian, S.; Martini, W.A.; Hodgson, N. *Vertical Patient Streaming in Emergency Departments*; HKS Working Paper No. RWP23-014; Harvard University: Cambridge, MA, USA, 2023. Available online: https://ssrn.com/abstract=4465161 (accessed on 1 April 2025).
6. Traub, S.J.; Stewart, C.F.; Didehban, R.; Bartley, A.C.; Saghafian, S.; Smith, V.D.; Silvers, S.M.; LeCheminant, R.; Lipinski, C.A. Emergency Department Rotational Patient Assignment. *Ann. Emerg. Med.* **2016**, *67*, 206–215. [CrossRef]
7. Breiman, L. Random Forests. *Mach. Learn.* **2001**, *45*, 5–32. [CrossRef]
8. Lundberg, S.M.; Lee, S.-I. A unified approach to interpreting model predictions. *Adv. Neural Inf. Process. Systems* **2017**, *30*, 4768–4777.
9. Kellermann, A.L. Waiting room medicine: Has it really come to this? *Ann. Emerg. Med.* **2010**, *56*, 468–471. [CrossRef]
10. Oskvarek, J.J.; Zocchi, M.S.; Black, B.S.; Celedon, P.; Leubitz, A.; Moghtaderi, A.; Nikolla, D.A.; Rahman, N.; Pines, J.M. Emergency Department Volume, Severity, and Crowding Since the Onset of the Coronavirus Disease 2019 Pandemic. *Ann. Emerg. Med.* **2023**, *82*, 650–660. [CrossRef]
11. Gorgens, S. They Are Dying in the Waiting Room. *Ann. Emeg. Med.* **2025**, *85*, 91. [CrossRef]
12. Han, J.H.; Zhou, C.; France, J.D.; Zhong, S.; Jones, I.; Storrow, A.B.; Aronsky, D. The effect of emergency department expansion on emergency department overcrowding. *Acad. Emerg. Med.* **2007**, *14*, 338–343. [CrossRef] [PubMed]
13. Anwar, M.R.; Rowe, B.H.; Metge, C.; Star, N.D.; Aboud, Z.; Kreindler, S.A. Realist analysis of streaming interventions in emergency departments. *BMJ Lead.* **2021**, *5*, 167–173. [CrossRef]
14. Hsieh, A.; Arena, A.; Oraha, A.; Cotarela, A.; McLean, M.; Hsieh, A.; Hsieh, I.C.; Chen, I.; Mok, N.; Milizia, R. Implementation of Vertical Split Flow Model for Patient Throughput at a Community Hospital Emergency Department—PubMed. *J. Emerg. Med.* **2023**, *64*, 77–82. [CrossRef]
15. Iscoe, M.S.; Venkatesh, A.K.; Holland, M.L.; Krumholz, H.M.; Sheares, K.D.; Melnick, E.R. Emergency Physician EHR Time per Encounter Based on Patient and Clinical Factors. *JAMA Netw. Open* **2024**, *7*, e2427389. [CrossRef]
16. Kachman, M.; Brennam, I.; Oskvarek, J.J.; Waseem, T.; Pones, J.M. How artificial intelligence could transform emergency care. *Am. J. Emerg. Med.* **2024**, *81*, 40–46. [CrossRef]
17. Kijpaisalratana, N.; Sanglertsinlapachai, D.; Techaratsami, S.; Musikatavorn, K.; Saoraya, J. Machine learning algorithms for early sepsis detection in the emergency department: A retrospective study. *Int. J. Med. Inform.* **2022**, *160*, 104689. [CrossRef]

18. Choi, A.; Choi, S.Y.; Chung, K.; Chung, H.S.; Song, T.; Choi, B.; Kim, J.H. Development of a machine learning-based clinical decision support system to predict clinical deterioration in patients visiting the emergency department. *Sci. Rep.* **2023**, *13*, 8561. [CrossRef]
19. Logothetis, S.B.; Green, D.; Holland, M.; Moibayed, N.A. Predicting acute clinical deterioration with interpretable machine learning to support emergency care decision making. *Sci. Rep.* **2023**, *13*, 13563.
20. Da'Costa, A.; Teke, J.; Origbo, J.E.; Osonuga, A.; Egbon, E.; Olawade, D.B. AI-driven triage in emergency departments: A review of benefits, challenges, and future directions. *Int. J. Med. Inform.* **2025**, *197*, 105838. [CrossRef] [PubMed]
21. Ivanov, O.; Wolf, L.; Brecher, D.; Lewis, E.; Masek, K.; Montgomery, K.; Andrieiev, Y.; McLaughlin, M.; Liu, S.; Dunne, R.; et al. Improving ED Emergency Severity Index Acuity Assignment Using Machine Learning and Clinical Natural Language Processing. *J. Emerg. Nurs.* **2021**, *47*, 265–278. [CrossRef]
22. Vântu, A.; Vasilescu, A.; Băicoianu, A. Medical emergency department triage data processing using a machine-learning solution. *Heliyon* **2023**, *9*, e18402. [CrossRef] [PubMed]
23. Xiaom, Y.; Zhang, J.; Chi, C.; Ma, Y.; Song, A. Criticality and clinical department prediction of ED patients using machine learning based on heterogeneous medical data. *Comput. Biol. Med.* **2023**, *165*, 107390.

Journal of
Personalized Medicine

MDPI

Article

Integrating Telemedical Supervision, Responder Apps, and Data-Driven Triage: The RuralRescue Model of Personalized Emergency Care

Klaus Hahnenkamp [1], Steffen Flessa [2,*], Timm Laslo [3] and Joachim Paul Hasebrook [4]

1 Clinic for Anaesthesia, Intensive Care, Emergency and Pain Medicine, University Medicine Greifswald, 17475 Greifswald, Germany; klaus.hahnenkamp@med.uni-greifswald.de
2 University Greifswald, 17489 Greifswald, Germany
3 University Greifswald, District Vorpommern-Greifswald, 17489 Greifswald, Germany; timm.laslo@kreis-vg.de
4 zeb business school, University Witten-Herdecke, 48153 Münster, Germany; jhasebrook@zeb-bs.de
* Correspondence: steffen.flessa@uni-greifswald.de

Abstract

Background/Objectives: This study aimed to evaluate a regional implementation project for rural emergency care (RuralRescue) and to examine how its components and outcomes may support personalized approaches in emergency medicine. While not originally designed as a personalized medicine intervention, the project combined digital, educational, and organizational innovations that enable patient-specific adaptation of care processes. **Methods**: Conducted in the rural district of Vorpommern-Greifswald (Mecklenburg–Western Pomerania, Germany), the intervention included (1) standardized cardiopulmonary resuscitation (CPR) training for laypersons, (2) a geolocation-based first responder app for medically trained volunteers, and (3) integration of a tele-emergency physician (TEP) system with prehospital emergency medical services (EMSs). A multi-perspective pre–post evaluation covered medical, economic, and organizational dimensions. Primary and secondary outcomes included bystander CPR rates, responder arrival times, telemedical triage decisions, diagnostic concordance, hospital transport avoidance, economic simulations, workload, and technology acceptance. **Results**: Over 12,600 citizens were trained in CPR and the responder app supported early intervention in hundreds of cases. TEPs remotely assisted 3611 emergency calls, including delegated medication in 17.8% and hospital transport avoidance in 24.3% of cases. Return of spontaneous circulation (ROSC) after out-of-hospital cardiac arrest (OHCA) was achieved in 35.6% of cases with early CPR. Diagnostic concordance reached 84.9%, and documentation completeness 92%. Centralized coordination of TEP units reduced implementation costs by over 90%. Psychological evaluation indicated variable digital acceptance by role and experience. **Conclusions**: RuralRescue demonstrates that digitally supported, context-aware, and regionally integrated emergency care models can contribute significantly to personalized emergency medicine and can be cost-effective. The project highlights how intervention intensity, responder deployment, and treatment decisions can be tailored to patient needs, professional capacity, and regional structures—even in resource-limited rural areas.

Keywords: emergency care; personalized medicine; tele-emergency physician; rural health; responder app; digital triage; EMS systems; context-aware care; implementation science; system integration

1. Introduction

The provision of timely, high-quality emergency medical services (EMSs) remains a major challenge in rural areas of Europe, where structural limitations such as long distances, staff shortages, and aging populations place disproportionate burdens on healthcare infrastructure. A recent systematic review found that rural populations in high-income countries experience significantly longer EMS response times and lower survival rates in time-critical emergencies such as cardiac arrest or stroke compared to urban populations [1].

In Germany, the district of Vorpommern-Greifswald, located in the northeastern state of Mecklenburg-Western Pomerania (Mecklenburg-Vorpommern), exemplifies this situation. With a land area of approximately 4000 square kilometers (1544 square miles) and a population density of just 60 inhabitants per square kilometer (155 inhabitants per square mile), it represents a structurally underserved rural region [2]. EMS provision in such regions is constrained by both geographical barriers and a shrinking pool of emergency physicians who are trained to deliver advanced prehospital interventions.

The German EMS follows a two-tier system: paramedics (with 3 years of training) attend all emergencies, and emergency physicians are dispatched separately under the "rendezvous system" when required for advanced interventions [3]. In practice, however, data show that physicians are dispatched in 46 percent of all EMS cases, but in up to one third of these deployments, no physician-specific intervention is ultimately needed [4]. This mismatch leads to inefficient resource use, delays in response, and regional disparities in care availability, particularly in rural areas [5].

In the district of Vorpommern-Greifswald, these problems are especially pronounced. According to project data, more than 60 percent of the district's territory lies beyond the 10 min emergency physician arrival time recommended in national guidelines, and long gaps in 24/7 physician coverage have been documented in several remote sub-regions [2,6]. These care deficits are not limited to this district: the official transfer recommendation by the Federal Joint Committee (G-BA) identifies similar challenges across multiple rural regions in Germany, including insufficient physician coverage, prolonged EMS response times, and gaps in advanced care provision [7].

To address these structural shortcomings, the RuralRescue (Land | Rettung) initiative piloted a comprehensive model for telemedicine-supported EMSs in Vorpommern-Greifswald, funded by the Innovation Fund of the Federal Joint Committee (Gemeinsamer Bundesausschuss, G-BA). At its core is the tele-emergency physician (TEP) system, which enables paramedics on site to receive real-time medical supervision via video, audio, and diagnostic data transmission. Between 2018 and 2020, over 9000 emergency cases were supported by tele-emergency physicians. In 24% of these, patient transport to hospital could be avoided, and in 18 percent, pharmacological interventions were delegated remotely [2,6].

Beyond remote supervision, the RuralRescue project integrates a smartphone-based first responder system, structured triage support, and role-specific training for EMS personnel, creating a flexible, data-driven model that aligns with the principles of personalized emergency medicine. Personalized emergency care is understood here as the dynamic adaptation of triage, treatment intensity, and care location to the real-time clinical, geographic, and contextual characteristics of each case [8,9].

This article introduces the RuralRescue project as a real-world implementation of personalized emergency medicine in rural environments. Drawing on data from over 250,000 EMS operations, it examines how telemedical innovation can improve equity, efficiency, and individualization in acute care.

1.1. Digital and Telemedical Solutions in Rural EMS: Evidence and Integration

Inequities in emergency medical care between urban and rural regions have been extensively documented in recent years. Multiple studies have shown that rural populations experience longer ambulance response times, limited access to advanced prehospital interventions, and lower survival rates in emergencies such as out-of-hospital cardiac arrest or stroke, compared to urban areas [10,11]. These disparities are particularly pronounced in geographically large and sparsely populated districts, where access to on-site emergency physicians is limited due to staff shortages and travel distances [10,12]. To address these systemic challenges, several regions have begun to implement telemedicine-based solutions in emergency services. These include tele-emergency physician systems, smartphone-based first responder alert applications, and digitally supported triage protocols. All of these have shown the potential to improve operational efficiency while enabling individualized medical decision-making at the point of care [12–14].

In the German context, tele-emergency physician systems have been piloted and evaluated in regions such as Aachen, Gütersloh, and others. These models enable emergency medical technicians and paramedics to connect remotely with a physician during an emergency. Vital parameters such as electrocardiogram (ECG), blood pressure, oxygen saturation, and high-definition video are transmitted in real time. Based on this data, the physician provides clinical decision support, authorizes pharmacological treatment, and may guide the selection of a destination hospital. In controlled evaluations, these systems have been associated with reduced unnecessary dispatches of on-site physicians, improved triage precision, and shorter delays to evidence-based interventions, particularly in acute myocardial infarction and polytrauma scenarios [15–17]. Furthermore, observational studies show high satisfaction and acceptance among paramedics, physicians, and patients, and demonstrate that delegated interventions such as analgesia or antihypertensive treatment can be delivered safely in the field under remote supervision [13].

Complementary to physician support systems, mobile first responder applications have been developed to engage trained laypersons and off-duty medical professionals in early resuscitation. Such systems rely on GPS-based activation of responders who are in close proximity to the emergency. These responders are alerted to suspected cardiac arrests or other life-threatening events, allowing them to initiate cardiopulmonary resuscitation (CPR) before the arrival of formal EMS teams. Studies report improved rates of bystander CPR and significant reductions in no-flow time for patients in rural areas where EMS response is delayed [18,19]. These systems represent a form of spatially and temporally adaptive response, in which the mobilization of human resources is tailored to each emergency's geographic and temporal context [12].

The RuralRescue project, implemented in the rural district of Vorpommern-Greifswald, represents the first fully integrated operational model in Germany that combines these technologies into a coherent system architecture (see Figure 1). Within the project, community-based first aid training, geolocation-based responder activation, real-time tele-emergency physician services, and tailored education for EMS professionals were systematically linked. This integration was not only technical but also procedural and organizational, allowing the participating actors to coordinate their actions across the emergency care chain. According to project evaluation data, over 9000 emergency cases were supported by the tele-emergency physician service between 2018 and 2020, with transport to hospital avoided in approximately 24 percent of cases, and delegated medication administered in 18 percent [6,12].

This combination of technologies and processes enables personalization of care in several respects. The involvement of the tele-emergency physician allows clinical decisions to be made based on real-time patient data, rather than standardized protocols alone. The mobile responder system adapts the alerting process to the location and qualifications of available individuals. Digital triage tools and structured communication protocols facilitate case-specific treatment escalation or de-escalation. The role-specific training programs for paramedics and dispatchers enhance collaborative competence and ensure that delegation and supervision are matched to individual team configurations and experience levels [20].

While each of these technologies has been deployed separately in earlier projects, the RuralRescue project is the first to evaluate their integration under real-world conditions in a structurally underserved rural area. As such, it provides both empirical insight and a transferable model for the implementation of personalized emergency medicine across the full span of the prehospital care pathway.

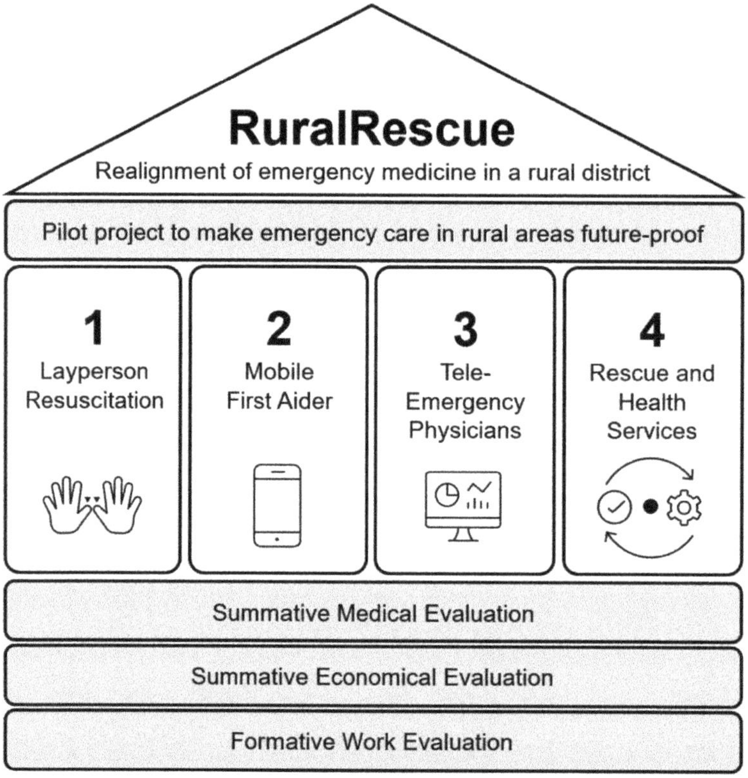

Figure 1. Structural framework of the RuralRescue (Land | Rettung) project.

1.2. Aim of the RuralRescue Project

The RuralRescue project was implemented in the rural district of Vorpommern-Greifswald between 2016 and 2020 under the Innovation Fund of the German Federal Joint Committee. The Innovation Fund was established to support implementation research for novel forms of care that go beyond existing standard provision. Its primary objective is to enable the transfer of evidence-based medical strategies into the statutory health insurance system, particularly in structurally underserved regions. In this context, RuralRescue aimed to redesign emergency medical services in rural areas through a coordinated four-pillar model: (1) public training in cardiopulmonary resuscitation (CPR), (2) smartphone-based activation of qualified first responders, (3) deployment of a tele-emergency physician (TEP) system, and (4) structural integration of emergency services with out-of-hours primary care [21].

The central aim of the project was to safeguard high-quality emergency medical care in rural areas by reducing the "therapy-free interval"—the time between the onset of an emergency and the beginning of effective intervention—while maintaining statutory response time thresholds [21]. Over 12,600 residents of the region were trained in CPR techniques, the RuralRescue mobile application was activated in hundreds of alerts, and more than 3600 emergency cases were supported remotely by a tele-emergency physician during the implementation phase [21]. These interventions were evaluated for their medical effectiveness, organizational feasibility, and potential for transferability to other rural districts [21].

Although the project was not originally conceptualized within the paradigm of personalized medicine, many of its key mechanisms are highly consistent with this approach. Real-time telemedical triage based on transmitted patient data allows for clinical decisions tailored to individual physiological profiles. The first responder system adapts emergency notifications based on geographic proximity and responder qualifications. Medication delegation, when conducted under remote supervision, is adjusted to the competencies of the on-scene personnel and the clinical needs of the patient. In the context of this study, personalized emergency medicine refers to the alignment of emergency medical interventions with individual patient needs, situational context, and regional infrastructure. This includes real-time tailoring of diagnostics, triage, and therapy based on clinical data, geographic conditions, and professional competencies, supported by digital tools and system-level adaptations.

This article evaluates the RuralRescue project as a model of digitally supported emergency medicine in a rural context and examines its alignment with the principles of personalized care. In doing so, it contributes to ongoing discussions about how data-driven, adaptive emergency services can improve individual outcomes while addressing systemic access gaps in structurally disadvantaged regions.

2. Materials and Methods

2.1. Intervention Design and Personalization Mechanisms

The RuralRescue project was implemented in the rural district of Vorpommern-Greifswald in northeastern Germany. It aimed to improve access to timely and high-quality emergency care in structurally underserved areas by shortening the "therapy-free interval"—the period between the onset of a medical emergency and the delivery of effective therapeutic intervention [22]. The intervention was based on a four-pillar model, of which three pillars were fully implemented and evaluated.

Pillar 1: Community-based layperson training in cardiopulmonary resuscitation (CPR). This component sought to increase first-aid competence in the general population by offering training courses in basic life support and the use of automated external defibrillators (AEDs). Over 12,600 residents participated in structured CPR training sessions, which were tailored to different age groups and learning settings [22]. This component indirectly contributed to personalized emergency response by expanding the pool of trained bystanders available for geolocation-based alerts (see Pillar 2), while also addressing community-specific preparedness levels.

Pillar 2: Smartphone-based first responder activation system. A mobile application called "Land | Retter" (German for "Rural Saver") was developed and deployed to alert nearby trained volunteers or off-duty healthcare professionals to time-critical emergencies, particularly out-of-hospital cardiac arrest (OHCA). The system used real-time GPS data to identify and notify individuals within a defined radius of the incident. In its later development stages, the alerting logic also considered responder qualifications (e.g., layperson, paramedic, physician), allowing contextual adaptation of mobilization strategies [22,23].

This geospatial and role-based personalization of emergency response enabled earlier intervention based on both the physical proximity and the skill profile of responders [23].

Pillar 3: Tele-emergency physician (TEP) system. To supplement and optimize the use of on-scene emergency physicians, a tele-emergency physician service was introduced. Paramedics were equipped with secure digital devices that enabled real-time transmission of clinical data—including ECGs, vital signs, and patient assessments—to a remotely located physician. Using a dedicated documentation interface (TeleDoc; see Figure 2), the tele-emergency physician could supervise diagnostics, delegate medication, and guide hospital triage decisions in accordance with standardized but situation-sensitive protocols [22,24]. This component allowed for clinical personalization of emergency care, with therapeutic decisions based on the real-time physiological and contextual information of the patient. Medication delegation was adapted to both the clinical profile of the patient and the training level of the on-scene personnel [24].

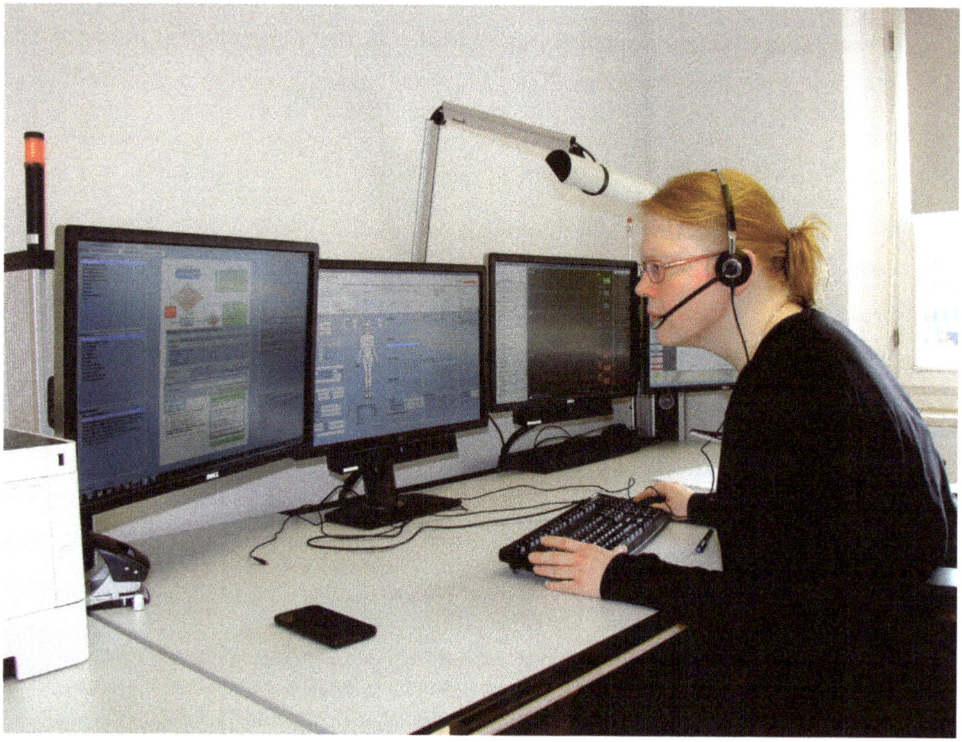

Figure 2. Working station of a tele-emergency physician (TEP; photo taken from [15]).

Pillar 4: Integration with out-of-hours primary care. The project's fourth conceptual pillar, closer coordination between EMS and on-call primary care physicians, was discussed with experts for regional adaptation as a part of the formative evaluation [22].

2.2. Evaluation Design

The evaluation of the RuralRescue project followed a multi-perspective, implementation science approach to assess the effectiveness, efficiency, and work–system integration of a digitally supported emergency medical model in a rural context. The RuralRescue evaluation employed a pre–post design without a control group, which is a widely used and accepted strategy in implementation research under real-world conditions where randomized allocation is neither feasible nor ethically appropriate. As emphasized in prior studies, such designs are particularly valuable for evaluating system-level innovations in complex, context-dependent settings, where the primary objective is to assess change under routine operational conditions rather than to isolate causal effects under controlled conditions [25,26]. Given the structural and technological complexity of the intervention, the evaluation was organized into three complementary domains: (1) a summative medical evaluation of clinical and operational outcomes, (2) a summative economic evaluation of resource use and cost-efficiency, and (3) a formative work psychological and organizational evaluation focused on digital acceptance, knowledge transfer, and collaborative practice adaptation.

2.2.1. Summative Medical Evaluation

The medical evaluation aimed to determine the clinical performance of the RuralRescue intervention using predefined tracer diagnoses and care pathway indicators. Key outcomes included the therapy-free interval (time from emergency onset to first therapeutic intervention), arrival times of EMS units and first responders, and effectiveness of TEP interventions, such as delegated medication and transport decisions [23]. For out-of-hospital cardiac arrest (OHCA) cases, return of spontaneous circulation (ROSC) served as a critical clinical endpoint [23].

Secondary indicators encompassed the rate of hospital admission versus non-transport, diagnostic accuracy in prehospital triage, and completeness and quality of digital documentation, including use of the dedicated TeleDoc system for physician–paramedic interaction logging. The evaluation used a matched-pairs design and time-series analysis, comparing TEP-supported cases to standard EMS contacts, and current performance to historical data from 2014 to 2017 [23].

Inclusion criteria encompassed all EMS operations in the district of Vorpommern-Greifswald between January 2018 and December 2021 where at least one RuralRescue component (CPR training, Land | Retter alerting, or TEP support) was activated and full clinical documentation was available. Exclusion criteria included pediatric emergencies (<6 years), trauma-related incidents, and cases with incomplete datasets. A total of 3611 TEP-supported cases and over 9000 app activations were analyzed, representing >85% of eligible cases after exclusion filtering. Recruiting followed a census-based approach using retrospective extraction from the central EMS IT system. Patient follow-up surveys and structured interviews were conducted using stratified convenience sampling with >600 completed cases. A post hoc power analysis for primary endpoints (e.g., ROSC, pain reduction) indicated power >0.80 at $\alpha = 0.05$ for medium effect sizes (Cohen's $d \geq 0.4$).

2.2.2. Summative Economic Evaluation

The economic evaluation of the RuralRescue model focused on the cost structure, utilization, and scalability of the TEP system in rural emergency medical services. Using operational data from Vorpommern-Greifswald and simulation modeling, this study assessed whether digitally supported, on-demand physician care could be delivered both effectively and efficiently under real-world conditions.

The economic evaluation examined the cost-effectiveness and systemic resource impact of the RuralRescue model compared to standard emergency care. Areas of focus included the implementation and operational costs of the TEP infrastructure, mobile responder alert system, and training programs, as well as savings from avoided on-scene physician deployments and unnecessary hospital admissions [24].

Economic modeling used full-cost accounting and queuing theory to simulate different TEP deployment strategies (centralized vs. decentralized) and assess effects on availability, capacity, and budgetary requirements. Primary data sources included complete deployment logs, billing data, and resource consumption reports from the emergency services IT platform. Stakeholder input was collected through ten semi-structured interviews with dispatch supervisors, EMS leads, and administrative staff. Cost structures were modeled based on full-cost accounting, differentiating between fixed and variable components (e.g., infrastructure, staff, licensing). The queue modeling (M/M/k structure with ∞, FIFO) simulated TED coverage scenarios under varying regional configurations. The analytical dataset covered all 3611 TEP interventions and was complemented by survey data on standby resource utilization and case complexity. Although no prospective recruitment occurred, the full case census provided sufficient data granularity to simulate system behavior across scalability tiers. Model fit was validated through sensitivity analyses. Test power was not relevant due to the deterministic nature of simulation outputs.

2.2.3. Formative Work Psychological and Organizational Evaluation

The formative evaluation addressed the subjective and behavioral adaptation of key stakeholders—paramedics, dispatchers, emergency physicians, and trained lay responders—to the digitally transformed care model. It assessed technology acceptance, perceived workload, knowledge transfer, and regional acceptance of the intervention.

The formative evaluation applied a triangulated mixed-methods design combining psychometric self-assessments, role-specific surveys, and expert workshops at two timepoints (pre- and post-implementation) [19]. Recruitment was purposive and role-stratified, targeting all 292 EMS professionals employed in the district during the project period, including paramedics, dispatchers, physicians, and administrative staff. The final sample included 164 fully completed surveys (response rate $\approx$ 56%), ensuring representativeness across roles and experience levels. The instruments included the NASA-TLX (for workload), TAM2 (for technology acceptance), and validated Likert-based scales for job satisfaction and knowledge transfer behavior. Test power was >0.80 for detecting small-to-medium effects (Cohen's $f \geq 0.20$, $\alpha = 0.05$) in repeated measures and interaction effects. Five moderated expert discussions involving 38 stakeholders applied the GEM Assay to analyze regional structural alignment and system readiness. Qualitative data were evaluated using thematic coding and triangulated with survey findings to identify barriers and enablers of system adaption.

Technology acceptance was measured focusing on perceived usefulness and ease of use of TEP systems and the Land | Retter application. Workload and job satisfaction were evaluated using the NASA Task Load Index (NASA-TLX), investigating the interrelationship of workload levels with willingness to adopt digital tools [27].

Knowledge transfer and the use of knowledge sources were examined using a framework based on the KODE® Competence Atlas, which distinguishes between explicit and implicit, as well as personal and organizational, knowledge domains. This approach was applied to better understand how work satisfaction influences both formal and informal knowledge sharing across professional boundaries [19].

Regional acceptance and structural compatibility were assessed using the GEM Assay, which evaluates system alignment across three domains: groundings (e.g., emergency infrastructure), enterprises and parties involved in EMS delivery, and the specific characteristics of the target region [23]. This method was applied to examine how well the RuralRescue model fits the local operational context and to assess its acceptance across different professional groups.

3. Results

Results are reported in alignment with the structure of the intervention and the three core domains of evaluation: medical effectiveness, economic feasibility, and work psychological and organizational adaptation. Together, these findings provide insight into the system-level impacts of digitally supported, regionally embedded emergency care models and their relevance for personalized medicine in rural settings.

3.1. Medical Results

The medical evaluation assessed the RuralRescue model's capacity to enhance prehospital emergency care through earlier, context-sensitive, and data-driven interventions. Results are reported along the three fully implemented pillars of the intervention: community-based CPR training (Pillar 1), activation of professional first responders via the Land | Retter app (Pillar 2), and tele-emergency physician support (Pillar 3). Each pillar contributed in different ways to advancing the principles of personalized emergency medicine—defined here as care that is responsive to individual clinical, geographic, and organizational context.

3.1.1. Pillar 1: Layperson CPR Training and Early Intervention

Over the course of the project, 12,600 citizens in the district of Vorpommern-Greifswald were trained in basic life support (BLS) using the nationally standardized "Prüfen-Rufen-Drücken" (Check–Call–Compress) model. Trainings were adapted to various community contexts, including schools, public events, and institutions, and included both in-person and digital learning components [28]. Post-training surveys indicated increased confidence and competence in handling emergency scenarios.

In out-of-hospital cardiac arrest (OHCA) cases with bystander CPR—triggered either by direct witnessing or informal proximity—the return of spontaneous circulation (ROSC) rate was 35.6 percent, exceeding the rural German average of 27 to 30 percent [26]. This demonstrates that early, community-based intervention significantly improves survival outcomes and exemplifies temporal and social individualization, enabling localized and non-professional response when formal care access is delayed.

3.1.2. Pillar 2: First Responder Activation via the Land | Retter App

During the implementation period, 9233 alerts were transmitted via the Land | Retter mobile application to a pool of professionally qualified responders, including off-duty emergency physicians, nurses, and paramedics. Each participant—referred to as a "Rural Saver" (LandRetter)—underwent standardized onboarding, including validation of clinical competencies and participation in an emergency readiness orientation [28].

The app's GPS-based alerting algorithm enabled dispatch centers to identify and notify the most suitable nearby responder based on both geographic proximity and professional qualification. In 44.3 percent of activations, a LandRetter arrived on scene before the EMS unit, achieving a median lead time of 4 min and 24 s [28]. This reduction in the therapy-free interval is especially relevant in remote areas where ambulance arrival may be delayed.

The Land | Retter system exemplifies spatial and operational personalization of emergency care. By matching responder profiles to emergency needs in real time, it enabled rapid deployment of medical support tailored to the situational geography and available human capital. Usability and acceptance surveys among participants yielded satisfaction ratings exceeding 4.2 on a 5-point scale, indicating high confidence in the system's reliability and effectiveness [28].

3.1.3. Pillar 3: Tele-Emergency Physician (TEP) Support

The tele-emergency physician (TEP) system was used in 3611 EMS cases across the project period. The system was deployed in cases where physician input was clinically indicated but direct on-site dispatch was either unnecessary or operationally unfeasible. Paramedics transmitted real-time clinical data—including vital signs, structured assessments, and ECGs—to the remotely located physician using the secure TeleDoc interface [23].

In 17.8 percent of TEP-supported cases, physicians delegated pharmacological treatment, most commonly involving analgesics, antihypertensives, and anti-epileptics. These interventions were made based on patient-specific data and symptom profiles transmitted from the field, allowing for individualized pharmacologic decision-making without requiring physical physician presence [23].

During the evaluation period, a total of 2935 patients were managed with the support of a tele-emergency physician (TEP). Of these, 362 patients (12.3%) reported a pain intensity of ≥7 on a numerical rating scale (NRS, range 0–10). Follow-up patient interviews indicated that effective pain relief was achieved in only 51.8 percent of comparable cases without TEP support, whereas the rate was significantly higher in the TEP-supported group at 66.3 percent ($p < 0.05$; see Figure 3; cf., [29]).

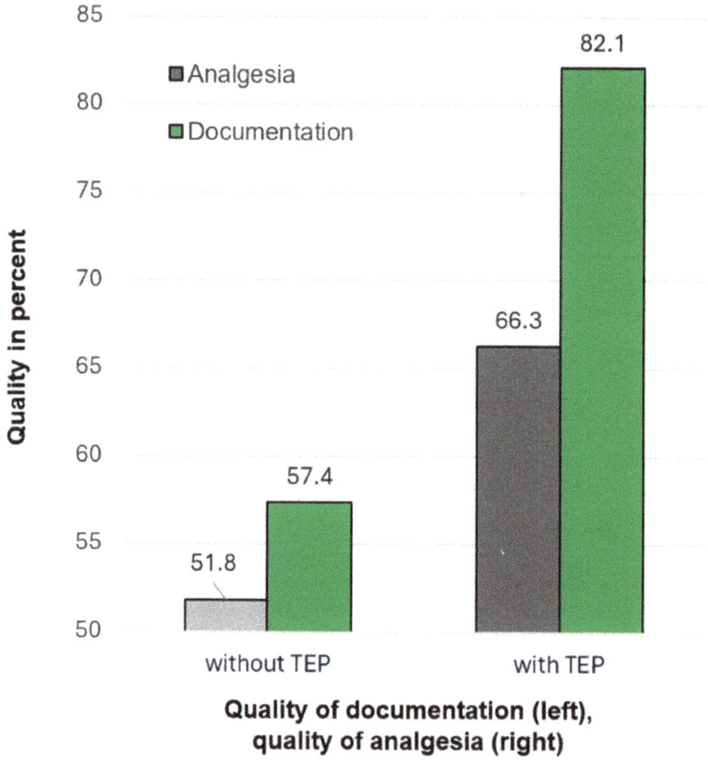

Figure 3. Comparison of analgesia effectiveness and documentation of hemodynamic baseline monitoring in prehospital emergency care with and without tele-emergency physician (TEP) support.

In addition, documentation quality was evaluated with respect to baseline hemodynamic monitoring, defined as the recording of key vital signs including blood pressure, heart rate, and peripheral oxygen saturation. This basic monitoring is essential for subsequent therapeutic decisions. It was documented in 57.4 percent of cases at the beginning of care and prior to hospital transfer in the non-TEP group, compared to 82.1 percent in TEP-supported cases ($p < 0.001$; cf., Figure 3). Importantly, 24.3 percent of all TEP-supported cases were resolved without hospital transport. In the majority of these cases (82%), the clinical presentation was deemed non-urgent and manageable by general practitioners or self-care. These case-specific triage decisions illustrate how telemedical supervision enables flexible, context-responsive routing of patients, thereby avoiding overtreatment and unnecessary resource consumption [23,30].

In terms of diagnostic accuracy, a comparison of prehospital assessments with hospital discharge data ($N = 323$) yielded an 84.9 percent diagnostic concordance rate across tracer conditions, including stroke, acute coronary syndrome, and COPD exacerbation [23]. Documentation completeness in TEP-supported cases was 92.1 percent driven by the structured data entry format of the TeleDoc system. This supports not only real-time decision-making but also retrospective quality assurance and system-level learning [30].

Together, these results show that the RuralRescue model improved clinical outcomes and optimized EMS workflows while embedding personalization at multiple levels. Through community engagement, professional responder matching, and remote physician support, care was tailored to the patient's clinical condition, location, and context-specific care options.

3.2. Economic Results

The analysis showed that decentralized TEP services improved system responsiveness while reducing overall operational costs, particularly in sparsely populated regions with long deployment routes [24]. The total annual full cost of operating a decentralized TEP unit on a 24/7 basis was calculated at EUR 696,949 (≈USD 766,600). This included EUR 148,876 (≈USD 163,800) in fixed costs (office infrastructure, administration) and EUR 548,073 (≈USD 602,800) in variable and jump-fixed costs, such as staff salaries, telemedicine equipment, and licenses [31]. While the system provided clinically valuable support, its average usage—3.96 cases per day with a mean service time of 24.6 min—resulted in idle time exceeding 90 percent, indicating substantial overcapacity in single-district settings [31].

To address this, a queuing system model (M/M/k; ∞, FIFO) was used to simulate alternative coordination scenarios. The modeling showed that one TED could effectively support up to 36 ambulances while keeping the probability of delayed physician contact below 5 percent, a level considered acceptable for most prehospital situations. Under a centralized model, where one TED supports 20 districts, the cost per district drops to EUR 57,300 (≈USD 63,000)—a reduction of over 90 percent compared to standalone district operation [31].

These findings confirm that personalized physician access—delivered based on real-time need, clinical data, and EMS telemetry—is not only medically feasible but also economically sustainable when scaled regionally. As Figure 4 shows, the unit cost depends strongly on the number of districts joining the tele-emergency center.

The system enables dynamic resource allocation, where expert supervision is activated for high-acuity cases and withheld in less critical scenarios, reflecting demand-sensitive personalization of care intensity. This approach supports both individualized patient management and strategic resource stewardship, aligning with core principles of value-based personalized emergency medicine.

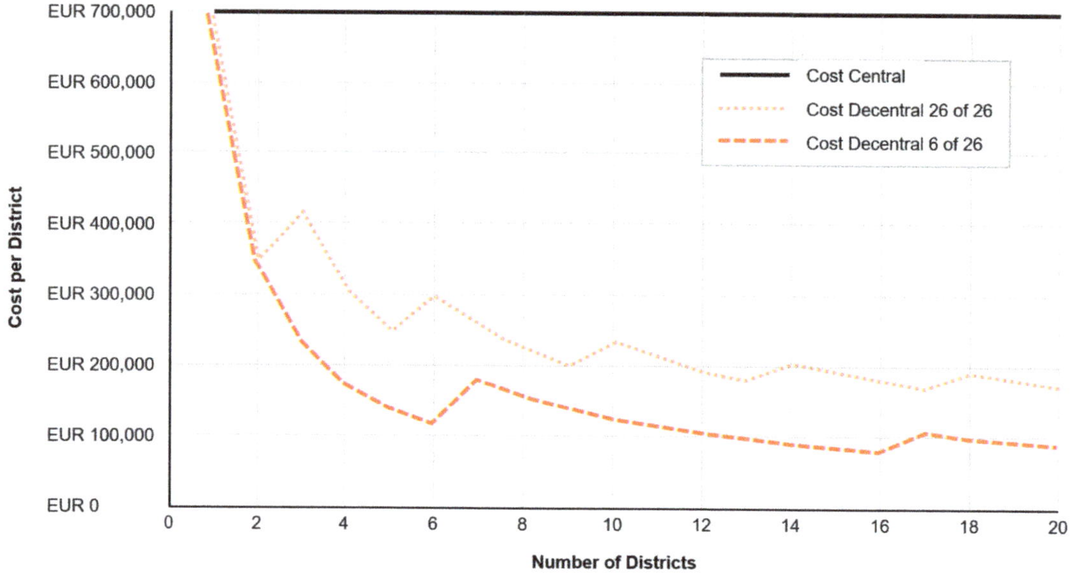

Figure 4. Cost functions of different scenarios of central or decentral tele-emergency services [11].

3.3. *Formative Work Psychological and Organizational Results*

The formative evaluation assessed how different professional groups within the Rural-Rescue model adapted to the digital and structural innovations introduced by the project. It focused on workload perception, job satisfaction, knowledge management, technology acceptance, and regional integration—factors that critically influence the success of personalized, data-enabled emergency care models in real-world settings.

3.3.1. Workload and Job Satisfaction

Workload was measured using the NASA Task Load Index (NASA-TLX) and job satisfaction via standardized Likert-based self-assessments. Results revealed differentiated patterns: Experienced EMS professionals, including long-serving paramedics and emergency physicians, reported increased job satisfaction following implementation of the new care model. In contrast, less experienced staff—especially newly trained paramedics—indicated heightened workload, transitional stress, and role uncertainty during the early phases of adoption [32,33]. The study also found that emergency teams with lower satisfaction scores reported higher degrees of informal knowledge sharing across professional boundaries [19].

Interestingly, the data also showed that higher workload levels were positively correlated with digital tool acceptance, particularly among dispatchers and field personnel. This suggests that digital supervision and documentation tools were perceived not as burdens, but as adaptive supports under pressure, reinforcing their value for role-specific adaptation [33].

Work satisfaction improvements were found to depend on prior digital experience. Work satisfaction was measured using a validated polarity scale from 1 (low satisfaction) to 10 (high satisfaction) [34]. The study found a significant interaction between time (pre vs. post digital transformation) and prior experience with telemedicine. While overall satisfaction increased after the implementation of tele-emergency physicians (TEPs), this effect was statistically significant only for participants with prior telemedical experience (pre = 3.98 vs. post = 5.27, F (1315) = 4.09, $p < 0.05$). In contrast, no comparable increase was observed among less experienced staff (pre = 4.01 vs. post = 4.24; see Figure 5). These results suggest that experience in digital systems moderates satisfaction gains during technology-driven innovation in emergency care.

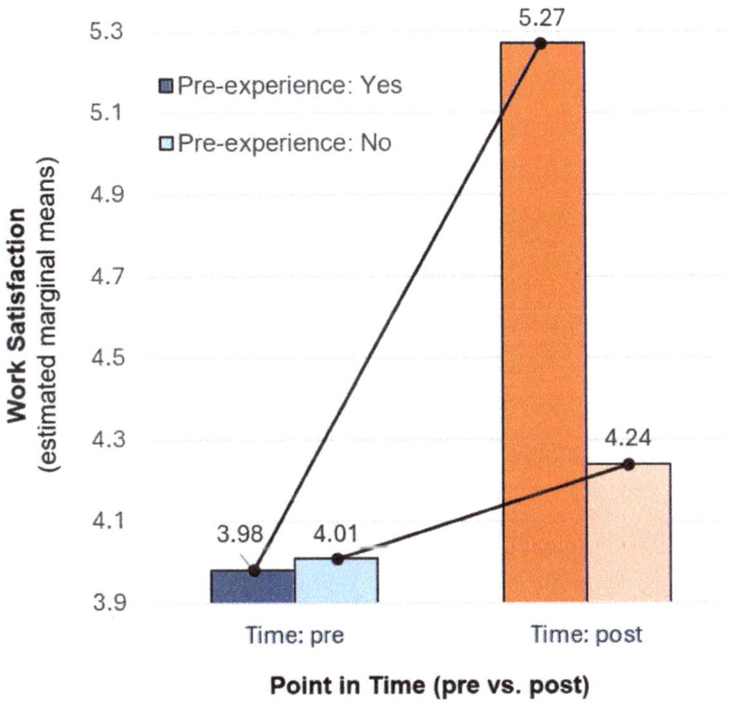

Figure 5. Interaction effect of time and prior telemedical experience on work satisfaction.

3.3.2. Knowledge Sources and Knowledge Transfer

Knowledge management was evaluated using the KODE® Competence Atlas framework, which classified sources of knowledge into four quadrants (personal/organizational × explicit/implicit). The evaluation found that informal knowledge transfer—including peer coaching, mentoring, and spontaneous collaborative problem-solving—was particularly high among staff with lower job satisfaction [31]. This indicates that interprofessional learning served as a compensatory mechanism, helping to bridge gaps in experience or protocol clarity.

The integration of telemedical feedback and digital case documentation further enabled context-sensitive learning loops, contributing to individualized professional development. These findings suggest that the system's learning infrastructure supports individualization not only for patients, but also for clinical decision-makers.

3.3.3. Technology Acceptance

Technology acceptance was measured using an adapted technical acceptance model (TAM), which included perceived usefulness, ease of use, and intention to adopt. Overall, acceptance of digital elements such as the tele-emergency physician interface and structured documentation systems was moderate to high, with notable variation across roles. Nurses and paramedics demonstrated the highest acceptance levels, followed by dispatchers; emergency physicians were more cautious, particularly regarding real-time decision transparency and medicolegal responsibility [30,31].

Notably, technology acceptance was strongly influenced by perceived task complexity and workload. Staff in high-stress roles were more likely to view digital tools as personally beneficial supports, reinforcing the idea that personalized system design should consider cognitive load and user-specific needs.

3.3.4. Regional and Structural Acceptance

The GEM Assay (adapted from the Global Entrepreneurship Monitor framework) was applied to assess regional attitudes toward innovation and structural change. The results showed broad support for the RuralRescue model among both frontline professionals and institutional stakeholders. Regional identity and a shared understanding of local healthcare challenges enhanced the acceptance of digitally supported models of care [30].

Stakeholders particularly appreciated the modular structure of the intervention, which allowed individual components (e.g., first responder system, TEPs) to be integrated based on regional capacity and readiness. This structural adaptability is a prerequisite for scalable personalized systems across diverse rural settings.

3.3.5. Relevance to Personalized Emergency Medicine

The formative evaluation demonstrates that personalization in emergency care extends beyond the patient to include providers, workflows, and digital interfaces. Variability in stress experience, technology acceptance, and knowledge behavior across professional roles underscores the need for context-aware implementation strategies. Tailoring support structures, training intensity, and digital onboarding to match professional background and regional infrastructure is essential for sustaining personalization at the system level. These findings align with the broader definition of personalization, encompassing not only clinical decision-making but also the social, psychological, and organizational factors that enable individualized care delivery in complex environments [29,30].

4. Discussion

The RuralRescue project demonstrated that personalized emergency care can be effectively implemented in rural regions through the coordinated use of digital technologies, targeted training, and adaptive care structures. The evaluation revealed improvements in clinical performance, resource efficiency, and organizational integration across all three implemented pillars of the model.

4.1. Summary of Main Findings

From a medical perspective, community-based CPR training (Pillar 1) significantly enhanced early intervention capacity, contributing to a 35.6% ROSC rate in OHCA cases—above the national rural average. The app-based responder activation system (Pillar 2) enabled geo-personalized mobilization of trained professionals, shortening the therapy-free interval by a median of over four minutes in nearly half of the activations. The TEP system (Pillar 3) supported remote diagnostics and delegated therapy in 3611 cases, with 17.8% involving physician-authorized medication and 24.3% avoiding unnecessary hospital transport. Diagnostic concordance with hospital data reached 84.9%, and digital documentation completeness exceeded 92%, demonstrating clinical precision and accountability.

Economically, decentralized TEP units proved effective but cost-intensive at the district level. Simulation models showed that centralized coordination could cut per-district costs by over 90%—from EUR 696,949 to EUR 57,300—without sacrificing service quality, assuming optimized TED-to-ambulance ratios. These results support the scalability of demand-sensitive personalization.

The organizational evaluation revealed divergent responses to digital transformation: experienced personnel reported greater job satisfaction, while less experienced staff indicated higher stress. Technology acceptance correlated positively with perceived workload and varied by role, with paramedics and nurses more receptive than physicians and dispatchers. Informal knowledge sharing emerged as a compensatory strategy, and stakeholder surveys confirmed broad regional support for the model's structural innovations.

Taken together, the findings demonstrate that personalized emergency care is feasible in rural areas when tailored to patient needs, regional infrastructure, professional diversity, and systemic constraints. RuralRescue offers a multi-dimensional proof of concept for integrating real-time clinical data, digital tools, and local capacity to enable individualized, value-based care in underserved regions.

4.2. Contributions to Personalized Emergency Medicine

The RuralRescue project demonstrates how personalized medicine can be operationalized in emergency care through the integration of digital tools, professional competencies, and real-time clinical data. Although not initially framed under the label of personalized medicine, the model supports key personalization mechanisms across the care continuum—from early intervention to triage, therapy, and system learning.

The tele-emergency physician (TEP) system exemplifies real-time clinical personalization. In over 3600 cases, remote physicians made diagnostic and therapeutic decisions using live ECGs, vital signs, structured assessments, and visual input. Nearly 18% involved delegated medication, tailored to both patient-specific data and the competencies of the on-site team. This situational, data-driven delegation aligned care intensity with clinical need rather than provider availability, enhancing precision in resource-limited rural areas.

TEP support also enabled context-aware triage: 24.3% of cases were managed without hospital transport, reflecting personalized decisions that minimized overtreatment, transport risks, and systemic strain.

The Land | Retter responder system implemented geo-personalized early intervention via a mobile app that alerted trained responders based on location and qualification. This real-time localization extended emergency coverage, adapting to local infrastructure, community layout, and responder distribution.

At the system level, over 250,000 EMS data points were collected, enabling longitudinal monitoring of outcomes, triage, and documentation. These data form the basis for adaptive learning and protocol refinement aligned with real-world trajectories.

Personalization was also advanced through role-specific training and workflow integration. Paramedics, dispatchers, and physicians received differentiated onboarding and developed collaborative competencies essential for tele-supervised care, supporting individualized professional development and smoother digital integration.

Formative findings highlight that implementation success depends on psychological and organizational factors. Technology acceptance varied by role, workload, and prior experience, underscoring the need to adapt tools and training to users' identities and stress profiles.

In sum, RuralRescue illustrates that personalized emergency medicine extends beyond molecular diagnostics to include dynamic alignment of care with patient status, professional readiness, regional resources, and digital infrastructure—a replicable framework for systems-level personalization in underserved regions.

4.3. Limitations

This article presents a secondary analysis of the RuralRescue project through the lens of personalized emergency medicine. The project was not originally designed to evaluate personalization but aimed at improving emergency care access and quality in a rural setting. Consequently, this re-analysis must be interpreted with caution.

The evaluation employed a pre–post design without a control group, consistent with common practice in implementation research under real-world constraints [25]. While this design ensured ecological validity, it limits causal attribution and increases vulnerability to confounding influences such as concurrent system changes, demographic shifts, or policy adjustments. Selection bias may have occurred due to non-random allocation of intervention components, with access to tele-emergency physician (TEP) support, responder alerts, or training programs influenced by dispatcher discretion, digital readiness, and geographic factors. Self-selection effects may also have influenced survey participation. Observer bias is a further limitation, particularly in self-reported outcomes related to work satisfaction, stress, and acceptance. These subjective measures are inherently prone to social desirability effects and role-dependent interpretation.

Confounding variables such as prior professional experience, local EMS infrastructure, and team composition may have moderated individual responses and organizational outcomes but were not fully controlled. Moreover, not all outcome indicators were available for the entire sample. Clinical metrics such as diagnostic concordance or triage decisions were analyzed only for subsets of cases, limiting generalizability.

Finally, integration with primary care—initially planned as a fourth intervention pillar—was not realized. As a result, the evaluation cannot address care continuity beyond the acute emergency phase or assess intersectoral personalization strategies. Despite these limitations, the RuralRescue project provides a robust, real-world foundation for understanding how personalization mechanisms can emerge from integrated emergency interventions in rural systems.

4.4. Recommendations for Further Research

While RuralRescue demonstrated the feasibility of personalized, digitally supported emergency care in rural regions, several areas merit further investigation to validate and extend these findings. Future research should apply controlled comparative designs, such as randomized or matched cohort studies, to strengthen causal claims. This is particularly relevant for assessing the impact of tele-delegated medication, triage accuracy, and diagnostic concordance under TEP supervision.

The extensive dataset generated by the project offers a foundation for predictive modeling and AI-based decision support. Tools such as adaptive triage algorithms and responder routing optimization could further personalize care and improve system responsiveness in real time. Studies should explore intersectoral integration, linking EMSs with out-of-hours care and hospital services to ensure continuity across the patient journey. While not realized in RuralRescue, this remains a critical area for delivering fully personalized, longitudinal emergency care.

Further research into the legal, ethical, and professional governance of remote clinical authority is essential. As tele-delegation increases, clear frameworks are needed to ensure safety, accountability, and acceptance by healthcare providers. Moreover, the variation in technology acceptance across roles suggests the need for personalized implementation strategies. Tailoring onboarding, digital training, and workflow redesign to staff roles, stress profiles, and institutional culture may enhance long-term adoption.

Lastly, disaggregated analysis of RuralRescue data could identify how personalization functions for underserved groups such as elderly patients or residents of isolated areas, helping refine equity-oriented design in rural EMS systems. These directions emphasize the need for interdisciplinary research that integrates clinical, technological, ethical, and organizational dimensions to advance system-level personalization in emergency medicine.

4.5. Practical Implications

The RuralRescue model demonstrates that personalized emergency care can be operationalized through digital infrastructure, tailored training, and adaptive policy—impacting clinical practice, organizational structures, and regulatory frameworks.

4.5.1. Individual and Clinical Practice Level

Customized digital workflows supported real-time TEP decision-making, enabling individualized diagnostics and therapy based on live clinical data. Paramedics delivered situation-specific care under remote oversight, particularly beneficial in high-acuity and resource-limited settings. The system's support for data-driven triage—24% of TEP-supervised cases managed without transport—aligns with value-based, risk-adjusted care models.

The Land | Retter app enabled geo-personalized responder mobilization based on proximity and verified competencies, improving early intervention in underserved areas. Role-specific training fostered telemedical integration and interprofessional collaboration, underscoring the role of personalized education in EMS transformation.

4.5.2. Organizational and System Level

RuralRescue's digital case documentation (over 250,000 records) provided a basis for longitudinal analysis, protocol refinement, and quality improvement. Technology acceptance varied by role, workload, and job satisfaction, highlighting the importance of context-aware implementation strategies tailored to human and organizational factors. Centralizing TEP coordination—as shown in simulation models—significantly reduced per-district costs while maintaining responsiveness, supporting economically sustainable personalization.

4.5.3. Policy, Legal, and Regulatory Implications

The project underscores the need for updated legal frameworks enabling remote medical delegation, digital consent, and real-time data protection. As a result, the state of Mecklenburg-Western Pomerania initiated the creation of a centralized tele-emergency center, following the project's economic recommendations. Long-term integration of TEP services with statutory on-call physicians and primary care could facilitate cross-sector continuity, advancing personalized emergency care as part of a cohesive, patient-centered system.

5. Conclusions

The RuralRescue project demonstrates that personalized emergency care is both feasible and effective in rural contexts when supported by digitally integrated, role-specific, and data-driven systems. Through real-time telemedical supervision, geo-personalized responder deployment, and adaptive workflows, the model advances core principles of personalized medicine—tailoring interventions not only to clinical presentation but also to geographic, organizational, and human resource factors. These findings offer a transferable framework for implementing individualized, value-based emergency services in structurally underserved regions and can be applied to other rural areas of hard-to-access environments.

Author Contributions: Conceptualization, J.P.H. and S.F.; methodology, K.H., S.F. and J.P.H.; validation, T.L., K.H. and S.F.; formal analysis, J.P.H. and S.F.; investigation, K.H., T.L., S.F. and J.P.H.; resources, K.H.; data curation, S.F. and J.P.H.; writing—original draft preparation, J.P.H.; writing—review and editing, K.H., S.F., T.L. and J.P.H.; visualization, J.P.H. and S.F.; supervision, K.H.; project administration, T.L.; funding acquisition, K.H. and J.P.H. All authors have read and agreed to the published version of the manuscript.

Funding: This research was funded by the Innovation Funds of the Joint Federal Committee (Gemeinsamer Bundesaussschuss, G-BA), grant number 01NVF16004.

Institutional Review Board Statement: The study was conducted in accordance with the Declaration of Helsinki, and approved by the Ethics Committee of the University Medicine Greifswald (protocol code approval BB 111/17, date of approval: 10 June 2017).

Informed Consent Statement: Informed consent was obtained from all subjects involved in the study.

Data Availability Statement: The full results including statistical data output, all surveys and tools as well the final report of the project, are open to the public at https://innovationsfonds.g-ba.de/projekte/neue-versorgungsformen/landrettung.63 (accessed on 7 February 2025).

Acknowledgments: We would like to thank our colleagues Bibiana Metelmann, Camilla Metelmann. Peter Brinkrolf, Lutz Fischer, Rebekka Süss, Julia Kuntosch and Dorothea Kohnen for their invaluable support and contribution to the implementation of the RuralRescue study.

Conflicts of Interest: The authors declare no conflicts of interest.

Abbreviations

The following abbreviations are used in this manuscript:

CPR	Cardiopulmonary Resuscitation
TEP	Tele-Emergency Physician
EMSs	Emergency Medical Services
ROSC	Return of Spontaneous Circulation
OHCA	Out-of-Hospital Cardiac Arrest
G-BA	Gemeinsamer Bundesausschuss (Federal Joint Committee)
AED	Automated External Defibrillator
FIFO	First-In-First-Out
M/M/k,∞, FIFO	M/M/k Infinity FIFO (Economical Queuing Model)

References

1. Bergrath, S.; Reich, A.; Rossaint, R.; Rörtgen, D.; Fischermann, H.; Beckers, S.K.; Felzen, M.; Hirsch, F.; Brokmann, J.C.; Czaplik, M. Implementation phase of a multicentre prehospital telemedicine system to support paramedics: Feasibility and limitations. *Scand. J. Trauma Resusc. Emerg. Med.* **2013**, *21*, 54. [CrossRef]
2. Felzen, M.; Beckers, S.K.; Kork, F.; Brokmann, J.C.; Czaplik, M.; Heussen, N.; Bergrath, S.; Rossaint, R. Utilization, safety, and technical performance of a telemedicine system for prehospital emergency care: Observational study. *J. Med. Internet Res.* **2019**, *21*, e14907. [CrossRef]
3. Skorning, M.; Bergrath, S.; Rörtgen, D.; Beckers, S.K.; Brokmann, J.C.; Gillmann, B.; Herding, J.; Protogerakis, M.; Fitzner, C.; Rossaint, R. Teleconsultation in pre-hospital emergency medical services: Real-time telemedical support in a prospective controlled simulation study. *Resuscitation* **2012**, *83*, 626–632.
4. Kozlowski, T. Die Einführung eines Telenotarztsystems in ländlichen Regionen. Dissertation, Universitätsmedizin Greifswald, Greifswald, Germany, 2020.
5. Prasser, C.; Süss, R.; Hahnenkamp, K.; Hasebrook, J.; Brinkrolf, P.; Fleßa, S. Der Telenotarzt als Innovation des Rettungsdienstes im ländlichen Raum-Kosten der Implementierung. *Gesundheitsökonomie & Qualitätsmanagement* **2020**, *25*, 150–156.
6. Felzen, M.; Beckers, S.K.; Kork, F.; Brokmann, J.C.; Czaplik, M.; Rossaint, R. Analgesia in the emergency medical service: Comparison between tele-emergency physician and callback procedure. *Anaesthesist* **2019**, *68*, 665–672.
7. Plum, R.; Felzen, M.; Beckers, S.K.; Bergrath, S.; Czaplik, M.; Rossaint, R. Patientenzufriedenheit im Rettungsdienst—Ein Vergleich nach Versorgung mit und ohne Telenotarzt. *Anästhesiol. Intensivmed.* **2020**, *61*, 40–45.
8. Simmons, K.M.; McIsaac, S.M.; Ohle, R. Impact of community-based interventions on out-of-hospital cardiac arrest outcomes: A systematic review and meta-analysis. *Sci. Rep.* **2023**, *13*, 10231.
9. Gross, B.; Schanderl, F.; Staedt, N.; Elsner, C. App-basierte Systeme zur Ersthelferalarmierung. *Notf. Rettungsmed.* **2019**, *22*, 483–491.
10. O'Meara, P.F.; Tourle, V.; Stirling, C.; Pedler, D. Extending the paramedic role in rural Australia: A story of flexibility and innovation. *Rural and Remote Health* **2012**, *12*, 1978.

11. Frichi, Y.; Aboueljinane, L.; Jawab, F. Ambulance location and relocation under budget constraints: Investigating coverage-maximization models and ambulance sharing to improve emergency medical services performance. *Health Care Manag. Sci.* **2025**, *28*, 274–297. [CrossRef]
12. Schröder, H.; Beckers, S.K.; Ogrodzki, K.; Borgs, C.; Ziemann, S.; Follmann, A.; Rossaint, R.; Felzen, M. Tele-EMS physicians improve life-threatening conditions during prehospital emergency missions. *Sci. Rep.* **2021**, *11*, 14366. [CrossRef] [PubMed]
13. Peters, G.A.; Ordoobadi, A.J.; Panchal, A.R.; Cash, R.E. Differences in out-of-hospital cardiac arrest management and outcomes across urban, suburban, and rural settings. *Prehospital emergency care.* **2023**, *27*, 162–169.
14. Metelmann, C.; Renzing, N.; Gräsner, J.-T.; Dölger, L.; Beckers, S.K.; Felzen, M.; Schröder, H.; Overheu, D.; Jacobsen, N.; Metelmann, B. Is a tele-emergency physician system a sensible addition in rural German regions? An analysis from a medical and economic perspective. *Prähospitale Telenotfallmedizin* **2020**, *15*, 381–395.
15. Koncz, V.; Kohlmann, T.; Bielmeier, S.; Urban, B.; Prückner, S. Telenotarzt. *Der Unfallchirurg* **2019**, *122*, 683–689.
16. Riva, G.; Ringh, M.; Jonsson, M.; Svensson, L.; Herlitz, J.; Claesson, A.; Djärv, T.; Nordberg, P.; Forsberg, S.; Rubertsson, S.; et al. Survival in out-of-hospital cardiac arrest after standard cardiopulmonary resuscitation or chest compressions only before arrival of emergency medical services: Nationwide study during three guideline periods. *Circulation* **2019**, *139*, 2600–2609. [CrossRef]
17. Groß, R.; Böttiger, B.W.; Wetsch, W.A. Laienreanimation in Deutschland: Das Nationale Aktionsbündnis Wiederbelebung (NAWIB). *Notf. Rettungsmed.* **2019**, *22*, 715–722. [CrossRef]
18. Goto, Y.; Funada, A.; Goto, Y. Relationship between emergency medical services response time and bystander intervention in patients with out-of-hospital cardiac arrest. *J. Am. Heart Assoc.* **2018**, *7*, e007568. [CrossRef]
19. Hasebrook, J.P.; Michalak, L.; Kohnen, D.; Metelmann, B.; Metelmann, C.; Brinkrolf, P.; Fleßa, S.; Hahnenkamp, K. Digital transition in rural emergency medicine: Impact of job satisfaction and workload on communication and technology acceptance. *PLoS ONE* **2023**, *18*, e0280956. [CrossRef]
20. Natafgi, N.; Shane, D.M.; Ullrich, F.; MacKinney, A.C.; Bell, A.; Ward, M.M. Using tele-emergency to avoid patient transfers in rural emergency departments: An assessment of costs and benefits. *J. Telemed. Telecare* **2018**, *24*, 193–201. [CrossRef]
21. Metelmann, C.; Metelmann, B.; Kohnen, D.; Prasser, C.; Süss, R.; Kuntosch, C.; Scheer, D.; Laslo, T.; Fischer, L.; Hasebrook, J.; et al. Evaluation of a Rural Emergency Medical Service Project in Germany: Protocol for a Multimethod and Multiperspective Longitudinal Analysis. *JMIR Res. Protoc.* **2020**, *9*, e14358.
22. Brinkrolf, P.; Kuntosch, J.; Metelmann, B.; Metelmann, C.; Hahnenkamp, K.; Süss, R.; Hasebrook, J.P.; Flessa, S. Is a tele-emergency physician system a sensible addition in rural German regions? An analysis from a medical and economic perspective. *Bundesgesundheitsblatt Gesundheitsforschung Gesundheitsschutz* **2022**, *65*, 1007–1015.
23. Marks, T.; Metelmann, B.; Gamberini, L.; Metelmann, C.; Schnaubelt, S.; Semeraro, F.; Hansen, C.M.; European Resuscitation Guidelines 2025 Systems Saving Lives Writing Group. Smartphone-based alert of community first responders: A multinational survey to characterise contemporary systems. *Resusc. Plus* **2025**, *24*, 100988. [CrossRef]
24. Ganter, J.; Busch, H.J.; Trummer, G.; Schmitz, D.; Pooth, J.S.; Steuber, T.; Brucklacher, T.; Mueller, M.P. Von der Smartphone-basierten Ersthelferalarmierung zum „lebensrettenden System". *Notfall. Rettungsmed.* **2024**, *30*, 1–9. [CrossRef]
25. Li, J.; Taljaard, M.; Van den Heuvel, E.R.; Levine, M.A.H.; Cook, D.J.; Wells, G.A.; Thabane, L. An introduction to multiplicity issues in clinical trials: The what, why, when and how. *Int. J. Epidemiol.* **2016**, *45*, 1551–1557. [CrossRef] [PubMed]
26. Glasgow, R.E.; Harden, S.M.; Gaglio, B.; Rabin, B.; Smith, M.L.; Porter, G.C.; Ory, M.G.; Estabrooks, P.A. RE-AIM planning and evaluation framework: Adapting to new science and practice with a 20-year review. *Front. Public Health* **2019**, *7*, 64. [CrossRef] [PubMed]
27. Lund, S.; Yan, M.; D'Angelo, J.; Wang, T.; Hallbeck, M.S.; Heller, S.; Zielinski, M. NASA-TLX assessment of workload in resident physicians and faculty surgeons covering trauma, surgical intensive care unit, and emergency general surgery services. *Am. J. Surg.* **2021**, *222*, 1158–1162. [CrossRef]
28. Metelmann, C.; Metelmann, B.; Schuffert, L.; Hahnenkamp, K.; Vollmer, M.; Brinkrolf, P. Smartphone apps to support laypersons in bystander CPR are of ambivalent benefit: A controlled trial using medical simulation. *Scand. J. Trauma Resusc. Emerg. Med.* **2021**, *29*, 76.
29. Kim, M.K.; Choi, G.J.; Oh, K.S.; Lee, S.P.; Kang, H. Pain Assessment Using the Analgesia Nociception Index (ANI) in Patients Undergoing General Anesthesia: A Systematic Review and Meta-Analysis. *J. Pers. Med.* **2023**, *13*, 1461. [CrossRef]
30. Astasio-Picado, Á.; Chueca, Y.C.; López-Sánchez, M.; Lozano, R.R.; González-Chapado, M.T.; Ortega-Trancón, V. Analysis of the Factors Intervening in the Prehospital Time in a Stroke Code. *J. Pers. Med.* **2023**, *13*, 1519. [CrossRef]
31. Fleßa, S.; Suess, R.; Kuntosch, J.; Brinkrolf, P.; Metelmann, B. Telemedical emergency services: Central or decentral coordination? *Health Econ. Rev.* **2021**, *11*, 7. [CrossRef]
32. Brinkrolf, P.; Scheer, D.; Hasebrook, J.; Hahnenkamp, K. Land | Rettung: Zukunftsfeste notfallmedizinische Neuausrichtung eines Landkreises. In *Innovationsfonds: Impulse für das Deutsche Gesundheitssystem*; MWVE: Richmond, VI, USA, 2017; pp. 140–145.

33. O'Sullivan, S.F.; Schneider, H. Developing telemedicine in Emergency Medical Services: A low-cost solution and practical approach connecting interfaces in emergency medicine. *J. Med. Access* **2022**, *6*, 1–12.
34. Hasebrook, J.; Hecke, J.; Volkert, T.; Singer, M.; Hinkelmann, J.; Michalak, L.; Hahnenkamp, K. Individual perspectives and mental maps of working conditions and intention to stay of physicians in academic medicine. *Front. Psychol.* **2023**, *14*, 1106501. [CrossRef] [PubMed]